This book is due for return on or before the l

PASS
THE PSA

Senior Content Strategist: *Pauline Graham*
Senior Content Development Specialist: *Ailsa Laing*
Project Manager: *Joanna Souch*
Designer: *Christian Bilbow*

PASS THE PSA

WILLIAM BROWN BSc MBBS MRCP(UK) FHEA
Academic Clinical Fellow, Department of Clinical Neurosciences, University of Cambridge & Addenbrooke's Hospital, Cambridge, UK

KEVIN LOUDON MBBS MRCP(UK) FHEA
Specialty Registrar Renal Medicine, Lister Hospital, Stevenage, UK

JAMES FISHER BSc MSc MBBS
Core Psychiatry Trainee, Central and North West London NHS Foundation Trust, London, UK

LAURA MARSLAND MPharm PGClinDip GPhC
Previous Lead Pharmacist for Neuroscience, Stroke and Rehabilitation at Addenbrooke's Hospital, Cambridge, UK, now studying medicine

Foreword by
Sam Leinster BSc MD FRCS SFHEA FAcadMEd
Emeritus Professor of Medical Education (formerly Inaugural Dean), Norwich Medical School, UK

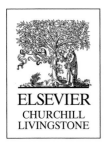

ELSEVIER
CHURCHILL
LIVINGSTONE

Edinburgh   London   New York   Oxford   Philadelphia   St Louis   Sydney   Toronto 2014

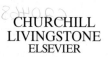

CHURCHILL
LIVINGSTONE
ELSEVIER

ISBN 978-0-7020-5518-8
eBook ISBN 978-0-7020-5517-1

British Library Cataloguing in Publication Data
A catalogue record for this book is available from the British Library.

Library of Congress Cataloging in Publication Data
A catalog record for this book is available from the Library of Congress.

Notices

Knowledge and best practice in this field are constantly changing. As new research and experience broaden our understanding, changes in research methods, professional practices, or medical treatment may become necessary.

Practitioners and researchers must always rely on their own experience and knowledge in evaluating and using any information, methods, compounds, or experiments described herein. In using such information or methods they should be mindful of their own safety and the safety of others, including parties for whom they have a professional responsibility.

With respect to any drug or pharmaceutical products identified, readers are advised to check the most current information provided (i) on procedures featured or (ii) by the manufacturer of each product to be administered, to verify the recommended dose or formula, the method and duration of administration, and contraindications. It is the responsibility of practitioners, relying on their own experience and knowledge of their patients, to make diagnoses, to determine dosages and the best treatment for each individual patient, and to take all appropriate safety precautions.

To the fullest extent of the law, neither the Publisher nor the authors, contributors, or editors, assume any liability for any injury and/or damage to persons or property as a matter of products liability, negligence or otherwise, or from any use or operation of any methods, products, instructions, or ideas contained in the material herein.

ELSEVIER your source for books,
journals and multimedia
in the health sciences
www.elsevierhealth.com

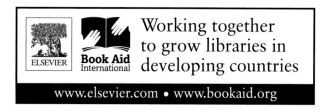

Working together
to grow libraries in
developing countries

www.elsevier.com • www.bookaid.org

The
Publisher's
policy is to use
paper manufactured
from sustainable forests

Printed in Italy

Contents

Foreword

One of the major tasks facing newly qualified doctors is prescribing drugs. Interviews with recent graduates suggest that this task takes up more of their time than taking medical histories and examining patients. Curiously, the emphasis in medical schools in the past has been on clerking and investigating patients in order to reach a diagnosis. Broad principles of management were, of course, taught and the science underlying the use of drugs was covered in clinical pharmacology and therapeutics courses, but the practicalities of safe prescribing were often omitted. Over the past 10 years there has been an increasing awareness of the frequency of prescription errors made by junior doctors in hospital.[1] Although many medical schools made changes to the curriculum in an attempt to address the problem, there was a continuing level of concern among the health care professions and the general public. In 2010 a committee was set up by the Medical School Council and the British Pharmacological Society with the aim of establishing a national prescribing assessment that all medical students would be required to pass before being allowed to register with the General Medical Council. The assessment has been extensively piloted and is due to go live in 2014.

This book has been written to help students prepare for the assessment. However, despite its title it is more than an examination crammer. The areas covered in the book mirror the examination but as a result it covers the major issues in practical prescribing. The mixture of demonstration scenario, theoretical discussion, useful mnemonics and practise questions with detailed feedback provides a sound educational tool. The advice is pragmatic and is clearly based on the real life experience of the authors in their day-to-day practice, but it is supported with appropriate evidence and relevant science.

Even if there were no Prescribing Safety Assessment, this book would be essential reading for all medical students prior to graduation.

Professor Sam Leinster BSc MD FRCS SFHEA FAcadMEd
Emeritus Professor of Medical Education (formerly Inaugural Dean)
Norwich Medical School, Norfolk, UK

---

[1] Dornan T, Ashcroft D, Heathfield H, et al. *An in depth investigation into causes of prescribing errors by foundation trainees in relation to their medical education. EQUIP study.* General Medical Council, London, 2009.

Preface

One of the key recommendations from *Tomorrow's Doctors* (2009) was to improve prescribing, and so the Prescribing Safety Assessment (PSA) was born. This exam, compulsory for full GMC registration, sets a minimum standard for prescribing, and aims to reduce the uncomfortably high number of prescription errors.

This book provides a practical, no-nonsense approach to prescribing, in a format written specifically for the exam. Each chapter addresses one exam section, and begins with a breakdown of the marking scheme, a summary of the knowledge required to pass, and then multiple questions covering scenarios common to the exam and foundation years, to make the reader a safe and excellent prescriber.

Good prescribing requires a firm grounding in data interpretation and the management of resultant diagnoses – two areas that students sometimes struggle with. We provide a pragmatic and concise summary of these in Chapters 3 and 4.

The authors include three doctors (WB, JF and KL) at the coalface of prescribing and teaching. Much as in clinical practice, we have toiled over this book and gained great satisfaction from producing it; and then gratefully and humbly watched it be markedly improved and corrected by a pharmacist (LM) who has contributed enormously. A word to the wise: befriending your ward pharmacist will be a greater investment than any medical insurance – accept that they know far more about prescribing and be grateful that they have your back.

We are indebted to those who have taught us, those who have worked with us and, most importantly, those who we have been privileged enough to care for. WB, JF and KL are particularly grateful to all staff at Norwich Medical School for their excellent teaching, particularly our outstanding pharmacology lecturer Dr Yoon Loke.

All that remains is to wish you the very best of luck.

Will Brown
Kevin Loudon
James Fisher
Laura Marsland

List of abbreviations

ABG — arterial blood gas
ACE — angiotensin converting enzyme
ACR — albumin–creatinine ratio
ACS — acute coronary syndrome
ADR — adverse drug reaction
AF — atrial fibrillation
AKI — acute kidney injury
ALP — alkaline phosphatase
ALT — alanine transaminase
AMT/AMTS — abbreviated mental test/score
AP — anterioposterior
aPTT — activated partial thromboplastin time
ARB — angiotensin receptor blocker
AST — aspartate aminotransferase
ATN — acute tubular necrosis

BBB — bundle branch block
BPAP — bi-level positive airway pressure
BTS — British Thoracic Society

CABG — coronary artery bypass graft
CCU — coronary care unit
CKD — chronic kidney disease
COPD — chronic obstructive pulmonary disease
CPAP — continuous positive airway pressure
CRP — C-reactive protein
CT — computerized tomography
CV — cardiovascular
CXR — chest X-ray

DC — direct current
DH — drug history
DIC — disseminated intravascular coagulation
DKA — diabetic ketoacidosis
DMARD — disease-modifying antirheumatic drug
DVT — deep vein thrombosis

ECG — electrocardiogram
ESR — erythrocyte sedimentation rate

FBC — full blood count
FEV1 — forced expiratory volume in 1 second
FFP — fresh frozen plasma

GAD — generalized anxiety disorder
GCS — Glasgow coma score
GTCS — generalized tonic–clonic seizures
GTN — glyceryl trinitrate

HAS — human albumin solution
HB — heart block
HONK — hyperosmolar nonketotic coma
Hx — history

ICS — inhaled corticosteroid
IHD — ischaemic heart disease
IM — intramuscular
INR — international normalized ratio
ITU — intensive therapy unit
IVI — intravenous infusion
IVIg — intravenous immunoglogulin

JVP — jugular venous pressure

LABA — long-acting beta-agonist
LAMA — long-acting muscarinic antagonist
LFT — liver function test
LMW — low molecular weight
LMWH — low molecular weight heparin
LP — lumbar puncture
LRTI — lower respiratory tract infection
LV — left ventricular
LVF — left ventricular failure
LVH — left ventricular hypertrophy

MAOIs — monoamine oxidase inhibitors
MAU — medical admissions unit
MCV — mean cell volume
MI — myocardial infarction
MMSE — mini-mental state examination
MSU — mid-stream urine

NAC — N-acetyl cysteine
NBM — nil by mouth
NEB — nebulized
NG — nasogastric
NICE — National Institute for Health and Care Excellence
NIV — noninvasive ventilation
NSTEMI — non-ST segment elevation myocardial infarction
NTD — neural tube defects

o/e — on examination
OSCE — objective structured clinical examination

PA — posterioanterior
PCI — percutaneous coronary intervention
PE — pulmonary embolism

PEF	peak expiratory flow
PMH	past medical history
PRN	as required
PT	prothrombin time
RUL	right upper lobe
SABA	short-acting β_2 agonist
SAMA	short-acting muscarinic antagonist
S/C	subcutaneous
SIADH	syndrome of inappropriate antidiuretic hormone
S/L	sublingual
SOB	shortness of breath
SR	sinus rhythm OR sustained release
SSRIs	selective-serotonin reuptake inhibitors
stat.	at once
STEMI	ST-segment elevation myocardial infarction
SVT	supraventricular tachycardia

TED	thromboembolism deterrent
TENS	transcutaneous electrical nerve stimulation
TFT	thyroid function text
THR	total hip replacement
TIA	transient ischaemic attack
TPMT	thiopurine S-methyl transferase
TSH	thyroid stimulating hormone
tx	treatment
U&E	urea and electrolytes
U/L	units per litre
UTI	urinary tract infection
VBG	venous blood gas
VTE	venous thromboembolism
WCC	white cell count

Basic principles of prescribing

Chapter objectives

- Understand the premise of this book and how it will help you to pass the Prescribing Safety Assessment (PSA).
- Learn how best to work your way through this book and how to follow the basic principles of safe prescribing.

INTRODUCTION

Drug prescribing is one of the most important parts of clinical practice. Yet it remains one of the most commonly failed components of undergraduate assessments and accounts for an uncomfortably high proportion of medical errors. To remedy this the PSA has been introduced. The General Medical Council expects that all UK undergraduates will pass this exam during their final year (though at the time of going to press, there is uncertainty over the date of such enforcement).

The exam comprises eight 'sections' within which different facets of prescribing are assessed (see Fig. 1.1). Students must complete the assessment within 2 hours. There are 200 marks available; the Prescribing and Prescription Review sections are assessed extensively and carry the most marks (112/200 marks in total).

HOW TO USE THIS BOOK

Pass the Prescribing Safety Assessment is written specifically for the exam, with one chapter dedicated to each PSA section. This chapter outlines the universal basic principles of prescribing for all sections and includes discussions of two common concepts applicable throughout. Chapter 2 introduces a simple, memorable and fail-safe approach to prescribing (the PReSCRIBER mnemonic) and each subsequent chapter builds on the previous, creating a robust prescribing method for both the PSA and foundation years. Each chapter also discusses the section's question structure and how to approach it. Questions (structured identically to the exam) conclude each chapter and cover all scenarios suggested for questioning in the PSA blueprint (2012). Finally, two mock exams (which should be completed within 2 hours each) enable consolidation of previous learning.

The chapter order imitates clinical practice and each chapter consolidates the work of previous ones. Knowing the correct diagnosis reflects accurate data interpretation (Chapter 3), which in turn enables the deduction of appropriate management strategies (Chapter 4). Some treatments require communication of specific information to patients (Chapter 5) and others require calculation skills (Chapter 6), before safely prescribing (Chapter 7). Finally, drug monitoring (Chapter 8) attempts to prevent some adverse drug reactions (Chapter 9).

A secondary aim of the book is to summarize the clinical knowledge required to pass the PSA. There is little merit in limiting learning to drug-related data interpretation or management while ignoring the substantial non-pharmacological remainder: this arbitrary distinction does not avail itself in clinical practice, and the PSA will include scenarios where a drug is not to blame. Consequently, Chapters 3 and 4 include concise, yet comprehensive, summaries of data interpretation and management algorithms, with the most common causes **emboldened**, and drug-related causes (which will of course be over-represented in the exam) ***emboldened/italicized***.

In the exam you will have access to the **British National Formulary** (BNF) for every section. If in doubt, look it up! Many questions will require even the most capable candidate to look up an answer, so you should become familiar with it during your preparations. The BNF will even tell you what to prescribe in common clinical situations (just look up the symptom or diagnosis in the index), but you will not have time to do this for each question. It is therefore advisable to learn the theory in each chapter and use the BNF as a backup. The BNF includes sections on antibiotic choice for different infections; you can use this or your local antibiotic policy while preparing, but you should know the first line antibiotic choices for common infections. Drug charts have been provided where written prescriptions are required (Chapter 7), so no additional materials beyond a BNF are needed whilst using this book.

BASIC PRINCIPLES FOR ALL PRESCRIBING

Every drug prescription must be:
- **Legible**
- **Unambiguous** (e.g. not a range of doses, such as 30–60 mg codeine which is a common error and entirely your fault if a patient is overdosed within your prescribed dosage range)
- An **approved** (generic) **name**, e.g. salbutamol not Ventolin®. See Box 1.1.
- **IN CAPITALS**
- **Without abbreviations**

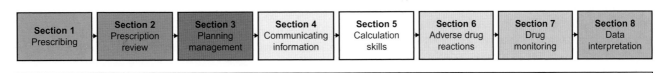

Section 1 Prescribing	Section 2 Prescription review	Section 3 Planning management	Section 4 Communicating information	Section 5 Calculation skills	Section 6 Adverse drug reactions	Section 7 Drug monitoring	Section 8 Data interpretation

Eight Sections = Total 200 marks, over 120 min

Figure 1.1 The Prescribing Safety Assessment structure.

- **Signed** (even when practising or in an exam, sign and make up a bleep number in order to get into this habit)
- If a drug is to be used 'as required' **provide two instructions**: (1) indication and (2) a maximum frequency (e.g. twice daily) or total dose in 24 hours (e.g. 1g)
- If an antibiotic is being prescribed include the **indication** and **stop/review date**
- Include of **duration** if the treatment is not long term (e.g. antibiotics) or if it is in a GP setting (e.g. 7 or 28 days).

Marks are awarded for each of these points.

Box 1.1   Generic versus trade drug names

There are a small number of exceptions when trade names should be used; one of the most important reflects the various preparations of tacrolimus (used for preventing the rejection of transplanted organs). The BNF states that trade names should be used for prescribing because switching between brands can result in toxicity (if relative levels increase) or rejection (if relative levels decrease). You will often see the brand name Tazocin® written instead of piperacillin with tazobactam – this is done for simplicity but is not acceptable, particularly because it masks the fact that the drug contains penicillin that is made obvious by the 'cillin' in piperacillin.

ENZYME INDUCERS AND INHIBITORS (See Chapters 8 and 9)

Most of this book concerns the effects of drugs on the body (pharmacodynamics). Conversely, what the body does to the drug (known as pharmacokinetics, including absorption, metabolism and excretion) is slightly less relevant in a practical guide to prescribing, as these processes are reasonably stable and thus a drug's effect is usually predictable. Problems arise, however, when other substances (in this case concomitantly administered drugs) unintentionally alter these complex systems resulting in increased or decreased drug levels and hence altered effects. Thus, from an early stage it is important to recognize that when you prescribe particular drugs (which are also enzyme inhibitors or enzyme inducers) they may affect seemingly unrelated drugs (Table 1.1).

Most drugs are metabolized to inactive metabolites by the cytochrome P450 enzyme system in the liver, preventing them exerting infinite effects. The activity of these enzymes, however, may in turn be altered by the presence of other particular drugs, known as enzyme inducers and inhibitors. An enzyme inducer will increase P450 enzyme activity, hastening metabolism of other drugs with the result that they exert a reduced effect (and thus a patient will require more of some other drugs in the presence of an enzyme inducer). Conversely, an enzyme inhibitor will decrease P450 enzyme activity and, subsequently, there will be increased levels of other drugs (which in the hands of a diligent physician require a reduced drug dose).

The classic example of this is the effect of newly introduced enzyme inhibitors on patients taking warfarin. In particular, the addition of erythromycin (an enzyme inhibitor) can sometimes and unpredictably cause a dangerous rise in international normalized ratio (INR) if the warfarin dose is not decreased; you should be aware of this in patients presenting with excessive anticoagulation (see Chapter 3).

Table 1.1: Most common enzyme inhibitors and inducers

Inducers	Inhibitors
↑ Enzyme Activity→ ↓ Drug Concentration	↓ Enzyme Activity→ ↑ Drug Concentration
PC BRAS: **P**henytoin, **C**arbamazepine, **B**arbiturates, **R**ifampicin, **A**lcohol (chronic excess), **S**ulphonylureas	**AODEVICES:** **A**llopurinol, **O**meprazole, **D**isulfiram, **E**rythromycin, **V**alproate, **I**soniazid, **C**iprofloxacin, **E**thanol (acute intoxication), **S**ulphonamides

---

PRESCRIBING FOR SURGERY

As a general rule for all surgery, most drugs should be continued during surgery (i.e. not stopped beforehand) because the risk of losing disease control outweighs the risk posed by drug continuation. Stopping some drugs may be detrimental intraoperatively too, particularly calcium-channel blockers and beta-blockers which must be continued. See Table 1.2 for the drugs that must be stopped before surgery.

DRUGS TO INCREASE DURING SURGERY

Patients on long-term corticosteroids (e.g. prednisolone) commonly have adrenal atrophy; they are therefore unable to mount an adequate physiological ('stress') response to surgery, resulting in profound hypotension if the steroids are discontinued. As with 'sick day rules' (where patients on steroids double their daily dose to counter this increased steroid requirement when ill), at induction of anaesthesia patients should be given IV steroids to prevent this.

Table 1.2: Drugs to stop before surgery

I LACK OP: **I**nsulin, **L**ithium, **A**nticoagulants/antiplatelets, **C**OCP/HRT, **K**-sparing diuretics, **O**ral hypoglycaemics, **P**erindopril and other ACE-inhibitors.

Drug	When to Stop
Combined oral contraceptive pill (COCP) and hormone replacement therapy (HRT)	4 weeks before surgery
Lithium	Day before
Potassium-sparing diuretics and ACE-inhibitors	Day of surgery
Anticoagulants (warfarin/heparin including prophylactic dose) Antiplatelets (aspirin/clopidogrel/dipyridamole)	Variable* (occasionally continued during surgery)
Oral hypoglycaemic drugs and insulin	Variable*,†

*Variable between hospitals and operations. Look at your local policy, but you will not be required to memorize these timescales for the PSA.
†Patients are 'nil by mouth' before surgery, thus metformin should be stopped because it will cause lactic acidosis. The other oral hypoglycaemics and insulin will cause hypoglycaemia unless stopped. In all cases, a sliding scale should be started instead where hourly blood glucose monitoring adjusts the hourly dose of insulin given to provide much tighter control.

Prescription review: a foolproof plan

Chapter objectives

- Learn a practical and reliable routine for all prescribing situations.
- Learn to identify the common traps in the Prescribing Safety Assessment (PSA, see 'Common trap' boxes).
- Reinforce your learning by using 10 scenarios with worked answers.

STRUCTURE OF THIS SECTION WITHIN THE PSA

The 'Prescription review' section will have 8 questions with 4 marks available per question and a possible total of 32 marks. You will be asked to identify which drug(s) from a list are causing a current problem, which may reflect a side effect, a contraindication, an interaction or ineffectiveness. (See Question 2.1 for a demonstration scenario.)

Question 2.1 Demonstration scenario
Prescription review item worth 4 marks

CASE PRESENTATION

James Dix, 74 years old, is admitted to hospital with a four-day history of shortness of breath, purulent sputum, haemoptysis and fever. He also complains of pleuritic chest pain. He is confused with an abbreviated mental test (AMT) score of 5/10.

His past medical history includes hypertension, diverticulosis and he had a transient ischaemic attack (TIA) last year. He has no history of renal failure, heart failure or dementia. He is allergic to penicillin. His current medications are as listed on the current prescriptions chart.

OBSERVATIONS

BP 130/72 mmHg; HR 118/min; RR 28/min; O_2 sat 82% (on air); Temperature 38.2°C.

	Value	Normal range
WCC	18×10^9/L	$(4–11 \times 10^9$/L)
Na	141 mmol/L	(135–145 mmol/L)
Hb	142 g/L	(135–175 g/L (male))
K	5.9 mmol/L	(3.5–5.0 mmol/L)
Ur	17 mmol/L	(3–7 mmol/L)
Cr	218 µmol/L	(60–125 µmol/L)

Chest x-ray (CXR): right lower lobe pneumonia.

He is started on antibiotics for severe community-acquired pneumonia.

Question: Select the drugs that should be stopped/temporarily withheld (with or without alternatives) with ticks in column A.

CURRENT PRESCRIPTIONS

Drug name	Dose	Route	Freq.	A
ASPIRIN	75 MG	ORAL	DAILY	☐
RAMIPRIL	5 MG	ORAL	DAILY	☐
BISOPROLOL	2.5 MG	ORAL	DAILY	☐
DRUGS STARTED ON ADMISSION				
CO-AMOXICLAV	1.2 G	IV	8-HOURLY	☐
PARACETAMOL	1 G	ORAL	4-HOURLY	☐
ENOXAPARIN	40 MG	S/C	DAILY	☐

INTRAVENOUS FLUID CHART

Date	Time	Fluid	Additive	Volume	Rate	Prescriber – sign + print	
01/02/13	17 00	0.9% SALINE	40 MMOL KCL	1 L	2 H	SIGNATURE	☐

Question 2.1 Answer, see ticks beside current prescriptions chart

1. This patient has haemoptysis (blood in sputum), so aspirin (an antiplatelet) and prophylactic enoxaparin (a low molecular weight (LMW) heparin) should be stopped.

2. This patient is hyperkalaemic, so the ACE-inhibitor (ramipril) should be stopped, which may also be contributing to his renal failure. The IV fluid containing potassium should also be stopped (and an alternative started).

3. This patient is allergic to penicillin, so co-amoxiclav (which contains amoxicillin, a penicillin) should be stopped and an alternative started.

4. This patient is receiving 6 g/day of paracetamol (i.e. 2 g more than the maximum dose): the frequency should be 6-hourly not 4-hourly.

Note: while representative of reality (and illustrative of the diversity of drug errors requiring identification), in the exam the number of errors will be specified.

CURRENT PRESCRIPTIONS

Drug name	Dose	Route	Freq.	A
ASPIRIN	75 MG	ORAL	DAILY	✓
RAMIPRIL	5 MG	ORAL	DAILY	✓
BISOPROLOL	2.5 MG	ORAL	DAILY	☐
DRUGS STARTED ON ADMISSION				
CO-AMOXICLAV	1.2 G	IV	8-HOURLY	✓
PARACETAMOL	1 G	ORAL	4-HOURLY	✓
ENOXAPARIN	40 MG	S/C	DAILY	✓

INTRAVENOUS FLUID CHART

Date	Time	Fluid	Additive	Volume	Rate	Prescriber – sign + print	
01/02/13	17 00	0.9% SALINE	40 MMOL KCL	1 L	2 H	SIGNATURE	✓

A SAFE ROUTINE FOR PRESCRIBING

Using the demonstration scenario (Question 2.1), we can identify and address the common pitfalls by:

- ensuring we have the **correct patient's** prescription/drug chart
- noticing and recording **allergies**
- **signing** the front of the chart
- considering the **contraindications** for each drug we prescribe
- considering the **route** for each drug we prescribe
- considering the need for **IV fluids**
- considering the need for **thromboprophylaxis**
- considering the need for **antiemetics**
- considering the need for **pain relief.**

This highlights just how many errors can be made and emphasizes the need for a comprehensive prescribing routine that may be followed every time you prescribe. The following mnemonic (PReSCRIBER) covers all these pitfalls and related traps within the PSA.

> ### Common trap
> Check the patient's name on each prescription: if they do not match up, do not prescribe it!

PReSCRIBER

This mnemonic will help you to remember the following essentials:

- **P**atient details
- **Re**action (i.e. allergy plus the reaction)
- **S**ign the front of the chart
- check for **C**ontraindications to each drug
- check **R**oute for each drug
- prescribe **I**ntravenous fluids if needed
- prescribe **B**lood clot prophylaxis if needed
- prescribe anti**E**metic if needed and
- prescribe pain **R**elief if needed.

PReSCRIBER explained

Patient details

- If working with a new chart then you must write three pieces of patient-identifying information on the front of the chart (e.g. patient name, date of birth and hospital number) or use a hospital addressograph sticker.
- If amending a chart then ensure that you have the correct patient's drug chart.

Reactions

- If working with a new chart then complete the allergy box including any drug reaction mentioned by the patient.
- If amending a chart then check the allergy box before prescribing.

> ### Common trap
> Do not forget that co-amoxiclav and Tazocin® both contain penicillin.

Sign chart

Most drug charts now have a section for all prescribers to sign. This is so that they may be contacted in the event of a query (or particularly poor prescribing!). Each individual prescription should be signed too.

Contraindications

For every drug prescribed, consider whether it is contraindicated. Realistically, at undergraduate level there are four groups of drugs for which you must know the contraindications (and less common examples are outlined in Chapter 8):

1. Drugs that increase bleeding (aspirin, heparin and warfarin) should not be given to patients who are bleeding, suspected of bleeding, or at risk of bleeding (e.g. those with a prolonged prothrombin time due to liver disease). Do not forget that prophylactic heparin is contraindicated in acute ischaemic stroke due to the risk of bleeding into the stroke. It is also important to remember that an enzyme inhibitor (such as erythromycin) can increase warfarin's effect (and thus the prothrombin time (PT) and international normalized ratio (INR)) despite a stable dose. This should be considered when patients present with excessive anticoagulation.

2. For steroids remember the side effects (and thus more loosely the contraindications) by using the mnemonic STEROIDS: **S**tomach ulcers, **T**hin skin, o**E**dema, **R**ight and left heart failure, **O**steoporosis, **I**nfection (including *Candida*), **D**iabetes (commonly causes hyperglycaemia and uncommonly progresses to diabetes), and Cushing's **S**yndrome.

3. With NSAIDs the following cautions and contraindications may be remembered with the mnemonic NSAID: **N**o urine (i.e. renal failure), **S**ystolic dysfunction (i.e. heart failure), **A**sthma, **I**ndigestion (any cause), and **D**yscrasia (clotting abnormality).
   While aspirin is technically a NSAID, it is not contraindicated in renal or heart failure, or in asthma.

4. For antihypertensives always think of the side effects in three categories:
   a. **Hypotension** (including postural hypotension) that may result from all groups of antihypertensives.
   b. Dividing the groups of antihypertensives into two mechanistic categories:
      1. Bradycardia may occur with beta-blockers and some calcium-channel blockers.
      2. Electrolyte disturbance can occur with angiotensin converting enzyme (ACE) inhibitors and diuretics (see Chapter 3).
   c. Individual drug classes have specific side effects:
      1. ACE-inhibitors can result in a dry cough.
      2. Beta-blockers can cause wheeze in asthmatics; worsening of acute heart failure (but helps chronic heart failure).
      3. Calcium-channel blockers can cause peripheral oedema and flushing.
      4. Diuretics can cause renal failure. Loop diuretics (e.g. furosemide) can also cause gout, and potassium-sparing diuretics (e.g. spironolactone) can cause gynaecomastia.

Route

If a patient is vomiting, antiemetics should be given by non-oral routes (i.e. IV/IM/SC). However, if vomiting is predicted to last a short time (which it usually is), changing the route of other prescribed medicine is usually not necessary (and can be difficult, especially in the case of drugs for which the non-oral dose is different). Conveniently, the doses of the common antiemetics are the same regardless of the route taken, e.g. cyclizine 50 mg 8-hourly, metoclopramide 10 mg 8-hourly.

It is very important to remember that a patient who is 'nil by mouth' should still receive their oral medication, including prior to surgery (see Chapter 1).

Intravenous fluids

There is no single 'right' answer in most fluid prescription questions; however, there are always 'wrong' answers, and the following rules should help you avoid them.

IV fluids are prescribed in two situations:

1. As **replacement** fluids for a dehydrated/acutely unwell patient.
2. As **maintenance** in a patient who is nil by mouth.

In both situations one must consider which fluid, how much to give, and how fast to give it.

Replacement: which fluid? Give all patients 0.9% saline (normal saline, a crystalloid) unless the patient:

- Is hypernatraemic or hypoglycaemic: give 5% dextrose instead.
- Has ascites: give human-albumin solution (HAS) instead. The albumin maintains oncotic pressure; furthermore, the higher sodium content of 0.9% saline will worsen ascites.
- Is shocked with systolic BP <90 mmHg: give gelofusine (a colloid) instead as it has a high osmotic content so stays intravascularly, thus maintaining BP for longer.
- Is shocked from bleeding: give blood transfusion, but a colloid first if no blood available.

Replacement: how much fluid and how fast? Start by assessing the HR, BP and urine output:

- If tachycardic or hypotensive give 500 mL bolus immediately (250 mL if heart failure) then reassess patient, especially HR, BP and urine output to assess response and speed of next bag of IV fluid.
- If only oliguric (and not due to urinary obstruction (e.g. an enlarged prostate)) then give 1 L over 2–4 h then reassess patient, especially and HR, BP and urine output to assess response and speed of next bag of IV fluid.
- It is possible to roughly predict how fluid-depleted an adult patient is by using their observations and knowing which are affected first:
  ▶ reduced urine output (oliguric if <30 mL/h; anuric if 0 mL/h) indicates 500 mL of fluid depletion
  ▶ reduced urine output plus tachycardia indicates 1 L of fluid depletion
  ▶ reduced urine output plus tachycardia plus shocked indicates >2 L of fluid depletion.
- As a general rule never prescribe more than 2 L of IV fluid for a sick patient. The effect on the patient and thus the rate of subsequent fluids should be reviewed regularly.
- You may see the symbol ° being used in clinical practice: this refers to the number of hours over which a bag of fluid should be given, e.g. 0.9% saline 1 L 2° means 1 L of 0.9% saline over 2 h. In the PSA (and indeed clinical practice) you should instead write '2 hours' or '2-hourly' or '2-hrly'.

Maintenance: which fluids and how much?

- As a general rule, adults require 3 L IV fluid per 24 hours and the elderly require 2 L.
- Adequate electrolytes are provided by 1 L of 0.9% saline and 2 L of 5% dextrose (1 salty and 2 sweet).
- To provide potassium, bags of 5% dextrose or 0.9% saline containing potassium chloride (KCL) can be used but this should be guided by urea and electrolyte (U&E) results; with a normal potassium level, patients require roughly 40 mmol KCl per day (so put 20 mmol KCl in two bags)

> **Common trap**
>
> IV potassium should not be given at more than 10 mmol/hour.

Maintenance: how fast to give fluids

- If giving 3 L per day = 8-hourly bags (24 ÷ 3).
- If giving 2 L per day = 12 hourly bags (24 ÷ 2).
  In the PSA it will not be possible to assess the patient; however, every time you prescribe fluids in real life, you must:
- Check the patient's U&E to confirm what to give them.
- Check that the patient is not fluid overloaded (e.g. increased jugular venous pressure (JVP), peripheral and pulmonary oedema).
- Ensure that the patient's bladder is not palpable (signifying urinary obstruction) if giving replacement fluids because of 'reduced urine output'.

Blood clot prophylaxis

The majority of patients admitted to hospital will receive prophylactic low molecular weight (LMW) heparin (e.g. dalteparin 5000 units daily s/c) and compression stockings for prevention of venous thromboembolism. To determine which patients should receive this treatment, almost all drug charts include an assessment tool and thus there is little point in learning the criteria. However, remember that if a patient is bleeding or at risk of bleeding (including due to a recent ischaemic stroke) they should not be prescribed warfarin or heparin. A patient with peripheral arterial disease (usually indicated by absent foot pulses) should not be prescribed compression stockings (which may cause acute limb ischaemia).

Antiemetics (see Table 2.1)

Table 2.1: Antiemetic choices

Situation	Prescribe
Nauseated	Regular antiemetic: • cyclizine 50 mg 8-hourly IM/IV/oral for most cases but causes fluid retention • metoclopramide 10 mg 8-hourly IM/IV if heart failure
Not nauseated	As-required antiemetic: • cyclizine 50 mg up to 8-hourly IM/IV/oral for most cases but causes fluid retention • metoclopramide 10 mg up to 8-hourly IM/IV if heart failure

Note: cyclizine is a good first-line treatment for almost all cases except cardiac cases (as it can worsen fluid retention), where metoclopramide 10 mg 8-hourly IM/IV is safer.

> **Common traps**
>
> Avoid metoclopramide (a dopamine antagonist) for:
> - Patients with Parkinson's disease due to the risk of exacerbating symptoms.
> - Young women due to the risk of dyskinesia, i.e. unwanted movements especially acute dystonia.

Pain relief (see Table 2.2)

Table 2.2: Analgesic choices

Situation	Prescribe regularly	Prescribe 'as required'
No pain	Nil	Paracetamol 1 g up to 6-hourly oral
Mild pain	Paracetamol 1 g 6-hourly oral	Codeine 30 mg up to 6-hourly oral*
Severe pain	Co-codamol 30/500, 2 tablets 6-hourly oral	Morphine sulphate 10 mg up to 6-hourly oral**

Tramadol is a suitable replacement.
***In order of increasing effectiveness, morphine sulphate may be given orally (as Oramorph®), subcutaneously or intravenously. Oramorph® is a liquid and comes in two strengths (the more concentrated is rarely used in hospitals) thus the strength must be specified and is usually 10 mg/5 mL.*

Common trap

Check how much paracetamol the patient is taking: they may often be on more than one preparation and thus over the daily maximum of 4 g (i.e. 8 tablets of 500 mg each), e.g. a patient taking 2 co-codamol 30/500 tablets (meaning 30 mg codeine and 500 mg paracetamol in each tablet) 6-hourly plus as required paracetamol is potentially taking too much. The underlying rule, when correcting this, is to ensure that no more than 4 g of paracetamol each day are given; whether this is through stopping the co-codamol or the paracetamol should be dictated by the patient's pain. Provided a safe paracetamol dose is prescribed, the exact choice is unlikely to lose you marks.

An NSAID (e.g. ibuprofen 400 mg 8-hourly) may be introduced at any stage regularly or 'as required' if not contraindicated (as discussed earlier under Contraindications). With **neuropathic pain** (i.e. pain arising from nerve damage or disease and usually described as 'shooting', 'stabbing' or 'burning') the first line of treatment is amitriptyline (10 mg oral nightly) or pregabalin (75 mg oral 12-hourly); duloxetine (60 mg oral daily) is indicated in painful diabetic neuropathy.

Question 2.2 Prescription review item worth 4 marks

CASE PRESENTATION

A 62-year-old man presents to A&E with nausea. After receiving an antiemetic he develops bradykinesia and rigidity. His medical history is notable for Parkinson's disease and hypertension. A copy of his usual medication is available (on the current prescriptions chart). The A&E doctor stops one of the drugs because his routine biochemistry shows potassium 2.4 mmol/L (normal 3.5–5.0 mmol/L) with normal sodium, urea and creatinine.

Question A: Select the *one* drug that was the most likely cause of the low potassium (and was stopped). Mark it with a tick in column A.

Question B: Select the *one* antiemetic responsible for the neurological deterioration with a tick in column B.

CURRENT PRESCRIPTIONS

Drug name	Dose	Route	Freq.	A	B
CO-BENELDOPA 12.5/50	2 TABLETS	ORAL	12-HOURLY	☐	☐
BISOPROLOL	10 MG	ORAL	DAILY	☐	☐
BENDROFLUMETHIAZIDE	2.5 MG	ORAL	DAILY	☑	☐
LISINOPRIL	10 MG	ORAL	DAILY	☐	☐
SELEGILINE	5 MG	ORAL	DAILY	☐	☐
PARACETAMOL	1 G	ORAL	AS REQUIRED UP TO 6-HOURLY	☐	☐
DOMPERIDONE	10 MG	ORAL	6-HOURLY	☐	☐
METOCLOPRAMIDE	10 MG	IV	8-HOURLY	☐	☑
CYCLIZINE	50 MG	IV	8-HOURLY	☐	☐

Question 2.2 Answers, see ticks beside current prescription chart

A	Bendroflumethiazide, a thiazide diuretic, causes hypokalaemia by increasing potassium excretion by the kidney. Lisinopril (an ACE-inhibitor) can cause hyperkalaemia.
B	Metoclopramide and domperidone are both dopamine antagonists. Metoclopramide crosses the blood-brain-barrier (BBB), and so exacerbates parkinsoninan symptoms by acting on central dopamine receptors. Domperidone does not cross the BBB, and so is safer to use in Parkinson's disease. Cyclizine is an anti-histamine antiemetic.

CURRENT PRESCRIPTIONS

Drug name	Dose	Route	Freq.	A	B
CO-BENELDOPA 12.5/50	2 TABLETS	ORAL	12-HOURLY	☐	☐
BISOPROLOL	10 MG	ORAL	DAILY	☐	☐
BENDROFLUMETHIAZIDE	2.5 MG	ORAL	DAILY	✓	☐
LISINOPRIL	10 MG	ORAL	DAILY	☐	☐
SELEGILINE	5 MG	ORAL	DAILY	☐	☐
PARACETAMOL	1 G	ORAL	AS REQUIRED UP TO 6-HOURLY	☐	☐
DOMPERIDONE	10 MG	ORAL	6-HOURLY	☐	☐
METOCLOPRAMIDE	10 MG	IV	8-HOURLY	☐	✓
CYCLIZINE	50 MG	IV	8-HOURLY	☐	☐

Question 2.3 Prescription review item worth 4 marks

CASE PRESENTATION

A 64-year-old patient presents to his GP complaining of a cough. He is not short of breath and denies chest pain. Examination is unremarkable. The GP sends routine bloods (see below) and a CXR is normal.

PAST MEDICAL HISTORY

Hypertension, hyperlipidaemia and gout. His current regular medicines are listed on the current prescriptions chart.

	Value	Normal range
Na	137 mmol/L	(135–145 mmol/L)
K	5.9 mmol/L	(3.5–5.0 mmol/L)
Ur	4.8 mmol/L	(3–7 mmol/L)
Cr	110 µmol/L	(60–125 µmol/L)
CRP	<3 mg/L	(<5 mg/L)

Question A: Select the *one* drug that is most likely to cause the cough with a tick in column A.

Question B: Select the *one* drug that is most likely to cause the electrolyte disturbance with a tick in column B.

CURRENT PRESCRIPTIONS

Drug name	Dose	Route	Freq.	A	B
SIMVASTATIN	10 MG	ORAL	NIGHTLY	☐	☐
BISOPROLOL	10 MG	ORAL	DAILY	☐	☐
ALLOPURINOL	100 MG	ORAL	DAILY	☐	☐
LISINOPRIL	10 MG	ORAL	DAILY	☑	☑
PARACETAMOL	1 G	ORAL	6-HOURLY	☐	☐
BENDROFLUMETHIAZIDE	2.5 MG	ORAL	DAILY	☐	☑

Question 2.3 Answers, see ticks beside current prescriptions chart

A	ACE-inhibitors cause a dry cough through accumulation of bradykinin via reduced degradation by ACE.
B	ACE-inhibitors cause hyperkalaemia through reduced aldosterone production and thus reduced potassium excretion in the kidneys. Remember that loop and thiazide diuretics (including bendroflumethiazide) cause hypokalaemia while aldosterone antagonists and ACE-inhibitors cause hyperkalaemia.

CURRENT PRESCRIPTIONS

Drug name	Dose	Route	Freq.	A	B
SIMVASTATIN	10 MG	ORAL	NIGHTLY	☐	☐
BISOPROLOL	10 MG	ORAL	DAILY	☐	☐
ALLOPURINOL	100 MG	ORAL	DAILY	☐	☐
LISINOPRIL	10 MG	ORAL	DAILY	✓	✓
PARACETAMOL	1 G	ORAL	6-HOURLY	☐	☐
BENDROFLUMETHIAZIDE	2.5 MG	ORAL	DAILY	☐	☐

Question 2.4 Prescription review item worth 4 marks

CASE PRESENTATION

A 56-year-old woman presents to A&E complaining of increasing indigestion for four weeks.

PAST MEDICAL HISTORY

Osteoarthritis, hypertension and ulcerative colitis. Her current regular medicines are listed on the current prescriptions chart. Examination reveals epigastric tenderness. Her bloods are as follows:

	Value	Normal range
Na	137 mmol/L	(135–145 mmol/L)
K	5.2 mmol/L	(3.5–5.0 mmol/L)
Ur	14 mmol/L	(3–7 mmol/L)
Cr	232 µmol/L	(60–125 µmol/L)
Hb	95 g/L	(120–150 g/L (female))

Question A: Select the *two* prescriptions most likely to be contributing to the indigestion with ticks in column A.

Question B: Select the *two* prescriptions most likely to be responsible for the renal failure with ticks in column B.

CURRENT PRESCRIPTIONS

Drug name	Dose	Route	Freq.	A	B
PARACETAMOL	1 G	ORAL	6-HOURLY	☐	☐
IBUPROFEN	200 MG	ORAL	8-HOURLY	☑	☑
PREDNISOLONE	30 MG	ORAL	DAILY	☑	☐
RAMIPRIL	2.5 MG	ORAL	DAILY	☐	☑
PENTASA (MESALAZINE)	2 G	ORAL	DAILY	☐	☐

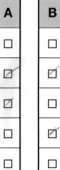

Question 2.4 Answer, see ticks beside current prescriptions chart

A	Ibuprofen inhibits prostaglandin synthesis needed for gastric mucosal protection from acid. It is therefore at risk of influencing inflammation and ulceration. Oral steroids inhibit gastric epithelial renewal thus predisposing to ulceration.
B	Ibuprofen inhibits prostaglandin synthesis which reduces renal artery diameter (and blood flow) and thereby reducing kidney perfusion and function. Ramipril, an ACE-inhibitor, reduces angiotensin-II production necessary for preserving glomerular filtration when the renal blood flow is reduced.

CURRENT PRESCRIPTIONS

Drug name	Dose	Route	Freq.	A	B
PARACETAMOL	1 G	ORAL	6-HOURLY	☐	☐
IBUPROFEN	200 MG	ORAL	8-HOURLY	✓	✓
PREDNISOLONE	30 MG	ORAL	DAILY	✓	☐
RAMIPRIL	2.5 MG	ORAL	DAILY	☐	✓
PENTASA (MESALAZINE)	2 G	ORAL	DAILY	☐	☐

Question 2.5 Prescription review item worth 4 marks

CASE PRESENTATION

A 78-year-old man is admitted by his GP following abnormal routine biochemistry results. He denies any pain and feels well in himself though he admits he has not opened his bowels for five days.

PAST MEDICAL HISTORY

Hypertension, osteoarthritis, hypercholesterolaemia. His medicines are listed on the current prescriptions chart.

	Value	Normal range
Na	133 mmol/L	(135–145 mmol/L)
K	2.7 mmol/L	(3.5–5.0 mmol/L)
Ur	4.2 mmol/L	(3–7 mmol/L)
Cr	73 µmol/L	(60–125 µmol/L)

Question A: Select the *one* prescription that is the most likely cause of the electrolyte disturbance with a tick in column A.

Question B: Select the *three* prescriptions which should be stopped with ticks in column B.

CURRENT PRESCRIPTIONS

Drug name	Dose	Route	Freq.	A	B
BENDROFLUMETHIAZIDE	2.5 MG	ORAL	DAILY	☑	☑
PARACETAMOL	500 MG	ORAL	6-HOURLY	☐	☐
SIMVASTATIN	20 MG	ORAL	NIGHTLY	☐	☐
AMLODIPINE	5 MG	ORAL	DAILY	☐	☑
CODEINE	30 MG	ORAL	6-HOURLY	☐	☑
LISINOPRIL	10 MG	ORAL	NIGHTLY	☐	☐
CO-CODAMOL 30/500	2 TABLETS	ORAL	AS REQUIRED UP TO 6-HOURLY	☐	☑

Question 2.5 Answer, see ticks beside current prescription chart

A	Bendroflumethiazide, a thiazide diuretic, causes hypokalaemia by increasing potassium excretion by the kidney. Lisinopril (an ACE-inhibitor) causes hyperkalaemia.
B	Bendroflumethiazide should be stopped due to hypokalaemia. As the patient is constipated, all opiate-derived drugs should be withheld (codeine and co-codamol). Note that the patient is also taking too much paracetamol (up to 6 g/day: 2 g regularly and up to 4 g PRN (within co-codamol), exceeding the daily maximum of 4 g). While one could have stopped the regular paracetamol instead of the co-codamol, this would be suboptimal because of the constipation. Further, the patient is pain free so minimal analgesics should be required.

CURRENT PRESCRIPTIONS

Drug name	Dose	Route	Freq.	A	B
BENDROFLUMETHIAZIDE	2.5 MG	ORAL	DAILY	✓	✓
PARACETAMOL	500 MG	ORAL	6-HOURLY	☐	☐
SIMVASTATIN	20 MG	ORAL	NIGHTLY	☐	☐
AMLODIPINE	5 MG	ORAL	DAILY	☐	☐
CODEINE	30 MG	ORAL	6-HOURLY	☐	✓
LISINOPRIL	10 MG	ORAL	NIGHTLY	☐	☐
CO-CODAMOL 30/500	2 TABLETS	ORAL	AS REQUIRED UP TO 6-HOURLY	☐	✓

Question 2.6 Prescription review item worth 4 marks

CASE PRESENTATION

A 24-year-old woman with rheumatoid arthritis and asthma is seen in A&E for dysuria, urinary frequency and nausea. A urine dipstick supports a diagnosis of urinary tract infection. A pregnancy test is negative. She is taking co-codamol, omeprazole and methotrexate 15 mg weekly (next dose due tomorrow). She is started on antibiotics and additional analgesia by a colleague who asks you to review the prescription before discharging her (see current prescriptions chart).

	Value	Normal range
CRP	139 mg/L	(<5 mg/L)

Question: Select the *four* prescriptions that should be stopped (with or without alternatives being prescribed) with ticks in column A.

CURRENT PRESCRIPTIONS

Drug name	Dose	Route	Freq.	A
CO-CODAMOL 8/500	2 TABLETS	ORAL	6-HOURLY	☐
METHOTREXATE	15 MG	ORAL	WEEKLY	☑
IBUPROFEN	200 MG	ORAL	12-HOURLY	☑
OMEPRAZOLE	20 MG	ORAL	DAILY	☐
PARACETAMOL	500 MG	ORAL	AS REQUIRED	☐
TRIMETHOPRIM	200 MG	ORAL	12-HOURLY	☑

Question 2.6 Answer, see ticks beside current prescription chart

1. Ibuprofen is an unwise choice of analgesic because the patient has a PMH of asthma; NSAIDs can cause bronchoconstriction in asthmatics and are therefore avoided unless strictly necessary (not in this case) and under close supervision (i.e. not at home).

2. The PRN paracetamol should be stopped: the patient is already taking the maximum daily dosage (4 g/day) within co-codamol (2 tablets, each containing 500 mg, four times per day). Furthermore, the paracetamol prescription is not valid because a maximum PRN frequency is not given.

3. Trimethoprim is a folate antagonist, and is a direct contraindication to patients taking methotrexate (another folate antagonist) due to the risk of bone marrow toxicity. This can lead to pancytopenia and neutropenic sepsis. The trimethoprim should therefore be stopped.

4. If a patient on methotrexate has sepsis this medication is withheld pending exclusion of neutropenic sepsis. Note that you are not told any haematology results to help determine whether she is neutropenic and, realistically, the patient would not be discharged until this was known, but certainly whilst septic, she should not receive the methotrexate. Therefore it should have been withheld. If in doubt, withhold!

CURRENT PRESCRIPTIONS

Drug name	Dose	Route	Freq.	A
CO-CODAMOL 8/500	2 TABLETS	ORAL	6-HOURLY	☐
METHOTREXATE	15 MG	ORAL	WEEKLY	✓
IBUPROFEN	200 MG	ORAL	12-HOURLY	✓
OMEPRAZOLE	20 MG	ORAL	DAILY	☐
PARACETAMOL	500 MG	ORAL	AS REQUIRED	✓
TRIMETHOPRIM	200 MG	ORAL	12-HOURLY	✓

Question 2.7 Prescription review item worth 4 marks

CASE PRESENTATION

A 76-year-old patient is on a rehabilitation ward recovering from an ischaemic stroke one week ago. Beyond hypertension, for which he was started on amlodipine and enalapril following admission, he has no other medical history. He was taking no drugs on admission. Three days ago he developed swollen ankles. He was started on furosemide and an echocardiogram was arranged.

You are asked so see him because his routine electrolytes are deranged. His echocardiogram shows no evidence of heart failure.

	Value	Normal range
Na	131 mmol/L	(135–145 mmol/L)
K	3.0 mmol/L	(3.5–5.0 mmol/L)
Ur	3.2 mmol/L	(3–7 mmol/L)
Cr	78 µmol/L	(60–125 µmol/L)

Question A: Select the drug which is most likely responsible for both the hyponatraemia and hypokalaemia with a tick in column A.

Question B: Select the *three* drugs which should be stopped with ticks in column B.

CURRENT PRESCRIPTIONS

Drug name	Dose	Route	Freq.	A	B
FUROSEMIDE	40 MG	ORAL	DAILY	☑	☑
PARACETAMOL	500 MG	ORAL	6-HOURLY	☐	☐
ASPIRIN	75 MG	ORAL	DAILY	☐	☐
ENALAPRIL	5 MG	ORAL	DAILY	☐	☑
AMLODIPINE	5 MG	ORAL	DAILY	☐	☑
ENOXAPARIN	40 MG	S/C	DAILY	☐	☐

Question 2.7 Answer, see ticks beside current prescription chart

A	All diuretics can cause hyponatraemia, although when they contribute to dehydration the sodium can increase too. However, loop diuretics (e.g. furosemide) and thiazide diuretics cause hypokalaemia, while potassium-sparing diuretics and ACE-inhibitors cause hyperkalaemia. Thus, the correct answer to this specific question is furosemide.
B	This patient has been started on a calcium-channel blocker (amlodipine) for hypertension. One side effect of this is peripheral oedema which he subsequently developed. The normal echo excludes heart failure as a cause. The oedema is incorrectly treated with furosemide rather than stopping the amlodipine, and this has caused the electrolyte disturbance. Thus, the furosemide and the amlodipine should be stopped. This patient suffered an acute stroke one week ago and should therefore not be taking heparin thromboprophylaxis for 2 months (duration varies throughout the UK). Stopping the enalapril would not be correct because it is indicated for hypertension and would typically cause hyperkalaemia.

CURRENT PRESCRIPTIONS

Drug name	Dose	Route	Freq.	A	B
FUROSEMIDE	40 MG	ORAL	DAILY	✓	✓
PARACETAMOL	500 MG	ORAL	6-HOURLY	☐	☐
ASPIRIN	75 MG	ORAL	DAILY	☐	☐
ENALAPRIL	5 MG	ORAL	DAILY	☐	☐
AMLODIPINE	5 MG	ORAL	DAILY	☐	✓
ENOXAPARIN	40 MG	S/C	DAILY	☐	✓

Question 2.8 Prescription review item worth 4 marks

CASE PRESENTATION

An 81-year-old patient is being treated for atrial fibrillation. He has a background of hypertension. He was initially started on warfarin and verapamil, but the ventricular rate remained above 100/min on maximum dose verapamil, so bisoprolol was added yesterday. The medical registrar also noticed peripheral oedema and so started furosemide. The patient has just had an echo performed which revealed a normal ejection fraction (i.e. no heart failure).

You have been asked to see him because HR is 52 b.p.m. and BP is 128/72 mmHg; all other observations are normal and he feels fine.

	Value	Normal range
Na	136 mmol/L	(135–145 mmol/L)
K	4.0 mmol/L	(3.5–5.0 mmol/L)
Ur	3.2 mmol/L	(3–7 mmol/L)
Cr	78 µmol/L	(60–125 µmol/L)
INR	7.8	(Target 2–3)

Question: Select the *four* drugs that should be stopped with ticks in column A.

CURRENT PRESCRIPTIONS

Drug name	Dose	Route	Freq.	A
FUROSEMIDE	20 MG	ORAL	DAILY	☐
WARFARIN	2-3 MG	ORAL	DAILY	☑
ENALAPRIL	10 MG	ORAL	DAILY	☐
VERAPAMIL	120 MG	ORAL	8-HOURLY	☑
BISOPROLOL	10 MG	ORAL	DAILY	☑
ENOXAPARIN	40 MG	S/C	DAILY	☑

Question 2.8 Answer, see ticks beside current prescription chart

Given the normal ejection fraction (and the presence of a calcium-channel blocker), the peripheral oedema can be considered drug-induced; thus the furosemide should stop, particularly as the culprit (the calcium-channel blocker) is being withdrawn (see below).

Enalapril is an ACE-inhibitor and not causing any side effects.

The patient's INR is very high (target 2-3); at this level warfarin should be stopped (see Chapter 2). Patients on warfarin (with an INR over 2 ('therapeutic')) should not be given prophylactic heparin as it increases the risk of bleeding unnecessarily. The enoxaparin should thus also be stopped.

Verapamil is a calcium-channel blocker, and can therefore cause peripheral oedema. Verapamil should not be used with beta-blockers due to the risk of bradycardia (or at worst asystole) and hypotension (unless under expert supervision). As the patient is mildly bradycardic one of the two rate-limiting drugs must be stopped; given the choice it makes sense to stop the drug that was ineffective at maximum dose and causing peripheral oedema (i.e. verapamil) rather than the beta-blocker.

While one could argue that both rate-limiting drugs should be stopped (as he is bradycardic, albeit mildly and asymptomatically) the other drug errors are a greater priority, and stopping both will likely produce a rebound tachycardia.

CURRENT PRESCRIPTIONS

Drug name	Dose	Route	Freq.	A
FUROSEMIDE	20 MG	ORAL	DAILY	✓
WARFARIN	2–3 MG	ORAL	DAILY	✓
ENALAPRIL	10 MG	ORAL	DAILY	☐
VERAPAMIL	120 MG	ORAL	8-HOURLY	✓
BISOPROLOL	10 MG	ORAL	DAILY	☐
ENOXAPARIN	40 MG	S/C	DAILY	✓

Question 2.9 Prescription review item worth 4 marks

CASE PRESENTATION

A 61-year-old patient is admitted following one week of shortness of breath and wheeze. His medical history includes asthma, gout and hypertension for which he started treatment a month ago. He is allergic to penicillin and does not smoke. His GP has given him antibiotics and analgesia believing his symptoms were due to a chest infection but this has not helped. When you see him his respiratory rate is 32/min, O_2 sat 91% (on air) and he is afebrile. He has a widespread expiratory wheeze and a new maculopapular rash over his legs.

His routine bloods and chest X-ray are unremarkable.

Question: Select the *four* drugs that should be stopped with ticks in column A.

CURRENT PRESCRIPTIONS

Drug name	Dose	Route	Freq.	A
ALLOPURINOL	100 MG	ORAL	DAILY	☐
AMLODIPINE	5 MG	ORAL	DAILY	☑
ASPIRIN	2 G	ORAL	8-HOURLY	☑
ENALAPRIL	10 MG	ORAL	DAILY	☐
PROPRANOLOL	40 MG	ORAL	8-HOURLY	☑
CO-AMOXICLAV	625 MG	ORAL	8-HOURLY	☑
IBUPROFEN	200 MG	ORAL	AS REQUIRED UP TO 8-HOURLY	☐

Question 2.9 Answer, see ticks beside current prescription chart

This patient has an exacerbation of asthma triggered by beta-blockers and then worsened by ibuprofen (both of which can precipitate bronchospasm; for this reason beta-blockers are contraindicated in asthmatics and NSAIDs should be used, if strictly necessary, with caution). If an asthmatic patient is already on an NSAID without worsening of asthma then it may be continued.

Despite being an NSAID, aspirin very rarely worsens asthma (less frequently than other NSAIDs), and is thus commonly (though cautiously) used. However, the usual cardioprotective dose is 75 mg daily, and in the treatment of acute coronary syndromes and stroke the dose is 300 mg daily; thus 2 g 8-hourly is clearly an error, and thus aspirin should be stopped.

The patient is allergic to penicillin; co-amoxiclav is a combination of amoxicillin (a penicillin) and clavulanic acid. This is probably the cause of the rash and it should be stopped because of the allergy and because it is not indicated anyway.

CURRENT PRESCRIPTIONS

Drug name	Dose	Route	Freq.	A
ALLOPURINOL	100 MG	ORAL	DAILY	☐
AMLODIPINE	5 MG	ORAL	DAILY	☐
ASPIRIN	2 G	ORAL	8-HOURLY	✓
ENALAPRIL	10 MG	ORAL	DAILY	☐
PROPRANOLOL	40 MG	ORAL	8-HOURLY	✓
CO-AMOXICLAV	625 MG	ORAL	8-HOURLY	✓
IBUPROFEN	200 MG	ORAL	AS REQUIRED UP TO 8-HOURLY	✓

Question 2.10 Prescription review item worth 4 marks

CASE PRESENTATION

The nurses have asked you to review the drug chart of a 56-year-old lady admitted yesterday with a stroke and a history of migraine with aura and diabetes. The pharmacist has found some errors on the drug chart, but, unfortunately, her instructions have gone missing.

Question: Please identify the *four* drug errors with ticks in column A.

CURRENT PRESCRIPTIONS

Drug name	Dose	Route	Freq.	A
METFORMIN	1 G	ORAL	12-HOURLY	☐
MICROGYNON ED®	ONE	ORAL	DAILY	☑
ENOXAPARIN	40 MG	S/C	DAILY	☐
CO-CODAMOL 30/500	2 TABLETS	ORAL	12-HOURLY	☑
BISOPROLOL	200 G	ORAL	DAILY	☑
NOVOMIX 30®	15 UNITS	IV	DAILY	☑
PARACETAMOL	1 G	ORAL	AS REQUIRED UP TO 12-HOURLY	☑
VERAPAMIL	40 MG	ORAL	8-HOURLY	☐

Question 2.10 Answer, see ticks beside current prescription chart

This is tricky!

Microgynon® is a combined oral contraceptive pill (COCP). Patients who have migraine with aura should not take the COCP as it significantly increases their risk of stroke (as perhaps illustrated here); therefore, it should be stopped. In addition, it would be worth confirming the indication given that the patient is 56 years old and likely post-menopausal. It could have been prescribed for the wrong patient.

Prophylactic enoxaparin is contraindicated following an acute stroke (for at least 2 months, but varies according to hospital).

The patient (unusually for these scenarios!) is taking an acceptable amount of paracetamol (4 g/24 h: 2 g from co-codamol and up to 2 g from PRN paracetamol). Neither paracetamol nor co-codamol needs to be stopped.

The bisoprolol dose is clearly incorrect (usually 10 mg daily) and, therefore, is a drug error. Remember that verapamil must not be used with beta-blockers; in this case the incorrect dose of bisoprolol means it (rather than the verapamil) should be stopped.

Novomix 30® (a combination of short and medium acting insulin) is never given IV; as a rule all insulin is s/c except for sliding scales using short-acting insulin (e.g. Actrapid® or NovoRapid®) given by IV infusion.

CURRENT PRESCRIPTIONS

Drug name	Dose	Route	Freq.	A
METFORMIN	1 G	ORAL	12-HOURLY	☐
MICROGYNON ED®	ONE	ORAL	DAILY	✓
ENOXAPARIN	40 MG	S/C	DAILY	✓
CO-CODAMOL 30/500	2 TABLETS	ORAL	12-HOURLY	☐
BISOPROLOL	200 G	ORAL	DAILY	✓
NOVOMIX 30®	15 UNITS	IV	DAILY	✓
PARACETAMOL	1 G	ORAL	AS REQUIRED UP TO 12-HOURLY	☐
VERAPAMIL	40 MG	ORAL	8-HOURLY	☐

Data interpretation

Chapter objectives

- Learn memorable and reliable methods of interpreting the most common test results.
- Learn how to interpret (and act on) drug-specific data.
- Use 10 scenarios with worked answers to reinforce these principles.

STRUCTURE OF THIS SECTION WITHIN THE PSA

The 'Data interpretation' section will have 6 questions with 2 marks available per question, so a possible total of 12 points. The questions will be of the multiple choice style and you will be asked to select the most appropriate answer from a list of five options (A–E). See Question 3.1 for a demonstration scenario.

Question 3.1 Demonstration scenario

Data interpretation item worth 2 marks

CASE PRESENTATION

A 27-year-old lady with a history of schizophrenia, migraine and asthma has routine blood tests performed. She feels well with occasional headaches and mild wheeze. She is currently taking clozapine, citalopram, propranolol, paracetamol and ibuprofen. Her GP is concerned about the results and refers her to the medical assessment unit for evaluation.

	Value	Normal range		Value	Normal range
WCC	1.3×10^9/L	$(4-11 \times 10^9$/L)	Ur	5 mmol/L	(3–7 mmol/L)
Neut.	0.01×10^9/L	$(2-8 \times 10^9$/L)	Cr	68 µmol/L	(60–125 µmol/L)
Lymph.	0.2×10^9/L	$(1-4.8 \times 10^9$/L)	Na	139 mmol/L	(135–145 mmol/L)
Hb	140 g/L	(120–150 g/L (female))	K	4.1 mmol/L	(3.5–5.0 mmol/L)
MCV	82 fL	(76–99 fL)	Glucose	4.8 mmol/L	

Option: Select the *most appropriate* decision option with regard to her management and mark it with a tick.

DECISION OPTIONS

A	STOP IBUPROFEN	☐
B	STOP PROPRANOLOL AND CITALOPRAM	☐
C	STOP CLOZAPINE, PROPRANOLOL AND IBUPROFEN	☐
D	STOP CLOZAPINE, PROPRANOLOL, IBUPROFEN AND PARACETAMOL	☐
E	STOP CLOZAPINE, PROPRANOLOL, IBUPROFEN AND CITALOPRAM	☐

Question 3.1 Answers

A	This patient is asthmatic and has a wheeze which might be attributable to ibuprofen (an NSAID), which should be stopped; however, there are other drugs to stop too.
B	Similarly, beta-blockers (in this case used for chronic migraine treatment) are contraindicated in asthmatics; this may be why she is mildly wheezy. However, citalopram (a selective serotonin reuptake inhibitor) is not contraindicated and need not be stopped.
C	**Correct:** clozapine is an antipsychotic. The most worrying side effect (for which all patients are monitored with at least monthly blood tests) is agranulocytosis resulting in neutropenia, as seen here. This requires immediate cessation of the drug and referral to a haematologist. The two drugs contraindicated in asthma should also be stopped. Note that if the question had not stated that the patient had a wheeze, the ibuprofen could be continued as it would suggest her asthma was not NSAID-sensitive.
D	There is no rationale to stop paracetamol.
E	There is no rationale to stop citalopram.

DECISION OPTIONS

A	STOP IBUPROFEN	☐
B	STOP PROPRANOLOL AND CITALOPRAM	☐
C	STOP CLOZAPINE, PROPRANOLOL AND IBUPROFEN	✓
D	STOP CLOZAPINE, PROPRANOLOL, IBUPROFEN AND PARACETAMOL	☐
E	STOP CLOZAPINE, PROPRANOLOL, IBUPROFEN AND CITALOPRAM	☐

INTRODUCTION

The 'Data interpretation' section requires knowledge of drug-specific data (such as paracetamol nomograms and drug monitoring) and general data interpretation (such as biochemistry and imaging).

An overview of common investigation abnormalities will be presented, with the drug related causes (to be particularly wary of in the exam) in **_bold italic,_** while the more common causes (in real life!) are **emboldened**.

GENERAL DATA INTERPRETATION

BLOOD TESTS: HAEMATOLOGY

The most important results of a full blood count (FBC) are the haemoglobin, the white cell count (WCC) and the platelets. The most commonly encountered abnormalities are shown in Tables 3.1–3.3.

Low haemoglobin (anaemia)

There are many causes of anaemia (see Table 3.1), so look at the mean cell volume (MCV) to narrow your differential.

BLOOD TESTS: BIOCHEMISTRY

Urea and electrolytes (U&E)

There are two principal abnormalities to glean from the U&E: high and low electrolytes (i.e. sodium or potassium), and the presence and type of kidney injury (i.e. through assessing the urea and creatinine).

Sodium (normal range 135–145 mmol/L)

- Hyponatraemia: to help narrow the (wide) differential for hyponatraemia assess the patient's fluid status (e.g. hypovolaemic/euvolaemic/hypervolaemic) (Table 3.4).
- Hypernatreamia: causes of this all begin with 'd':
  dehydration;
  drips (i.e. too much IV saline);
  drugs (e.g. effervescent tablet preparations or intravenous

preparations with a high sodium content);
diabetes insipidus (which is effectively the opposite of syndrome of inappropriate anti-diuretic hormone (SIADH).

Potassium (normal range 3.5–5.0 mmol/L)

Hypokalaemia and hyperkalaemia are particularly important because they cause fatal cardiac arrhythmias. Their causes may thus be remembered with the mnemonics DIRE and DREAD (Table 3.5).

Table 3.2: High and low white blood cells

	Causes
High neutrophils (neutrophilia)	**Bacterial infection** Tissue damage (inflammation/infarct/ malignancy) Steroids
Low neutrophils (neutropenia)	**Viral infection** Chemotherapy or radiotherapy* **_Clozapine (antipsychotic)_** **_Carbimazole (antithyroid)_**
High lymphocytes (lymphocytosis)	**Viral infection** Lymphoma Chronic lymphocytic leukaemia

*Patients undergoing chemotherapy or radiotherapy may become neutropenic (or even pancytopenic) in response to infection ('neutropenic sepsis'). This carries a much higher mortality rate so they must be given urgent IV broad-spectrum antibiotics (the choice is hospital specific).

Table 3.3: Causes of thrombocytosis and thrombocytopenia

	Causes
Low platelets (thrombocytopenia)	Reduced production: • infection (usually viral) • **_drugs (esp. penicillamine (e.g. in rheumatoid arthritis treatment))_** • myelodysplasia, myelofibrosis, myeloma Increased destruction: • **_heparin_** • hypersplenism • disseminated intravascular coagulation (DIC) • idiopathic thrombocytopenic purpura (ITP) • haemolytic uraemic syndrome/ thrombotic thrombocytopenic purpura
High platelets (thrombocytosis)	Reactive: • bleeding • tissue damage (infection/ inflammation/malignancy) • post-splenectomy Primary: • myeloproliferative disorders

Table 3.1: Causes of anaemia

Type of anaemia	Causes
Microcytic (low MCV)	**Iron deficiency anaemia** Thalassaemia Sideroblastic anaemia
Normocytic (normal MCV)	**Anaemia of chronic disease** **Acute blood loss** Haemolytic anaemia Renal failure (chronic)
Macrocytic (high MCV)	**B_{12}*/folate deficiency ('megaloblastic anaemia')** **Excess alcohol** **Liver disease (including nonalcoholic causes)** Hypothyroidism Haematological diseases beginning with 'M': myeloproliferative, myelodysplastic, multiple myeloma

*B_{12} deficiency includes pernicious anaemia.

Table 3.4: Causes of hyponatraemia

Fluid status	Causes of hyponatraemia
Hypovolaemic	**Fluid loss (especially diarrhoea/ vomiting)** Addison's disease ***Diuretics (any type)***
Euvolaemic	SIADH* Psychogenic polydipsia Hypothyroidism
Hypervolaemic	**Heart failure** **Renal failure** Liver failure (causing hypoalbuminaemia) Nutritional failure (causing hypoalbuminaemia) Thyroid failure (hypothyroidism; can be euvolaemic too)

*Causes of SIADH can be remembered with the mnemonic SIADH: **S**mall cell lung tumours, **I**nfection, **A**bscess, **D**rugs (especially carbamazepine and antipsychotics), and **H**ead injury.*

Table 3.5: Causes of hypokalaemia and hyperkalaemia

	Causes
Hypokalaemia (DIRE)	***Drugs (loop and thiazide diuretics)*** **I**nadequate intake or intestinal loss (diarrhoea/vomiting) **R**enal tubular acidosis **E**ndocrine (Cushing's and Conn's syndromes)
Hyperkalaemia (DREAD)	***Drugs (potassium-sparing diuretics and ACE-inhibitors)*** **R**enal failure **E**ndocrine (Addison's disease) **A**rtefact (very common, due to clotted sample) **D**KA (note that when insulin is given to treat DKA the potassium drops requiring regular (hourly) monitoring +/− replacement)

Acute kidney injury (AKI)

See Table 3.6 for the causes of AKI (which was previously called acute renal failure).

Common trap

Raised urea indicates kidney injury **or upper gastrointestinal (GI) haemorrhage.** A raised urea usually indicates renal failure; however, because it is a breakdown product of amino acids (such as globin chains in haemoglobin), it can also reflect an upper GI bleed where haemoglobin has been broken down by gastric acid into urea, which is subsequently absorbed into the blood. The same phenomenon occurs if you eat a big (and bloody) steak. Thus, a raised urea with normal creatinine in a patient who is not dehydrated (i.e. does not have prerenal failure) should prompt a look at the haemoglobin; if this has dropped then the patient probably has an upper GI bleed.

Table 3.6: Causes of acute kidney injury

Type of AKI	Biochemical disturbance	Causes
Prerenal (70%)	Urea rise >> creatinine rise, e.g.: Urea 19 (3–7.5 mmol/L) Creatinine 110 (35–125 μmol/L)	Dehydration (or if severe, shock) of any cause, e.g. sepsis, blood loss. Renal artery stenosis (RAS)*
Intrinsic renal (10%)	Urea rise << creatinine rise, bladder or hydronephrosis not palpable, e.g.: Urea 9 (3–7.5 mmol/L) Creatinine 342 (35–125 μmol/L)	**INTRINSIC:** **I**schaemia (due to prenal AKI, causing acute tubular necrosis) ***Nephrotoxic antibiotics****** **Tablets (ACEI, NSAIDs)** **R**adiological contrast **I**njury (rhabdomyolysis) **N**egatively birefringent crystals (gout) **S**yndromes (glomerulonephrides) **I**nflammation (vasculitis) **C**holesterol emboli
Postrenal (20%) (obstructive)	Urea rise << creatinine rise, bladder or hydronephrosis may be palpable depending on level of obstruction, e.g.: Urea 9 (3–7.5 mmol/L) Creatinine 342 (35–125 μmol/L)	In lumen: stone or sloughed papilla In wall: tumour (renal cell, transitional cell), fibrosis External pressure: benign prostatic hyperplasia, prostate cancer, lymphadenopathy, aneurysm

Note: the creatinine can rise with severe prerenal AKI; to differentiate this from intrinsic and obstructive AKI, multiply the urea by 10; if it exceeds the creatinine (showing a relatively greater increase in urea compared to creatinine) then this suggests a prerenal aetiology.
AKI in RAS is often triggered by drugs (ACEI or NSAIDs**) and effectively causes hypoperfusion of the kidneys and thus a prerenal picture.*
***Especially **gentamicin, vancomycin** and **tetracyclines**.*

LIVER FUNCTION TESTS (LFTs)

One can assess the liver by looking at markers of:
- Hepatocyte injury or cholestasis such as:
  ▸ bilirubin
  ▸ alanine aminotransferase (ALT) and the less commonly measured aspartate aminotransferase (AST)
  ▸ alkaline phosphatase (alk phos or ALP).
- Synthetic function (i.e. the proteins it makes):
  ▸ albumin
  ▸ vitamin K-dependent clotting factors (II, VII, IX and X) measured via PT/INR.

LFTs help to narrow the causes of raised bilirubin (which may cause jaundice) (Table 3.7). A raised bilirubin on its own indicates prehepatic jaundice (see later in this chapter) that is rarely due to any liver problem itself (in the same way a raised urea on its own (i.e. prerenal AKI) rarely indicates an intrinsic renal problem); rather, because bilirubin is a breakdown product of haemoglobin, a solitary raised bilirubin usually indicates haemolysis.

Clinical hint

A raised alk phos does not necessarily indicate posthepatic jaundice; common causes may be remembered using the mnemonic ALKPHOS: **A**ny fracture, **L**iver damage (posthepatic), **K** (for kancer), **P**aget's disease of bone and **P**regnancy, **H**yperparathyroidism, **O**steomalacia, and **S**urgery.

THYROID FUNCTION TESTS (TFT)

TFTs assess the thyroid stimulating hormone (TSH) and T4; Table 3.8 shows the most common abnormal patterns and causes. In the PSA, students may be asked to change a levothyroxine dose according to TFT results for patients with hypothyroidism (Table 3.9). The trick to this is to use the TSH as a guide: target range ~0.5–5 mIU/L and, unless grossly hypo/hyperthyroid, change by the smallest increment offered.

Table 3.9: How to interpret and change levothyroxine dose following TFT results

TSH range (mIU/L)	Change to thyroxine
<0.5	Decrease dose
0.5–5	Nil action – same dose
>5	Increase dose

Table 3.7: Causes of deranged liver function tests

	Pattern of LFT derangement	Causes
Prehepatic	Bilirubin ⇑	**Haemolysis** Gilbert's and Crigler–Najjar syndromes
Intrahepatic	Bilirubin ⇑ and AST/ALT ⇑	Fatty liver **Hepatitis*** **Cirrhosis*** **Malignancy** (primary or secondary) Metabolic: Wilson's disease/haemochromatosis Heart failure (causing hepatic congestion)
Posthepatic (obstructive)	Bilirubin ⇑ and ALP ⇑	In lumen: **stone (gallstone),** *drugs causing cholestasis*** In wall: tumour (cholangiocarcinoma), primary biliary cirrhosis, sclerosing cholangitis Extrinsic pressure: **pancreatic or gastric cancer**, lymph node

*Hepatitis and cirrhosis may be due to (1) **alcohol**, (2) **viruses** (Hepatitis A–E, CMV and EBV), (3) **drugs (paracetamol overdose, statins, rifampicin)**, and (4) autoimmune (primary biliary cirrhosis, primary sclerosing cholangitis and autoimmune hepatitis).*
Flucloxacillin, coamoxiclav, nitrofurantoin, steroids** and **sulphonylureas

Table 3.8: Abnormal thyroid function tests (image at right from GeekyMedics.com, with permission).

	TFT	
Primary hypothyroidism (⇓ T4 from thyroid causing compensatory ⇑ TSH) *Causes:* Hashimoto's thyroiditis, drug-induced hypothyroidism	T4 ⇓, TSH ⇑	
Secondary hypothyroidism (⇓ TSH from pituitary causing ⇓ T4) *Causes:* Pituitary tumour or damage	T4 ⇓, TSH ⇓	
Primary hyperthyroidism (⇑ T4 from thyroid causing ⇓ TSH*) *Causes:* Grave's disease, toxic nodular goiter, drug-induced hyperthyroidism	T4 ⇑, TSH ⇓	
Secondary hyperthyroidism (⇑ TSH from pituitary causing ⇑ T4) *Causes:* Pituitary tumour	T4 ⇑, TSH ⇑	

Through negative feedback from increased T4 levels.

CHEST X-RAYS

As with all data, a routine must be followed to prevent questions catching you out. The most likely scenarios in the PSA will be **pulmonary oedema** or **pneumonia**. CXR interpretation involves assessing the quality of the film, the structures and the difficult areas.

Quality of film

It is important to check that the film is PRIM:
- **P**rojection (e.g. posterioanterior (PA) (normally) or anterioposterior (AP). If AP the heart will appear larger. If no markings then it is PA)
- **R**otation (e.g. if distance between spinous process and clavicles is equal then no rotation)
- **I**nspiration (e.g. if the seventh anterior (down-sloping) rib transects the diaphragm then adequate)
- **M**arkings (if additional markings, e.g. 'red marks', then the radiographer has spotted an abnormality).

Structures

The main structures to be considered are the:
- Heart which should be less than 50% of the width of the lungs (in PA film); if more then cardiomegaly should be considered.*
- Lungs where if a white area is present then effusion (seen as unilateral and solid), pneumonia (seen as unilateral and fluffy), oedema (seen as bilateral and fluffy*) or fibrosis (seen as bilateral and honeycomb) should be considered.
- Trachea which should be central and if not consider collapse (i.e. towards affected side) or pneumothorax (i.e. away from affected side).
- Mediastinum which if widened consider right upper lobe collapse (with tracheal deviation) or aortic dissection (without tracheal deviation).
- Bones where it is important to look for rib fractures or lytic lesions (i.e. usually suggesting metastases).

Difficult areas

- Are the costophrenic angles sharp? If not then this suggests pleural effusion(s).*
- Is there air under the right hemidiaphragm? This suggests bowel perforation or recent surgery. Under the left side is the gastric air bubble (which is normal).
- Is there a triangle behind the heart (i.e. sail sign)? This suggests left lower lobe collapse.
- Are the apices clear? If not, consider tuberculosis or an apical tumour.

Clinical hint

*If any of these signs are present, look for the ABCDE signs of **pulmonary oedema: A**lveolar oedema (bat wings), Kerley **B** lines (interstitial oedema), **C**ardiomegaly, **D**iversion of blood to upper lobes (where vessels in upper zone are larger than in lower zone), and pleural **E**ffusions.

ARTERIAL BLOOD GASES

It is important to follow a routine:
- **Check inspired oxygen concentration** (FiO_2). This is important because one expects a patient on oxygen to have a higher PaO_2 than one on air, i.e. a patient on 100% oxygen with a PaO_2 of 13 kPa is grossly hypoxic despite having a 'normal range' PaO_2. One can calculate a normal PaO_2 for a patient on oxygen in two ways: accurately (using the arterial–alveolar gradient which is beyond the scope of this book) or approximately by subtracting 10 from the FiO_2 and if the PaO_2 exceeds this calculated number then the patient is not hypoxic; if the PaO_2 is lower, then the patient is hypoxic. For example, a patient on 60% oxygen with an FiO_2 of 30 kPa is actually hypoxic because one would expect a PaO_2 of 50 kPa or above (i.e. 60 minus 10).
- **Check for the presence of respiratory failure** (i.e. is the PaO_2 low or inappropriately normal as explained above). If present then distinguish the type using the $PaCO_2$:
  - Type 1 (most common): low or normal $PaCO_2$ (i.e. **fast/normal breathing**) and can be caused by anything that damages the heart or lungs causing SOB.
  - Type 2 (less common): high $PaCO_2$ (i.e. **slow/shallow breathing**) and can be caused by 'blue-bloaters' subtype of COPD, and less commonly neuromuscular failure or restrictive chest wall abnormalities.
- **Check acid-base status** by looking at pH: if low this indicates acidosis and if high this indicates alkalosis. Look at the $PaCO_2$ and HCO_3 to determine whether this is respiratory or metabolic:
  - If only $PaCO_2$ is abnormal this indicates a respiratory cause.
  - If only HCO_3 is abnormal this indicates a metabolic cause.
  - If both are increased or both decreased this indicates compensation; if the pH is normal then it is fully compensated; if pH remains abnormal then it is partially compensated.
  - If both $PaCO_2$ and HCO_3 are abnormal but in opposite directions then there is coexistent metabolic and respiratory disease.
  - For confirmation remember that CO_2 is an acid and HCO_3 is an alkali; thus in respiratory acidosis, the CO_2 must be high (to explain the acidosis), and in metabolic acidosis, the HCO_3 must be low (to explain the acidosis) and vice versa.
- **Think about the causes** of each abnormality:
  - *Respiratory alkalosis* caused by rapid breathing, whether due to disease or anxiety.
  - *Respiratory acidosis* has the same causes as type 2 respiratory failure.
  - *Metabolic alkalosis* caused by vomiting, diuretics and Conn's syndrome.
  - *Metabolic acidosis* has multiple causes and the most frequent are lactic acidosis, DKA, renal failure and ethanol/methanol/ethylene glycol intoxication. One can use the anion gap to narrow the cause (but this is beyond the scope of this book).

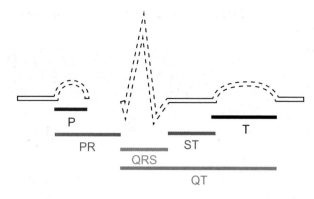

Figure 3.2 ECG measurements.

Table 3.10: QRS Complex deflections: use the mnemonic william morrow to remember these

1st deflection of QRS in V1	Type of BBB			1st deflection of QRS in V6
Down like letter **W**	**i**	LL	**ia**	**M**: up like in letter M
Up like letter **M**	**o**	RR	**o**	**W**: down like in letter W

ECG

Again, follow a practised routine:

- **Rate** (divide 300 by the number of large squares between each QRS complex): normal 60–100 b.p.m., < 60 b.p.m. indicates bradycardia, >100 b.p.m. indicates tachycardia.
- **Rhythm:**
  - ▸ Are there P-waves? If yes then sinus rhythm (SR). If PR interval (Fig. 3.2) is constant and <1 large square then SR without heart block (HB). If SR but PR not constant or over 1 large square then this is **HB.** If PR interval is:
- constant but >1 large square then **first degree HB**
- increasing, then missing QRS, then increasing again indicates **second degree HB (type 1),**
- two or three P-waves for every QRS then **second degree HB (type 2),**
- random (no relationship between P and QRS) then **third degree (i.e. complete HB).**
  - ▸ If no P-waves (and irregular QRS complexes) then the rhythm is **atrial fibrillation (AF).**
- QRS complex:
  - ▸ Width: if QRS <3 small squares wide then there is no **bundle branch block (BBB)**; if QRS >3 small squares wide then BBB is present; to determine which subtype assess QRS shape (see Table 3.10):
    - □ if in V1 the first deflection of the QRS is ⇓ (w-shape) and in V6 the first deflection is ⇑ (m-shape) then this is **left** BBB;
    - □ if in V1 the first deflection of the QRS ⇑ (m-shape) and in V6 the first deflection is ⇓ (w-shape) then this is **right** BBB.
  - ▸ Height: add the largest deflection of the QRS in V1 to that in V6 (in terms of large squares) and if the sum exceeds 3.5 large squares then **left ventricular hypertrophy** (LVH) is present. If there are small complexes throughout then consider a **pericardial effusion**.
- ST segment (see Fig. 3.3):
  - ▸ If elevated then:
    - □ **infarction** (ST segment flat and only raised in some leads), or

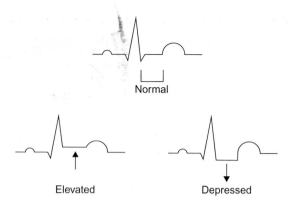

Figure 3.3 Abnormalities of the ST segment.

- □ **pericarditis** (ST segment convex and raised in all leads).
  - ▸ If depressed then:
    - □ **ischaemia** (ST segment flat and only depressed in some leads);
    - □ *digoxin* treatment (ST segment down-sloping in all leads).
- T-waves:
  - ▸ Height: if more than two-thirds of the QRS height throughout the ECG then **hyperkalaemia** is likely present.
  - ▸ Inversion: normal in aVR and I (top middle two) leads; in other leads suggests **old infarction/LVH.**

DRUG-SPECIFIC DATA

AN INTRODUCTION TO DRUG MONITORING

The practicalities of drug monitoring are covered in Chapter 8. However, a general framework for how to interpret and manage abnormal results will be addressed here.

Drugs with a narrow therapeutic index (i.e. where there is a small difference in blood concentration between therapeutic and toxic effects) usually require monitoring. The most common of these are digoxin, theophylline, lithium, phenytoin and certain antibiotics (gentamicin (see later in chapter) and vancomycin).

Monitoring requires assessment of the clinical state (i.e. patient response to the drug and evidence of drug toxicity) plus measurement of serum drug levels. The dose (or frequency) may then be altered if necessary:

- If inadequate response to the drug and low serum drug level then increase dose. In general increase the dose by the smallest possible increment. This is especially important if the drug exhibits zero-order kinetics (such as phenytoin), as a small dose increase will lead to a large clinical effect (with higher risk of toxicity).
- If adequate response to the drug and normal or low serum drug level then no change to the dose is required, i.e. clinical response is more important. There is no point in increasing the dose just to get the patient into what is generally considered a 'therapeutic' range – it's already therapeutic!
- If adequate response to the drug and high serum drug level then decrease the dose. If there is evidence of toxicity (see later in chapter) and clearly if the level is very high then omitting the drug for a few days is appropriate. The only exception to this is gentamicin, where a high serum level (without signs of toxicity) should pre-empt a decrease in frequency by 12 h rather than reducing the dose, e.g. changing from every 24 h (daily) to every 36 h (see below for explanation).

Table 3.11: Signs of commonly encountered drug toxicity

Drug	Features of toxicity
Digoxin	Confusion, nausea, visual halos and arrhythmias
Lithium	Early: tremor Intermediate: tiredness Late: arrhythmias, seizures, coma, renal failure and diabetes insipidus
Phenytoin	Gum hypertrophy, ataxia, nystagmus, peripheral neuropathy and teratogenicity
Gentamicin	Ototoxicity and nephrotoxicity
Vancomycin	Ototoxicity and nephrotoxicity

Table 3.12: Gentamicin monitoring for divided daily dosing regimens

	Normal range in infective endocarditis (5 mg/L)	Normal range in everything else (mg/L)	Action if out of range
Peak (1 h post dose)	3–5	5–10	Adjust dose
Trough (just before next dose)	<1	<2	Adjust dose interval

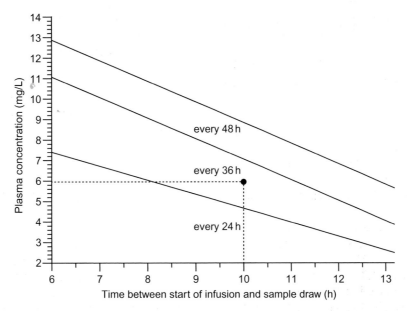

Figure 3.4 Gentamicin treatment nomogram. (From Nicolau DP, et al. Experience with a once-daily aminoglycoside program administered to 2,184 adult patients. *Antimicrobial Agents and Chemotherapy* 1995;39(3):650–655.)

- If evidence of toxicity (see Table 3.11), regardless of drug levels then there are three treatments: (1) stop drug (+/− alternative if required); (2) supportive measures (usually IV fluids); (3) give antidote (if one is available).

Gentamicin monitoring

Gentamicin is an IV aminoglycoside antibiotic used for severe infections. Doses are calculated according to the patient's weight and renal function. Most patients are treated with a **high-dose regimen of 5–7 mg/kg once-daily**; patients with severe renal failure (creatinine clearance <20 mL/min) or endocarditis may receive a **divided daily dosing (1 mg/kg)** 12-hourly (in renal failure) or 8-hourly (in endocarditis) depending on individual hospital policy.

Once-daily regimen monitoring

Monitoring is vital because of the high risk of ototoxicity and nephrotoxicity. For the once-daily regimen the exact monitoring will be determined locally, but usually involves:
- Measuring gentamicin levels at particular times such as 6–14 h after the last gentamicin infusion is started (i.e. the time of the sample must be recorded).

- Using a nomogram (e.g. Hartford if 7 mg/kg dose (Fig. 3.4) or Urban and Craig if 5 mg/kg dose (similar principles)) to determine whether the level is too high: plot the blood concentration (y-axis) against the time between starting last infusion and taking the blood (x-axis). If the resultant point on the graph falls within the 24 h area (q24h) then continue at the same dose; if it falls above the q24h area then change the dosing interval as follows:
  ▸ if point falls in the q36h area change to 36-hourly dosing
  ▸ if point falls in the q48h area change to 48-hourly dosing
  ▸ if point rests above the q48h area repeat the gentamicin level and only re-dose when the concentration <1 mg/L.

This adjustment of the frequency of the dose (rather than the dose itself) reflects the need for a sufficient dose to provide the required peak to hit the minimum inhibitory concentration of the organism.

Divided daily dosing

A nomogram exists for divided daily dosing (Table 3.12), although usually daily peak and trough levels are used instead.

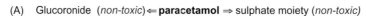

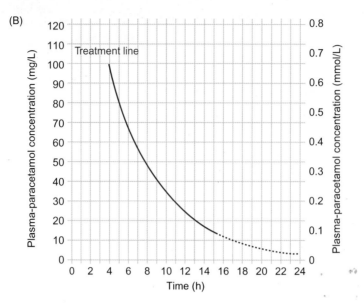

Figure 3.5 **(A)** Paracetamol metabolism and (**B**) the paracetamol nomogram. The paracetamol nomogram is simple to use: at least 4 h after ingestion, if the plasma paracetamol level is below the line, the patient does not require NAC; if the plasma level is above the line, they do. If a staggered overdose was taken, or the time of ingestion is unknown, treatment with NAC is advised. Previous use of a 2-line graph has been replaced by this simpler version. (Nomogram with kind permission of the MHRA.)

Paracetamol nomograms

To understand how to treat a paracetamol overdose one must be able to interpret a paracetamol nomogram. The management for paracetamol overdose involves:

- Specific management (*N*-acetyl cysteine (NAC)) if appropriate (see later in chapter).
- Supportive management (particularly IV fluids) (see Chapter 4, pp. 55).

Paracetamol is normally metabolized by the liver (see Fig. 3.5) in a process reliant on the antioxidant known as glutathione. In paracetamol overdose the limited hepatic stores of glutathione are quickly depleted, leading to accumulation of the toxic metabolite NAPQI. Accumulation of NAPQI is the cause of acute liver damage in paracetamol overdose. NAC replenishes the stores of glutathione, and so reduces the formation of NAPQI, therefore protecting against liver damage.

Warfarin (excessive anticoagulation with warfarin)

Warfarin inhibits synthesis of vitamin K-dependent clotting factors (II, VII, IX and X). This prolongs the prothrombin time (PT) from which the international normalized ratio (INR) is derived: the higher the PT, the higher the INR.

The INR may be viewed as a ratio of the patient's PT compared to the background (normal) population, and is calculated to overcome subtle differences in measurement between labs to enable international comparison – therefore the normal INR is 1. It is only useful for monitoring warfarin (i.e. use the PT instead for those with liver disease or disseminated intravascular coagulation (DIC)).

Target INRs for most patients on warfarin are 2.5 unless there is recurrent thromboembolism while on warfarin or metal replacement heart valves where the INR would be 3.5.

If there is a major bleed (i.e. causing hypotension or bleeding into a confined space (i.e. brain or eye)):

- stop warfarin
- give 5–10 mg IV vitamin K
- give prothrombin complex (e.g. Beriplex®).

Otherwise, use the parameters outlined in Table 3.13 and as found in the BNF.

Table 3.13: How to manage over anticoagulation

INR	Action
<6*	Reduce warfarin dose
6–8*	Omit warfarin for 2 days then reduce dose
>8*	Omit warfarin and give 1–5 mg oral vitamin K
if minor bleeding with INR > 5 give IV instead of oral vitamin K 1–3 mg.	

Question 3.2 Data interpretation item worth 2 marks

CASE PRESENTATION

A 72-year-old man presents to hospital complaining of weakness and malaise. One week earlier he started regular ibuprofen (400 mg oral 8-hourly) for osteoarthritis. His only other history is hypertension, for which he takes ramipril 5 mg daily and amlodipine 10 mg daily. Blood tests find a recent change:

	Today	Last month	Normal range
WCC	6.2×10^9/L	6.0×10^9/L	($4–11 \times 10^9$/L)
Hb	136 g/L	134 g/L	(135–175 g/L (male))
MCV	96.2 fL	96.2 fL	(76–99 fL)
Na	135 mmol/L	135 mmol/L	(135–145 mmol/L)
K	6.9 mmol/L	3.6 mmol/L	(3.5–5.0 mmol/L)
Ur	13.5 mmol/L	5.6 mmol/L	(3–7 mmol/L)
Cr	210 µmol/L	90 µmol/L	(60–125 µmol/L)

Option: Select the *most appropriate* decision option with regard to his current prescription based on this data and mark it with a tick.

DECISION OPTIONS

A	STOP IBUPROFEN	☐
B	STOP AMLODIPINE	☐
C	START SPIRONOLACTONE	☐
D	STOP ACE-INHIBITOR + IBUPROFEN	☑
E	STOP ACE-INHIBITOR	☐

Question 3.3 Data interpretation item worth 2 marks

CASE PRESENTATION

You are called about a 67-year-old woman with an INR of 6.1 (target range is 2–3). She appears well and examination reveals no bleeding. She has completed a course of erythromycin for a chest infection one week ago.

PAST MEDICAL HISTORY

Myocardial infarction and atrial fibrillation.

DRUG HISTORY

Bisoprolol (2.5 mg oral daily) and warfarin (usual dose is 3 mg oral daily). She is allergic to penicillin.

Option: Select the *most appropriate* decision option with regard to her anticoagulation based on this data and mark it with a tick.

DECISION OPTIONS

A	STOP BISOPROLOL 2.5 MG DAILY	☐
B	GIVE VITAMIN K 5 MG IV	☐
C	REDUCE DOSE OF WARFARIN TO 2 MG DAILY	☐
D	INCREASE WARFARIN TO 5 MG, DAILY AND RECHECK INR	☐
E	OMIT WARFARIN AND RECHECK INR	☐

Question 3.2 Answers

A	Ibuprofen decreases renal blood flow by inhibiting prostaglandins that normally dilate blood vessels flowing into the kidney, especially if the patient has renal artery stenosis. Reduced blood flow to the kidney mimics hypotension and prerenal failure, which if prolonged causes intrarenal failure with raised urea, creatinine and potassium. While this is one of the correct drugs to stop, there is another drug that should also be stopped – see option D.
B	Amlodipine is a calcium-channel blocker; it has no effect on electrolyte levels nor renal function and thus does not need to be stopped.
C	Spironolactone is a potassium-sparing diuretic and can cause hyperkalaemia; therefore, it should not be started.
D	**Correct:** see explanation A+E: both should be stopped. Note that while his renal function and potassium were within normal limits whilst on ramipril (suggesting it is not to blame for the acute kidney injury and subsequent hyperkalaemia) the dangerously high potassium means the ACE-inhibitor, which can cause hyperkalaemia, should be stopped (and it can always be re-started later).
E	ACE-inhibitors may cause hyperkalaemia directly (through reduced aldosterone production due to inhibition of ACE) and/or cause renal failure. Renal failure occurs because efferent vessels leaving the kidney rely on angiotensin II to constrict, thereby increasing blood pressure in the kidney. Thus, ACE-inhibitors which decrease angiotensin II production reduce pressure and cause renal damage (e.g. renal failure). This is most marked in patients with renal artery stenosis in whom renal blood flow is reduced anyway.

DECISION OPTIONS

A	STOP IBUPROFEN	☐
B	STOP AMLODIPINE	☐
C	START SPIRONOLACTONE	☐
D	STOP ACE-INHIBITOR + IBUPROFEN	✓
E	STOP ACE-INHIBITOR	☐

Question 3.3 Answers

A	Bisoprolol is a beta-blocker used to treat hypertension, chronic heart failure and arrhythmias. It has no effect on clotting so should not be stopped.
B	Vitamin K reverses the effect of warfarin by allowing synthesis or factors II, VII, IX, X (which warfarin indirectly inhibits). It should be given intravenously if there is minor or major bleeding (with any raised INR) or orally if the INR exceeds 8 without bleeding. If major bleeding occurs, prothrombin complex (e.g. Beriplex®) should also be administered. With an INR <8 and no bleeding then vitamin K is not indicated. Vitamin K administration complicates the reintroduction of warfarin, and hence it is only undertaken in the presence of bleeding or an INR exceeding 8.
C	Reducing the dose would only be appropriate if the INR was less than 6. When over 6, it should be omitted for two days then re-started at a lower dose.
D	An increase in warfarin would further disrupt vitamin K-dependent clotting and therefore further increase the INR.
E	**Correct:** omitting two doses of warfarin should see a therapeutic decline in INR levels. She is anticoagulated for AF with a target INR of 2–3. This has been disrupted because erythromycin is an enzyme inhibitor, i.e. reduces warfarin breakdown and thereby increases its plasma level. Warfarin interrupts vitamin K-dependent clotting (II, VII, IX, X) impairing various parts of the clotting cascade and prolonging the PT (and thus the INR).

DECISION OPTIONS

A	STOP BISOPROLOL 2.5 MG DAILY	☐
B	GIVE VITAMIN K 5 MG IV	☐
C	REDUCE DOSE OF WARFARIN TO 2 MG DAILY	☐
D	INCREASE WARFARIN TO 5 MG DAILY AND RECHECK INR	☐
E	OMIT WARFARIN AND RECHECK INR	✓

Question 3.4 Data interpretation item worth 2 marks

CASE PRESENTATION

A 64-year-old woman with lymphoma and hypertension presents to casualty with a 1-week history of cough productive of green sputum, pleuritic chest pain and fever of 38.5°C. She is currently taking lisinopril and as required codeine. She has recently completed a cycle of chemotherapy. She has no allergies. A CXR confirms pneumonia and her blood results are listed below.

	Value	Normal range		Value	Normal range
WCC	1.2×10^9/L	$(4-11 \times 10^9$/L)	Ur	12.2 mmol/L	(3–7 mmol/L)
Neut.	0.20×10^9/L	$(2-8 \times 10^9$/L)	Cr	92 µmol/L	(60–125 µmol/L)
Lymph.	0.8×10^9/L	$(1-4.8 \times 10^9$/L)	Na	137 mmol/L	(135–145 mmol/L)
Hb	153 g/L	(120–150 g/L (female))	K	6.3 mmol/L	(3.5–5.0 mmol/L)
MCV	92 fL	(76–99 fL)			

She is keen to go home.

Option: Select the *most appropriate* decision option with regard to her management and mark it with a tick.

DECISION OPTIONS

A	START ORAL AMOXICILLIN AND DISCHARGE HOME	☐
B	START ORAL AMOXICILLIN; STOP LISINOPRIL	☐
C	START PIPERACILLIN WITH TAZOBACTAM IV AND GENTAMICIN IV	☐
D	START PIPERACILLIN WITH TAZOBACTAM IV, GENTAMICIN IV AND PARACETAMOL; STOP LISINOPRIL	☐
E	START PIPERACILLIN WITH TAZOBACTAM IV, GENTAMICIN IV AND PARACETAMOL	☐

Question 3.5 Data interpretation item worth 2 marks

CASE PRESENTATION

A 62-year-old male presents to A&E with confusion and a first seizure lasting 30 seconds. His medical history includes congestive cardiac failure (for which he takes bisoprolol and furosemide) and bipolar disorder (for which he takes lithium and more recently carbemazepine). BP 132/64; HR 72/min. His chest is clear on auscultation and JVP is not raised. A CT of the head is normal. Blood results are shown below:

	Value	Normal range		Value	Normal range
WCC	5×10^9/L	$(4-11 \times 10^9$/L)	Ur	6 mmol/L	(3–7 mmol/L)
Neut.	3×10^9/L	$(2-8 \times 10^9$/L)	Cr	72 µmol/L	(60–125 µmol/L)
Lymph.	1.2×10^9/L	$(1.4-4.8 \times 10^9$/L)	Na	113 mmol/L	(135–145 mmol/L)
Hb	153 g/L	(135–175 g/L (male))	K	4.0 mmol/L	(3.5–5.0 mmol/L)
MCV	82 fL	(76–99 fL)	Li	0.5 mmol/L	(0.4–0.8 mmol/L)

Option: Select the *most appropriate* decision option with regard to his management and mark it with a tick.

DECISION OPTIONS

A	STOP FUROSEMIDE	☐
B	STOP FUROSEMIDE AND GIVE IV LORAZEPAM	☐
C	STOP FUROSEMIDE AND BISOPROLOL	☐
D	STOP FUROSEMIDE AND LITHIUM	☐
E	STOP FUROSEMIDE AND CARBEMAZEPINE	☐

Question 3.4 Answers

A	This patient has neutropenic sepsis (i.e. any source of sepsis (in this case pneumonia) with neutrophils <1). The chemotherapy predisposes to this. Oral antibiotics are never adequate in neurotropenic sepsis which (in patients with cancer) caries a 30% mortality rate.
B	As above. It would, however, be important to stop the lisinopril (an ACE-inhibitor) because of the hyperkalaemia.
C	The combination of piperacillin with tazobactam and gentamicin is the most common regimen for neutropenic sepsis; in this question, it is the only IV regimen. However, option C does not address either the cause of the hyperkalaemia (the ACE-inhibitor which should be stopped) nor the fever and pain (for which an antipyretic/analgesic such as paracetamol should be prescribed).
D	**Correct:** this option provides an appropriate antibiotic regimen, stops the ACE-inhibitor responsible for the hyperkalaemia and provides symptomatic relief from the fever and pleuritic chest pain through paracetamol.
E	This option fails to address hyperkalaemia (by continuing the lisinopril).

DECISION OPTIONS

A	START ORAL AMOXICILLIN AND DISCHARGE HOME	☐
B	START ORAL AMOXICILLIN; STOP LISINOPRIL	☐
C	START PIPERACILLIN WITH TAZOBACTAM IV AND GENTAMICIN IV	☐
D	START PIPERACILLIN WITH TAZOBACTAM IV, GENTAMICIN IV AND PARACETAMOL; STOP LISINOPRIL	✓
E	START PIPERACILLIN WITH TAZOBACTAM IV, GENTAMICIN IV AND PARACETAMOL	☐

Question 3.5 Answers

A	This patient is confused and has had a seizure due to hyponatraemia. Furosemide, a loop diuretic, is likely to be contributing to the hyponatraemia and should therefore be stopped. However, carbamazepine can also cause hyponatraemia (through SIADH) – given that this has recently been started it would be sensible to stop this too.
B	While lorazepam is an appropriate choice for a seizure lasting longer than 5 minutes (when seizures last more than 30 minutes the term status epilepticus is used, though treatment should begin after 5 minutes), it is not indicated in a postictal patient as they are not currently fitting.
C	Bisoprolol, a beta-blocker, is indicated as a first-line treatment of chronic heart failure. Its side effects are bronchospasm (which would cause wheeze), hypotension and bradycardia; none of which are present. Thus, it should be continued.
D	Lithium toxicity is very unusual with therapeutic plasma levels (i.e. a level within the normal range): whilst it can cause confusion and even seizures, one would expect tremor and diarrhoea too.
E	**Correct:** while the carbemazapine may be the trigger for the hyponatraemia in this case, the furosemide is likely to also be contributing and should therefore be stopped too (though it may be re-started after the sodium has normalized).

DECISION OPTIONS

A	STOP FUROSEMIDE	☐
B	STOP FUROSEMIDE AND GIVE IV LORAZEPAM	☐
C	STOP FUROSEMIDE AND BISOPROLOL	☐
D	STOP FUROSEMIDE AND LITHIUM	☐
E	STOP FUROSEMIDE AND CARBEMAZEPINE	✓

Question 3.6 Data interpretation item worth 2 marks

CASE PRESENTATION

An 18-year-old woman has been complaining of malaise and urinary frequency for three days. She smokes 10 cigarettes a day, takes the combined contraceptive pill, and has no known allergies. Her blood results are below.

	Value	Normal range		Value	Normal range
WCC	12.9×10^9/L	$(4–11 \times 10^9$/L)	Ur	4.3 mmol/L	(3–7 mmol/L)
Neut.	10.6×10^9/L	$(2–7.5 \times 10^9$/L)	Cr	92 μmol/L	(60–125 μmol/L)
Lymph.	1.2×10^9/L	$(1.3–3.5 \times 10^9$/L)	Na	137 mmol/L	(135–145 mmol/L)
Hb	153 g/L	(120–150 g/L (female))	K	4.4 mmol/L	(3.5–5.0 mmol/L)
MCV	98.2 fL	(76–99 fL)			

Urinary pregnancy test: bHCG +ve

Urinalysis:

Nitrite	+	Leukocytes	++
Blood	–	Protein	+

Option: Select the *most appropriate* decision option with regard to her drug management and mark it with a tick.

DECISION OPTIONS

A	START TRIMETHOPRIM 200 MG TWICE DAILY FOR 7 DAYS	☐
B	STOP ALL MEDICATION	☑
C	START TRIMETHOPRIM 200 MG TWICE DAILY FOR 7 DAYS AND FOLIC ACID SUPPLEMENTATION	☐
D	START CO-AMOXICLAV 625 MG 8-HOURLY FOR 3 DAYS	☐
E	START CO-AMOXICLAV 625 MG 8-HOURLY FOR 3 DAYS AND STOP ALL OTHER MEDICATION	☐

Question 3.6 Answers

A	Trimethoprim is a folate antagonist, and is thus contraindicated in pregnancy because it predisposes to neural tube defects. Further, the typical microbiology advice for uncomplicated UTIs in women limits treatment to 3–5 days.
B	This woman has a UTI in early pregnancy. She should stop her contraceptive, but needs a further prescription to treat the UTI.
C	Folate supplementation is routine in pregnancy anyway. While this may limit the risk of neural tube defects, it may also limit trimethoprim's effectiveness and is an inappropriate risk to take when other (non-teratogenic) antibiotics are offered.
D	This is correct in part. The patient is not penicillin allergic, so co-amoxiclav is a good choice (although sensitivities from a swab/MSU would be useful). However, she remains on a contraceptive during pregnancy which is clearly contraindicated!
E	**Correct:** see options B + D for explanation. Of course, she should be referred for routine antenatal care to include smoking cessation, but the question specifically asks for drug management. Local antibiotic policies should always be consulted; for example some hospitals give longer courses of antibiotics in pregnancy.

DECISION OPTIONS

A	START TRIMETHOPRIM 200 MG TWICE DAILY FOR 7 DAYS	☐
B	STOP ALL MEDICATION	☐
C	START TRIMETHOPRIM 200 MG TWICE DAILY FOR 7 DAYS AND FOLIC ACID SUPPLEMENTATION	☐
D	START CO-AMOXICLAV 625 MG 8-HOURLY FOR 3 DAYS	☐
E	START CO-AMOXICLAV 625 MG 8-HOURLY FOR 3 DAYS AND STOP ALL OTHER MEDICATION	✓

Question 3.7 Data interpretation item worth 2 marks

CASE PRESENTATION

A 52-year-old lady with diabetes, Addison's disease and atrial fibrillation presents to A&E with increasing dizziness and dysuria. Her investigation results are shown below. There is no drop in lying-standing blood pressures (95/74 mmHg on both). She is currently taking digoxin, gliclazide, hydrocortisone and aspirin and has no allergies.

	Value	Normal range		Value	Normal range
WCC	13×10^9/L	(4–11×10^9/L)	Ur	6 mmol/L	(3–7 mmol/L)
Neut.	11×10^9/L	(2–8×10^9/L)	Cr	72 µmol/L	(60–125 µmol/L)
Lymph.	1.2×10^9/L	(1–4.8×10^9/L)	Na	136 mmol/L	(135–145 mmol/L)
Hb	140 g/L	(120–150 g/L (female))	K	4.8 mmol/L	(3.5–5.0 mmol/L)
MCV	82 fL	(76–99 fL)	Glucose	5.8 mmol/L	

Urinalysis:

Protein	+	Nitrite	+
Blood	–	Leukocytes	++

Slow Bradycardia

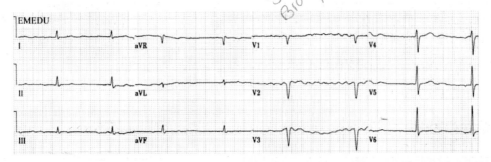

Option: Select the *most appropriate* decision option with regard to her management and mark it with a tick.

DECISION OPTIONS

A	STOP DIGOXIN AND GIVE TRIMETHOPRIM	☐
B	GIVE TRIMETHOPRIM, AND STOP HYDROCORTISONE AND DIGOXIN	☐
C	INCREASE HYDROCORTISONE AND GIVE TRIMETHOPRIM	☐
D	GIVE TRIMETHOPRIM, INCREASE HYDROCORTISONE AND STOP DIGOXIN	☑
E	STOP GLICLAZIDE AND START TRIMETHOPRIM	☐

Question 3.7 Answers

A	This patient has a UTI. Therefore trimethoprim (or another suitable antibiotic) will be needed. The ECG shows slow AF. (To calculate the rate divide 300 by the number of large squares between complexes – ranges from 42 to 58 on tracing, i.e. bradycardic.) Thus, digoxin should be withheld.
B	When addisonian patients become sick they should increase their intake of steroids (so-called 'sick day rules') to provide adequate cortisol for the stress response, i.e. stopping the steroid is wrong. (Note: the absence of a postural drop in BP does not circumvent the need for increased steroids – it simply indicates that the patient is not severely hydrocortisone depleted at present.)
C	This option is almost correct, but does not take account of the bradycardia which is the likely cause of the presentation (i.e. dizziness).
D	**Correct:** this option addresses the bradycardia, steroid requirements and infection.
E	The blood glucose is normal, so stopping gliclazide is unnecessary and fails to address the need for a steroid and the bradycardia.

DECISION OPTIONS

A	STOP DIGOXIN AND GIVE TRIMETHOPRIM	☐
B	GIVE TRIMETHOPRIM, AND STOP HYDROCORTISONE AND DIGOXIN	☐
C	INCREASE HYDROCORTISONE AND GIVE TRIMETHOPRIM	☐
D	GIVE TRIMETHOPRIM, INCREASE HYDROCORTISONE AND STOP DIGOXIN	✓
E	STOP GLICLAZIDE AND START TRIMETHOPRIM	☐

Question 3.8 Data interpretation item worth 2 marks

CASE PRESENTATION

A 58-year-old patient attends A&E with wheeze and dyspnoea. He has a PMH of osteoarthritis, hypertension and asthma. His current medications are listed below. He has widespread polyphonic wheeze on auscultation but is speaking in full sentences with normal BP and pulse rate. The admitting doctor has started treatment for a non-infective exacerbation of asthma with regular salbutamol and ipratropium nebs plus oral prednisolone. His investigations confirm a normal WBC and CRP and no consolidation on CXR. You are asked to write up his regular medications as the A&E doctor has forgotten.

1. Paracetamol 1 g 6-hourly as required
2. Ibuprofen 400 mg 8-hourly
3. Amlodipine 5 mg daily
4. Bisoprolol 2.5 mg daily
5. Salbutamol 100 inhaler as required 2 puffs

Option: Select the *most appropriate* decision option with regard to his management and mark it with a tick.

	DECISION OPTIONS	
A	STOP AMLODIPINE	☐
B	STOP AMLODIPINE AND IBUPROFEN	☐
C	STOP IBUPROFEN AND BISOPROLOL	☐
D	STOP IBUPROFEN AND WITHHOLD SALBUTAMOL INHALER	☐
E	STOP IBUPROFEN AND BISOPROLOL; WITHHOLD SALBUTAMOL INHALER	☐

Question 3.9 Data interpretation item worth 2 marks

CASE PRESENTATION

A 70-year-old female is admitted with worsening breathlessness and leg swelling for the last three days. She has no medical history and is taking no regular medications. She has crepitations to both mid-zones with a raised JVP (4 cm) and pitting oedema to the knees. SaO$_2$ 85% (on air). Respiratory rate 30/min. BP: 150/70 mmHg

Blood (including FBC, CRP, U&E and D-dimer) are normal.

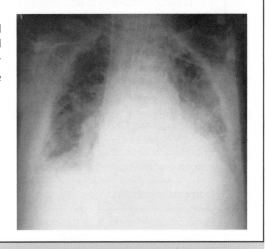

Option: Select the *most appropriate* acute treatment option and mark it with a tick.

	DECISION OPTIONS	
A	FUROSEMIDE 20 MG ORAL	☐
B	CO-AMOXICLAV 625 MG ORAL	☐
C	BUMETANIDE 1 MG ORAL	☐
D	FUROSEMIDE 40 MG IV	☑
E	BENDROFLUMETHIAZIDE 2.5 MG ORAL	☐

Question 3.8 Answers

A	Amlodipine is a calcium-channel blocker which has no ill effects on asthma. As the BP and HR are normal there is no need to stop this.
B	Ibuprofen is an NSAID which can trigger an asthma attack and is therefore contraindicated. However, the inclusion of stopping amlodipine precludes this option.
C	Bisoprolol is a beta-blocker. Its side effects are bronchospasm (which would cause wheeze), hypotension and bradycardia. It should therefore be stopped with the ibuprofen.
D	The salbutamol inhaler should be stopped whilst he is being given the same drug by the (more effective) nebulised route (as denoted in the question body).
E	**Correct:** as explained above, the two drugs likely to be responsible for the asthma exacerbation (bisoprolol and ibuprofen) should be stopped, and the salbutamol inhaler withheld while using nebulised salbutamol.

DECISION OPTIONS

A	STOP AMLODIPINE	☐
B	STOP AMLODIPINE AND IBUPROFEN	☐
C	STOP IBUPROFEN AND BISOPROLOL	☐
D	STOP IBUPROFEN AND WITHHOLD SALBUTAMOL INHALER	☐
E	STOP IBUPROFEN AND BISOPROLOL; WITHHOLD SALBUTAMOL INHALER	✓

Question 3.9 Answers

A	There is evidence of right-sided heart failure (i.e. peripheral oedema and raised JVP) and left-sided heart failure (i.e. bilateral crepitations and breathlessness) collectively giving a diagnosis of congestive cardiac failure (left and right heart failure together). The CXR shows two of the five signs of pulmonary oedema: cardiomegaly and bilateral pleural effusions. With such a small picture it is difficult to identify upper lobe diversion, bat-wing appearance or Kerley-B lines. Furosemide is the mainstay of treatment in acute heart failure; however, in the acute setting it should be administered intravenously.
B	The normal CRP and WBC make pneumonia unlikely. Unless bilateral, pneumonia usually gives unilateral crepitations and CXR abnormalities.
C	Bumetanide is another loop diuretic, though it is usually reserved for patients resistant to furosemide. This is also an oral medication and thus not suitable in this case.
D	**Correct:** see above.
E	Bendroflumethiazide is a thiazide diuretic used in the treatment of hypertension and uncommonly used in managing chronic heart failure.

DECISION OPTIONS

A	FUROSEMIDE 20 MG ORAL	☐
B	CO-AMOXICLAV 625 MG ORAL	☐
C	BUMETANIDE 1 MG ORAL	☐
D	FUROSEMIDE 40 MG IV	✓
E	BENDROFLUMETHIAZIDE 2.5 MG ORAL	☐

Question 3.10 Data interpretation item worth 2 marks

CASE PRESENTATION

An 85-year-old female is admitted with breathlessness for four weeks. Except asthma, for which she takes seretide 250 two puffs 12-hourly and salbutamol as required, she has no medical history. BP 140/70 mmHg, saturations 100% on air and heart rate noted to be 138 b.p.m. Other than some peripheral oedema, examination is unremarkable. Bloods including FBC, CRP, U&E magnesium, TSH and D-dimer are normal. You perform an ECG which is below.

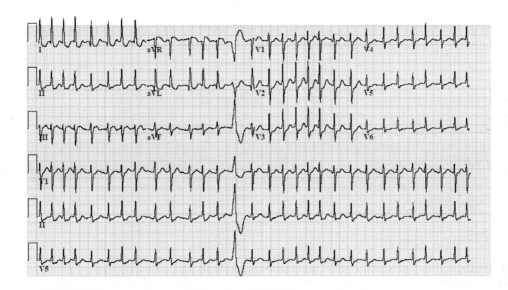

Option: Select the *most appropriate* acute treatment option and mark it with a tick.

DECISION OPTIONS

A	D/C CARDIOVERSION	☑
B	BISOPROLOL	☐
C	AMLODIPINE	☐
D	DIGOXIN	☐
E	DILTIAZEM	☐

Question 3.10 Answers

A	The patient has fast AF as shown by a rapid, irregular ECG without P-waves. (If <100 b.p.m. AF does not require rate control and is not termed fast.) The absence of adverse features (i.e. chest pain, heart failure (no crepitations or oedema/raised JVP), low blood pressure or syncope) means that DC cardioversion is not required in the acute setting. Furthermore, DC cardioversion cannot be performed in AF if it has been present for over 48 hours due to the risk of intracardiac thrombus and subsequent stroke with reversion to sinus rhythm. In this instance, formal anticoagulation and cardiac echo to exclude thrombus would be warranted.
B	Bisoprolol is a beta-blocker and is thus contraindicated in asthmatics.
C	Amlodipine is a calcium-channel blocker. While this may slow the heart, diltiazem is the only commonly used calcium-channel blocker in AF; however, the presence of peripheral oedema should steer one away from calcium-channel blockers as they worsen fluid retention.
D	**Correct:** digoxin is an appropriate choice in this instance, although mainly because of the contraindications to the other two commonly used drugs in AF (i.e. beta-blockers and diltiazem).
E	While a first line drug in AF this may worsen fluid retention and should thus be avoided.

DECISION OPTIONS

A	D/C CARDIOVERSION	☐
B	BISOPROLOL	☐
C	AMLODIPINE	☐
D	DIGOXIN	✓
E	DILTIAZEM	☐

Planning management

Chapter objectives

- Learn management algorithms for the most common acute scenarios, chronic diseases and symptoms.
- Use 10 scenarios with worked answers to reinforce these principles.

STRUCTURE OF THE SECTION WITHIN THE PSA

The 'Planning management' section will have 8 questions with 2 marks available per question, so a possible total of 16 marks. You will be asked to identify the most appropriate prescription (which may be preventative, curative, symptomatic or palliative) from a list of five for each scenario (see Question 4.1).

Question 4.1 Demonstration scenario
Planning management item worth 2 marks

CASE PRESENTATION

A 45-year-old man is admitted to a general medical ward with severe lower back pain radiating into his right buttock. He works as a bricklayer and reports long-standing back pain for many years. An MRI scan of his thoracolumbar spine shows generalized spondylitis but no obvious nerve root compression or disc prolapse. The neurosurgical team feels that no surgical intervention is required.

He is prescribed regular paracetamol 1 g four times daily, morphine sulphate modified release 15 mg twice daily and 'as required' morphine sulphate (Oramorph® (10 mg/5 mL)) 5 mg every 4 hours. Despite this, he describes ongoing back pain, and in particular shooting pain into his buttock.

Question: Select the *most* appropriate management option at this stage and mark it with a tick.

	DECISION OPTIONS	
A	ADD AMITRIPTYLINE 10 MG NIGHTLY	☑
B	ADD CO-CODAMOL (8/500) 2 TABLETS FOUR TIMES DAILY	☐
C	ADD PREDNISOLONE 40 MG, DAILY FOR 21 DAYS	☐
D	INCREASE 'AS REQUIRED' MORPHINE SULPHATE (ORAMORPH® 10 MG/ 5 ML) TO 10 MG EVERY 4 HOURS.	☐
E	TOPICAL LIDOCAINE PATCH 5%	☐

Question 4.1 Answer

A	**Correct:** tricyclic antidepressant, effective in the treatment of neuropathic pain, which appears to be this patient's main complaint.
B	Co-codamol contains paracetamol and must not be used along with single preparation paracetamol due to the risk of excessive paracetamol administration (i.e. more than 4 G per day). Adding a weak opiate would not be sensible (as he is already on a strong opiate).
C	This is incorrect. Although corticosteroids may have a role in the management of spondylitis, it would certainly not be as a first line treatment.
D	'As required' doses of morphine sulphate (in this case Oramorph®) are usually calculated as one sixth of the total daily dose (in this case one sixth of 30 mg, i.e. 5 mg) given up to every 4 to 6 hours. If a patient in chronic pain is requiring higher 'as required' doses, it follows that the regular dose requires adjustment.
E	Neither very useful nor licensed for use for back pain with neuropathic pain. Typically used in postherpetic neuralgia.

DECISION OPTIONS

A	ADD AMITRIPTYLINE 10 MG NIGHTLY	✓
B	ADD CO-CODAMOL (8/500) 2 TABLETS FOUR TIMES DAILY	☐
C	ADD PREDNISOLONE 40 MG, DAILY FOR 21 DAYS	☐
D	INCREASE 'AS REQUIRED' MORPHINE SULPHATE (ORAMORPH® 10 MG/ 5 ML) TO 10 MG EVERY 4 HOURS.	☐
E	TOPICAL LIDOCAINE PATCH 5%	☐

INTRODUCTION

In this chapter, we have divided the likely exam scenarios up into three sections: management of acute conditions, management of common chronic conditions and symptom control.

As with Chapter 2, the practical summaries in each of the three sections incorporate common scenarios in clinical practice and medical examinations, while encompassing those most likely to be seen in the PSA exam.

MANAGEMENT OF ACUTE CONDITIONS

The management of any sick patient must always begin with a practised routine of assessing their airway, breathing, circulation, disability and exposure. Realistically, for the PSA most answers will be from the specific management, but do not forget the obvious solutions such as oxygen for the hypoxic patient, or fluids for the hypotensive patient.

CARDIOVASCULAR (CV) EMERGENCIES (FIG. 4.1)

In all these treatment algorithms, the standard PSA abbreviations of Hx, o/e, inv. and Δ for history, on examination, investigations and diagnosis, respectively, are used.

TACHYCARDIA > 125 B.P.M.

Remember that many tachycardias > 125 b.p.m. will reflect a sick patient with non-cardiac disease (e.g. sinus tachycardia), but always consider the algorithm in Figure 4.2 when not a sinus rhythm.

ST-segment-elevation myocardial infarction (STEMI)

| ABC and O$_2$ (15L) by non-rebreather mask (unless COPD) | Hx, o/e, inv. Δ STEMI | Aspirin 300 mg oral | Morphine 5–10 mg IV with metoclopramide 10 mg IV | GTN spray/tablet | Primary PCI (preferred) or thrombolysis | β-blocker e.g. atenolol 5 mg oral (unless LVF/asthma) | Transfer CCU |

Non-ST-segment-elevation myocardial infarction (NSTEMI) (note 7 of 8 boxes are the same as for STEMI)

| ABC and O$_2$ (15L) by non-rebreather mask (unless COPD) | Hx, o/e, inv. Δ NSTEMI | Aspirin 300 mg oral | Morphine 5–10 mg IV with metoclopramide 10 mg IV | GTN spray/tablet | Clopidogrel 300 mg oral and LMW heparin (e.g. enoxaparin 1 mg/kg bd SC) | β-blocker, e.g. atenolol 5 mg (unless LVF/asthma) | Transfer CCU |

Acute left ventricular failure (LVF) (note 5 of 8 boxes are the same as for STEMI)

| ABC and O$_2$ (15L) by non-rebreather mask (unless COPD) | Hx, o/e, inv. Δ LVF +/– cause | Sit patient up | Morphine 5–10 mg IV with metoclopramide 10 mg IV | GTN spray/tablet | Furosemide 40–80 mg IV | If inadequate response, isosorbide dinitrate infusion +/– CPAP | Transfer CCU |

Figure 4.1 Cardiovascular emergencies. GTN, glyceryl trinitrate; PCI, percutaneous coronary intervention; CCU, coronary care unit; CPAP, continuous positive airway pressure.

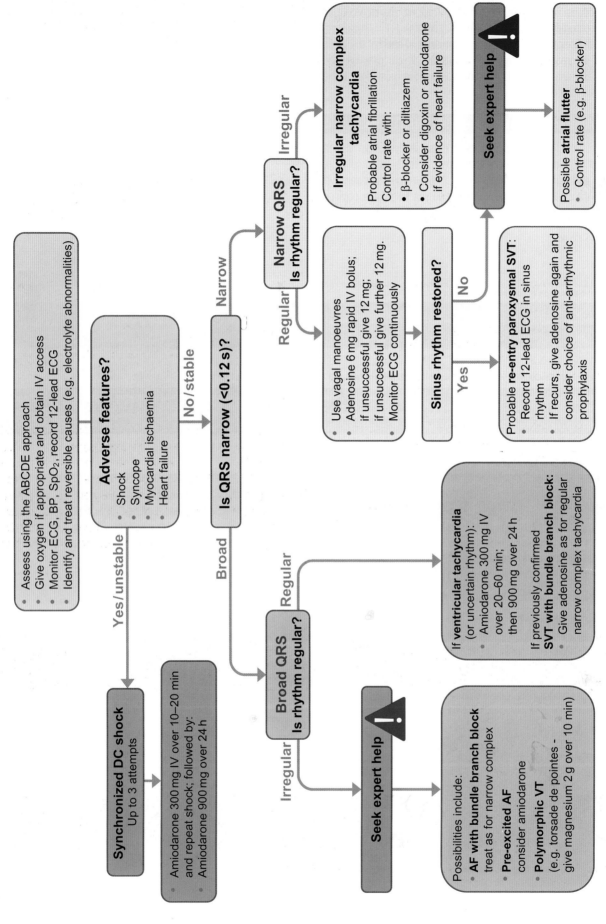

Figure 4.2 Treatment algorithm for adult tachycardia (with pulse). (Resuscitation Council (UK), with permission.)

ANAPHYLAXIS (FIG. 4.3)

ABC and O₂ (15 L) by non-rebreather mask (unless COPD)	Hx, o/e, inv. Δ anaphylaxis	Remove the cause ASAP e.g. blood transfusion	Adrenaline 500 micrograms of 1:1000 IM	Chlorphenamine 10 mg IV	Hydrocortisone 200 mg IV	Asthma tx if wheeze	Amend drug chart allergies box

Figure 4.3   Anaphylaxis treatment, including anaphylactic transfusion reaction.

RESPIRATORY EMERGENCIES

Acute exacerbation of asthma (Fig. 4.4)

ABC	Hx, o/e, inv. Δ acute asthma	100% O₂ by non-rebreather mask	Salbutamol (5 mg NEB)	Hydrocortisone 100 mg IV (if severe/life threatening) or prednisolone 40–50mg oral (if moderate)	Ipratropium (500 micrograms NEB)	Theophylline (only if life threatening)

Figure 4.4   Acute asthma treatment.

Acute exacerbation of chronic obstructive pulmonary disease (COPD)

Same treatment as asthma (see Fig. 4.4), but add antibiotics if infective exacerbations. Patients are also more likely to have type 2 respiratory failure, so use high-flow oxygen with care. Remember, hypoxia will kill much quicker than hypercapnia. Therefore, in the acute setting, even if a very sick patient has known COPD, apply high-flow oxygen then review it quickly after an arterial blood gas (ABG). This is the same in the PSA: providing the patient is not peri-arrest (in which case high-flow should be applied), 28% oxygen is a safe starter in patients with COPD with ABG 30 min later to assess the effect.

Pneumothorax

● If **secondary** (i.e. patient has lung disease) then always needs treatment: chest drain if >2 cm or patient SOB or if >50 years old; otherwise aspirate.
● If **tension pneumothorax** (i.e. clinical distinction but often tracheal deviation +/− shock) then emergency aspiration required, but will need chest drain quickly.

● Otherwise (i.e. if **primary**) determine whether the patient needs treatment:
  ▶ if <2 cm rim and not SOB then discharge with outpatient follow-up in 4 weeks.
  ▶ if >2 cm rim on CXR or feels SOB then aspirate and if unsuccessful aspirate again, and if still unsuccessful then chest drain.

Pneumonia

See Figure 4.5 for treatment algorithm. Use mnemonic CURB65 to assess severity of community-acquired pneumonia and hence treatment: Confusion (abbreviated mental test score (AMTS) ≤ 8/10), Urea >7.5 mmol/L, Respiratory rate >30/min, Blood pressure (systolic) <90 mmHg and age ≥65 years. For the patient with none or one of these then home treatment is possible; with two or more of these then hospital treatment with oral or IV antibiotics according to policy and severity is required; and with more than three of these then consider ITU admission.

ABC	Hx, o/e, inv. Δ pneumonia	High-flow oxygen	Antibiotics (e.g. amoxicillin or co-amoxiclav)	Paracetamol	If low BP: or raised HR IV fluids as normal

Figure 4.5   Pneumonia treatment.

Pulmonary embolism (PE, Fig. 4.6)

ABC	Hx, o/e, inv. Δ PE	High-flow oxygen	Morphine 5–10 mg IV, metoclopramide 10 mg IV	LMWH e.g. tinzaparin 175 units/kg SC daily	If low BP: IV gelofusine-> noradrenaline-> thrombolysis

Figure 4.6   Pulmonary embolism treatment. LMWH, low molecular weight heparin.

GASTROENTEROLOGY EMERGENCIES

Gastrointestinal bleeding (Fig. 4.7)

ABC and O₂ (15 L by non-rebreather mask unless COPD)	Hx, o/e, inv. Δ acute GI bleed	Cannulae (x2 large bore)	Catheter (and strict fluid monitoring)	Crystalloid/colloid*	Cross-match 6 units blood	Correct clotting abnormalities**	Camera (Endoscopy)	Stop culprit drugs (NSAIDs, aspirin, warfarin, heparin)	Call the surgeons if severe

*See Chapter 1: in general give a crystalloid (e.g. 0.9% saline) if BP normal/high, or a colloid (e.g. gelofusine) if BP low; once cross-matched, give blood.

If PT/aPTT more than 1.5×normal range ⇒ give fresh frozen plasma (unless** due to warfarin ⇒ give prothrombin complex (e.g. Beriplex®)); if platelets <50 × 10⁹/L (and actively bleeding) give platelet transfusion.

Figure 4.7 The eight 'C's of treating gastrointestinal bleeding.

NEUROLOGICAL EMERGENCIES

Bacterial Meningitis

A GP will normally have given the patient 1.2 g benzylpenicillin if there is any suspicion of meningitis (see Fig. 4.8). A computerized tomography (CT) scan of the head is not always required before lumbar puncture (LP); scanning the patient can delay the LP and hence antibiotics.

ABC	Hx, o/e, inv. Δ meningitis	High-flow oxygen	IV fluid	Dexamethasone IV unless severely immunocompromised	LP (+/− CT head)	2 g cefotaxime IV (give pre-LP if having CT head or prolonged LP)	Consider ITU

Figure 4.8 Bacterial Meningitis.

Seizures and status epilepticus

If the patient is having a seizure then (1) ensure the airway is patent, (2) put in recovery position to prevent aspiration if patient vomits and (3) check for provoking factors (e.g. plasma glucose, electrolytes, drugs and sepsis). If the patient is having a seizure for more than 5 minutes, then drugs must be given to stop the seizure as outlined in Figure 4.9. Note that status epilepticus technically means a seizure lasting >30 minutes.

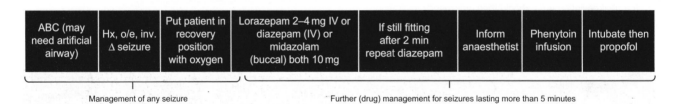

ABC (may need artificial airway)	Hx, o/e, inv. Δ seizure	Put patient in recovery position with oxygen	Lorazepam 2–4 mg IV or diazepam (IV) or midazolam (buccal) both 10 mg	If still fitting after 2 min repeat diazepam	Inform anaesthetist	Phenytoin infusion	Intubate then propofol

Management of any seizure ⎵ Further (drug) management for seizures lasting more than 5 minutes

Figure 4.9 Management of seizures.

Stroke (Fig. 4.10)

If CT shows haemorrhage (of any type) discuss with neurosurgery unit immediately and do not give aspirin or thrombolysis.

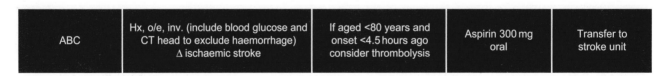

ABC	Hx, o/e, inv. (include blood glucose and CT head to exclude haemorrhage) Δ ischaemic stroke	If aged <80 years and onset <4.5 hours ago consider thrombolysis	Aspirin 300 mg oral	Transfer to stroke unit

Figure 4.10 Management of ischaemic stroke.

METABOLIC EMERGENCIES

Hyperglycaemia (DKA and HONK, Fig. 4.11)

In general, hyperglycaemia in type 1 diabetes can cause diabetic ketoacidosis (DKA) and hyperglycaemia in type 2 diabetes can cause hyperosmolar nonketotic (HONK) coma.

Diabetic ketoacidosis

To diagnose DKA consider the following:
- Diabetic (i.e. hyperglycaemia – BM often >30 mmol/L)
- Keto (i.e. check urine or blood ketone levels)
- Acidosis (i.e. low pH on ABG). Also watch out for increased potassium.

Hyperglycaemic HONK coma

To diagnose hyperglycaemic HONK consider the following:
- Hyperglycaemia (usually >35 mmol/L)
- HO (hyperosmolar: osmolality over 340 mmol/L (calculated by (x2 Na + x2 K) + urea + glucose)
- NK (nonketotic, i.e. no ketones in blood or urine).
  HONK management is the same as DKA management (see Fig. 4.11), except half the rate of fluids is required.

Hypoglycaemia (BM blood glucose <3 mmol/L)

If the patient is able to eat then give a sugar-rich snack, e.g. orange juice and biscuits. However, if unable to eat (i.e. drowsy/vomiting) give IV glucose via a cannula, e.g. 100 mL 20% glucose (traditionally 50 mL 50% glucose IV but can cause extravasation). If unable to eat and no cannula give IM glucagon 1 mg.

ABC	Hx, o/e, inv. Δ DKA	IV fluid: 1 L stat then 1 L over 1 hour, then 2 hours, then 4 hours, then 8 hours	Sliding scale insulin	Hunt for trigger (infection, MI, missed insulin)	Monitor BM, K and pH

Figure 4.11 Management of hyperglycaemia.

Acute kidney injury (AKI, previously known as acute renal failure) (Fig. 4.12)

ABC	Hx, o/e, inv. Δ acute renal failure	Cannula and catheter, strict fluid monitoring	IV fluid: 500 ml stat. then 1 L 4 hourly	Hunt for cause* and complications**	Moniter U&E, and fluid balance

*The causes are as in Chapter 2: at a minimum request routine bloods, ABG, urinalysis, US kidneys and check drug chart for nephrotoxic medications.
**The complications are fluid overload, hyperkalaemia and acidosis.

Figure 4.12 Management of acute renal failure.

Acute poisoning (Fig. 4.13)

ABC	Hx, o/e, inv. Δ acute poisoning	Cannula and catheter, strict fluid balance	Supportive measures*	Correct electrolyte distrubance	Reduce absorption**	Increase elimination***	Psychiatric management

*The supportive measures are IV fluids and analgesia (but only if appropriate, i.e. do not give paracetamol to someone who has just overdosed on it!).
**Reduce absorption if within 1 hour by carrying out (1) gastric lavage (i.e. 'stomach pumping' unless caustic/acid content), (2) whole bowel irrigation (if lithium/iron), (3) charcoal (dx-dependent).
***Increase elimination by giving generous IV fluids plus:
  • N-acetyl cysteine (if paracetamol level at 4 hours or more is over the line on treatment nomogram (see Chapter 2).
  • Naloxone (if opiates have been taken and there is now slow breathing or low GCS).
  • Flumazenil (if benzodiazepines have been taken).

Figure 4.13 Management of acute poisoning.

MANAGEMENT OF CHRONIC CONDITIONS

Junior doctors are more likely to manage acute conditions (on wards) than chronic conditions (generally in primary care and clinics), and the PSA should reflect this. Questions on common diseases with clear guidelines are likely to come up in the exam. The 12 most likely scenarios for chronic management are detailed below. The scenarios are exam focussed and exclude psychosocial management.

CARDIOVASCULAR CONDITIONS

Hypertension

When to treat (see Fig. 4.14)

NICE now recommends ambulatory or home BP monitoring to minimize white coat hypertension; hence, the below values are lower than with clinic-based measurements.

- Treat if BP >150/95 mmHG or >135/85 mmHg if any of the following are also present:
  - ▶ Existing or high risk of vascular disease (ischaemic heart disease (IHD), stroke and peripheral vascular disease).
  - ▶ Hypertensive organ damage (intracerebral bleed, chronic kidney disease, left ventricular hypertrophy and retinopathy).

Target blood pressures on treatment

- In patients aged less than 80 years, aim for <140/85 mmHg (for measurements taken at a clinic) and <135/85 mmHg (for ambulatory or home measurements).
- In patients aged over 80 add 10 mmHg to the systolic values.

Chronic heart failure (adapted from NICE guideline CG108, 2010)

The following treatment is recommended to manage chronic heart failure:

- ACE-inhibitor (e.g. lisinopril 2.5 mg daily) plus beta-blocker (e.g. bisoprolol 1.25 mg daily).
- If inadequate increase doses as tolerated.
- If still inadequate then add according to the severity:
  - ▶ Mild–moderate: add angiotensin receptor blocker (e.g. candesartan 4 mg daily).
  - ▶ Moderate–severe (African–Caribbean patients): add hydralazine 25 mg 8-hourly and isosorbide mononitrate 20 mg 8-hourly.
  - ▶ Moderate–severe (other patients): add spironolactone 25 mg daily.

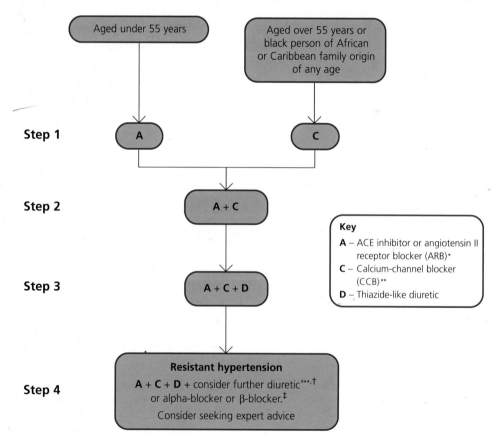

Figure 4.14 Treatment of hypertension (from NICE CG127, 2011, with permission).
*Choose a low-cost ARB. **A CCB is preferred but consider a thiazide-like diuretic if a CCB is not tolerated or the person has oedema, evidence of heart failure or a high risk of heart failure. ***Consider a low dose of spironolactone† or higher doses of a thiazide-like diuretic. †At the time of publication (August 2011), spironolactone did not have a UK marketing authorisation for this indication. Informed consent should be obtained and documented. ‡Consider an alpha-blocker or beta-blocker if further diuretic therapy is not tolerated, or is contraindicated or ineffective.

Atrial fibrillation (adapted from NICE guideline CG36, 2006)

Treatment has two aims. The first is to prevent stroke (as turbulent blood flow can lead to an atrial clot, which can pass to the carotid arteries particularly when sinus rhythm is restored). The second aim is to control the rhythm or rate of the heart. For most patients, rate-control is initiated using beta-blockers or calcium-channel blockers. Note that the presence of adverse features should trigger the use of the Resuscitation Council tachycardia algorithm (see Figure 4.2).

Stroke prevention

- Calculate the CHA2DS2-VASc (previously CHAD) score where each factor contributes one point unless indicated:
  Congestive heart failure (or left heart failure alone)
  Hypertension
  Age >75 (contributing 2 points)
  Diabetes mellitus
  Stroke or TIA before (contributing 2 points)
  Vascular disease (e.g. peripheral arterial disease or IHD)
  Age 65–74
  Sex (female).
- Generally if:
  - Score 0 then consider aspirin 75 mg daily
  - Score 1 use either aspirin or warfarin (aiming for INR 2.5)
  - Score 2 or more give warfarin aiming for INR 2.5

Determine the aim of the treatment according to the patient:

- Rhythm control:
  - Who? – if young/symptomatic AF/first episode of AF/AF due to treated precipitant (e.g. sepsis or electrolyte disturbance).
  - How? – cardioversion: electrical or pharmacological (amiodarone 5 mg/kg IV over 20–120 mins). The patient will require anticoagulation if more than 48 hours since onset.
- Rate
  - Who?: everyone else with heart rate >90 b.p.m.
  - How?: start with (depending on the contraindications) either (1) beta-blocker, e.g. propranolol 10 mg 6-hourly or (2) rate-limiting calcium-channel blocker, e.g. diltiazem 120 mg daily. Verapamil can be used instead but avoid with beta-blockers due to the complication of profound bradycardia.
  - Then add digoxin if needed (or use first line if beta-blockers and calcium-channels are contraindicated). Load then start 62.5–125 micrograms daily.

Stable angina (angina pectoris)

Management of stable angina (adapted from NICE clinical guideline CG126, 2011)

- There are three facets to first line management:
  - GTN spray 'as required' (for symptomatic relief when required).
  - Secondary prevention: consider aspirin, statin and cardiovascular risk factor modification.

Clinical hints

Ensure the patient does have stable angina rather than an acute coronary syndrome (ACS) (the term ACS incorporates unstable angina and both types of myocardial infarction (MI)).

All patients usually present with the same type of chest pain (central, crushing and sometimes radiating to the jaw/arm) but certain factors help to distinguish the causes:
CLINICAL FEATURES
- The presence of sweating or vomiting ⇒ likely ST-segment elevation myocardial infarction (STEMI)/ non-ST segment elevation myocardial infarction (NSTEMI).
- The nature of onset: (1) if it occurs on exertion/emotion and ceases within 15 min then likely stable angina, (2) if it occurs at rest and lasts more than 15 min then likely ACS.
- The response to GTN spray: if this resolves the pain then most likely stable angina.

SIMPLE INVESTIGATIONS
ECG, troponin and 12 h troponin level) provide confirmation:
- If troponin raised = STEMI/NSTEMI ⇒ look at ECG to determine which:
  - If ST elevated ⇒ STEMI
  - If ST depressed or normal ⇒ NSTEMI.
  Note that ST depression in anterior leads (V1–4) may be anterior ischaemia (i.e. stable/unstable angina) or posterior infarction: add leads V7–9 posteriorly to confirm ST elevation for the latter.
- If first troponin not raised then use ECG:
  - If normal/ST depression then stable angina if typical onset (see the nature of onset described above); otherwise unstable angina, but need to exclude NSTEMI with 12 h troponin.
  - If ST elevation then STEMI and troponin will be raised even if having to await 12 h troponin.

- One anti-anginal drug and, dependent on contraindications, either (1) beta-blocker (e.g. atenolol) (contraindications: hypotension, bradycardia, asthma and acute heart failure), or (2) calcium-channel blocker (e.g. amlodipine or diltiazem) (contraindications: hypotension, bradycardia and peripheral oedema).
- If still experiencing stable angina increase dose of beta-blocker or calcium-channel blocker as tolerated.
- If still experiencing stable angina add second anti-anginal therapy. If not contraindicated add the other option (i.e. beta-blocker or calcium-channel blocker). Otherwise add (1) long-acting nitrate, e.g. isosorbide mononitrate, or (2) potassium channel activator, e.g. nicorandil.
- If uncontrolled on two anti-anginal drugs refer for urgent revascularization therapy (percutaneous coronary intervention (PCI) or coronary artery bypass graft (CABG)).

Even if controlled with medical management, patients should be referred routinely for consideration of revascularization.

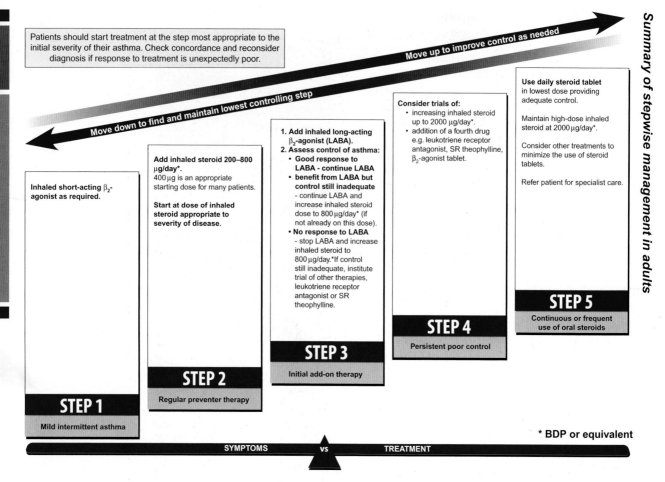

Patients should start treatment at the step most appropriate to the initial severity of their asthma. Check concordance and reconsider diagnosis if response to treatment is unexpectedly poor.

Move up to improve control as needed

Move down to find and maintain lowest controlling step

Inhaled short-acting β₂-agonist as required.

Add inhaled steroid 200–800 μg/day*.
400 μg is an appropriate starting dose for many patients.

Start at dose of inhaled steroid appropriate to severity of disease.

1. **Add inhaled long-acting β₂-agonist (LABA).**
2. **Assess control of asthma:**
   - **Good response to LABA - continue LABA**
   - **benefit from LABA but control still inadequate**
     - continue LABA and increase inhaled steroid dose to 800 μg/day* (if not already on this dose).
   - **No response to LABA**
     - stop LABA and increase inhaled steroid to 800 μg/day.*If control still inadequate, institute trial of other therapies, leukotriene receptor antagonist or SR theophylline.

Consider trials of:
- increasing inhaled steroid up to 2000 μg/day*.
- addition of a fourth drug e.g. leukotriene receptor antagonist, SR theophylline, β₂-agonist tablet.

Use daily steroid tablet in lowest dose providing adequate control.

Maintain high-dose inhaled steroid at 2000 μg/day*.

Consider other treatments to minimize the use of steroid tablets.

Refer patient for specialist care.

STEP 5
Continuous or frequent use of oral steroids

STEP 4
Persistent poor control

STEP 3
Initial add-on therapy

STEP 2
Regular preventer therapy

STEP 1
Mild intermittent asthma

* **BDP or equivalent**

SYMPTOMS — vs — TREATMENT

Figure 4.15 SIGN asthma guidelines (from the British Thoracic Society and Scottish Intercollegiate Guidelines Network's 'British Guideline on the Management of Asthma' (2011), with permission).

RESPIRATORY CONDITIONS

Chronic asthma (see Fig. 4.15)

COPD

- Patients will require smoking cessation advice and therapy including referral to a smoking cessation clinic, nicotine replacement therapy and bupropion or varenicline to reduce cravings.
- Inhaled therapy (see Fig. 4.16).

DIABETES

Management of both type 1 and 2 diabetes

This management must include four components (adapted from NICE guidelines CG15 and CG87, 2009):
1. Education and dietary/exercise advice.
2. CV risk factor management:
   a. aspirin 75 mg daily if any significant CV risk factors (or over age 50 in type 2 diabetes)
   b. simvastatin 20–40 mg daily if any significant CV risk factor (or over age 40 in type 2 diabetes).
3. Annual review of complications. For the PSA this includes checking an albumin–creatinine ratio (ACR) as (1) an early indicator of diabetic nephropathy, and (2) a predictor of cardiovascular disease, e.g. microalbuminuria (ACR ≥ 3 mg/mmol) indicates the need for

an ACE-inhibitor. Ironically, ACE-inhibitors can worsen acute kidney injury but in the chronic setting (with careful monitoring) offer significant cardiovascular and renal protection.
4. Blood glucose-lowering therapy.

Blood glucose lowering therapy in type 1 diabetes

Start with insulin* (and never use oral hypoglycaemic drugs).

Blood glucose lowering therapy in type 2 diabetes

If HbA1c ≥48 mmol/mol (after trial of diet and exercise) use the following steps:
1. Metformin 500 mg with breakfast orally; however, if low/normal weight or creatinine >150 μmol/L use sulphonylurea instead (e.g. gliclazide 40 mg with breakfast orally).
2. If HbA1c ≥48 mmol/mol then increase the drug dose to the maximum as tolerated.
3. If HbA1c still ≥ 48 mmol/mol with
   a. metformin then add sulphonylurea (e.g. gliclazide)
   b. sulphonylurea then add a gliptin (DPP-4 inhibitor), e.g. sitagliptin.
4. If HbA1c still ≥48 mmol/mol add insulin.*

---

*Insulin is best started by a diabetologist, but usually long-acting analogues (e.g. glargine) or NPH insulin (e.g. humulin) are the first choices.

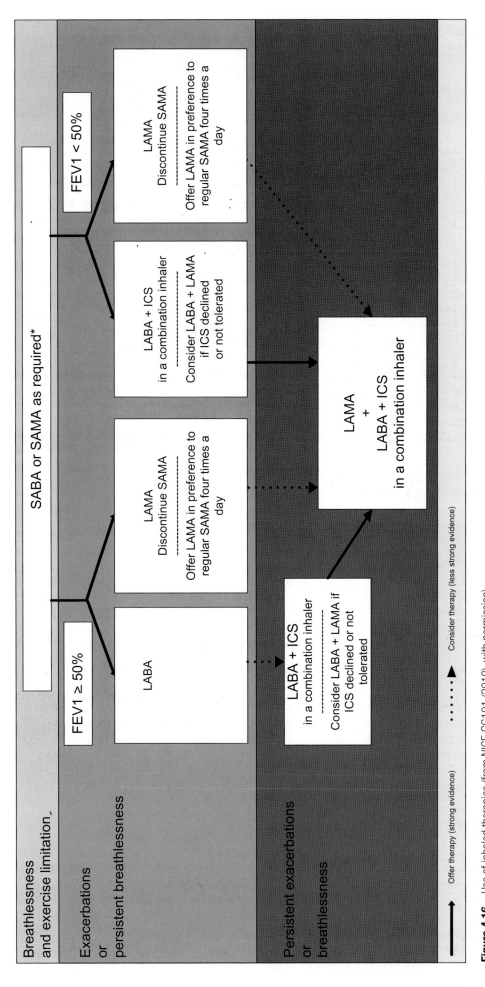

Figure 4.16 Use of inhaled therapies (from NICE CG101 (2010), with permission).
*SABA (as required) may continue at all stages

NEUROLOGICAL CONDITIONS

Parkinson's disease

Most treatments for Parkinson's disease increase the depleted dopamine levels in the basal ganglia.

There is disagreement about first-line therapy in Parkinson's disease. The authors propose that PSA candidates plump for the most commonly used regimen: co-beneldopa or co-careldopa (i.e. levodopa combined with a peripheral dopa decarboxylase inhibitor (benserazide or carbidopa respectively)), unless the question presents a patient with very mild Parkinson's disease who is particularly concerned about the finite period of benefit from levodopa. In this case a dopamine agonist (such as ropinirole) or MAO-inhibitor (such as rasagiline) may be more appropriate.

Epilepsy

Remember, epilepsy means two or more seizures; most first seizures are not treated with antiepileptic drugs.

The choice of antiepileptic drug (NICE CG137, 2012) reflects the type of seizures:

- Generalized tonic–clonic seizures – sodium valproate
- Absence seizures – sodium valproate or ethosuximide
- Myoclonic seizures – sodium valproate
- Tonic seizures – sodium valproate
- Focal seizures – carbamazepine or lamotrigine.

Each drug has multiple side effects, but for the purposes of selecting a drug when a choice of two is presented then valproate's teratogenicity and the lamotrigine rash should help select the most appropriate (Table 4.1).

Table 4.1: Common side effects of antiepileptic medications

Antiepileptic drug	Common side effects
Lamotrigine	Rash, rarely Stevens–Johnson syndrome
Carbamazepine	Rash, dysarthria, ataxia, nystagmus, ⇓Na
Phenytoin	Ataxia, peripheral neuropathy, gum hyperplasia, hepatotoxicity
Sodium valproate	Tremor, teratogenicity, tubby (weight gain)

Alzheimer's disease

- If mild/moderate dementia then treat with acetylcholinesterase (AChE) inhibitors. However, note the following:
  - treatment may only be started by specialist doctors
  - there are three licenced drugs: donepezil, rivastigmine and galantamine.
- If moderate/severe dementia then treat with NMDA antagonist (memantine).

CROHN'S DISEASE (ADAPTED FROM NICE CG152, 2012)

Distinguish whether the question refers to inducing remission (i.e. treating a flare) or maintaining remission (i.e. preventing a flare).

Inducing remission

Treat a mild flare with prednisolone 30 mg daily orally, and treat a severe flare with hydrocortisone 100 mg 6-hourly IV and supportive care (e.g. IV fluid, nil by mouth and antibiotics). In either case, if the patient has rectal disease, use rectal hydrocortisone too.

Maintaining remission

Azathioprine or 6-mercaptopurine

Azathioprine is a pro-drug, metabolized by the liver to the active agent 6-mercaptopurine. In turn, 6-mercaptopurine is metabolized to inactive components by the enzyme thiopurine S-methyl transferase (TPMT). In 10% of the population there is congenitally low activity of TPMT, which would lead to abnormal accumulation of 6-mercaptopurine when azathioprine is given in normal doses. This would increase the risk of liver and bone marrow toxicity. It is therefore important to check TPMT levels before starting either drug. If TPMT is found to be low, consider starting methotrexate instead.

RHEUMATOID ARTHRITIS

- Treat with a combination of methotrexate plus one other disease-modifying antirheumatic drug (DMARD: usually sulfasalazine or hydroxychloroquine) as soon as possible.
- During a flare the following treatments are appropriate:
  - short-term glucocorticoids, e.g. IM methylprednisolone 80 mg
  - short-term NSAIDs, e.g. ibuprofen 400 mg 8-hourly with gastro-protection (e.g. lansoprazole)
  - re-instate DMARDs if dose previously reduced.
- After failure to respond to two DMARDs, severely active rheumatoid arthritis may be managed with TNF-α inhibitors, e.g. infliximab.

SYMPTOMS

Management of pain and nausea has been reviewed in Chapter 2.

FEVER

Beyond treating the underlying cause (usually infection) prescribe paracetamol as an antipyretic (i.e. same dose as for analgesia, maximum 4 g in 24 h).

CONSTIPATION

Beyond treating the underlying cause (e.g. cancer, hypercalcaemia, etc.) prescribe a laxative depending on the cause of constipation and any known contraindications (Table 4.2). Never give a laxative if there is evidence of obstruction.

DIARRHOEA

The commonest cause of diarrhoea is gastrointestinal infection (particularly norovirus and *Clostridium difficile* gastroenteritis). The quick removal of such infectious agents (via diarrhoea) should not be intentionally inhibited by drugs. However, chronic diarrhoea (that has been proven to be non-infectious with negative stool cultures and microscopy) may be treated with loperamide 2 mg oral up to 3-hourly or codeine 30 mg oral up to 6-hourly (which will also provide relief of pain).

INSOMNIA

Many patients will complain of poor sleep in hospital: it is an unfamiliar, noisy and often an unpleasant environment. They may be on drugs that prevent sleep (for example corticosteroids which should be given in the morning to prevent this), and they may nap during the day. These aspects should be dealt with where possible before reaching for a hypnotic, despite requests from nurses. Patients not used to such drugs, particularly the elderly, may become very drowsy and their risk of falling if visiting the toilet, for example, is high. For the purposes of the exam, if you do give a hypnotic, start with zopiclone 7.5 mg oral nightly in adults (and 3.75 mg nightly in the elderly).

Table 4.2: Treatment options for constipation

	Example	Contraindications	Comments
Stool softener	Docusate sodium* Arachis oil (rectal)	Arachis oil: nut allergy	Good for faecal impaction
Bulking agents	Isphagula husk	Faecal impaction Colonic atony	Can take days to develop effect
Stimulant laxatives	Senna Bisacodyl	Bisacodyl: acute abdomen	May exacerbate abdominal cramps
Osmotic laxatives	Lactulose Phosphate enema	Phosphate enema: acute abdomen	May exacerbate bloating

*Stimulant at higher doses.

QUESTIONS

Question 4.2 Planning management item worth 2 marks

CASE PRESENTATION

An 18-year-old man has been using a salbutamol 100 micrograms inhaler (2 puffs 12-hourly) since being diagnosed with asthma 6 months ago. He reports a worsening of his nocturnal cough and a tremor over the last month accompanied by a 20% drop in peak expiratory flow. The cough has responded to an increased frequency of use of salbutamol.

PAST MEDICAL HISTORY

The patient has allergic rhinitis and eczema, managed with cetirizine 10 MG oral, daily) and topical agents.

Question: Select the *most appropriate* treatment option with regard to his asthma management and mark it with a tick.

DECISION OPTIONS

A	STOP SALBUTAMOL 100 MICROGRAMS INHALER	☐
B	INCREASE SALBUTAMOL INHALER TO 2 PUFFS 6-HOURLY	☐
C	ADD PREDNISOLONE 40 MG, DAILY FOR 21 DAYS	☐
D	ADD INHALED BECLOMETHASONE 200 MICROGRAMS, 1 PUFF TWICE DAILY INHALED	☐
E	COUNSEL ABOUT SALBUTAMOL OVERUSE AND ADD INHALED STEROID (BECLOMETHASONE 200 MICROGRAMS, 1 PUFF TWICE DAILY INHALED)	☐

Question 4.2 Answers

A	Salbutamol causes bronchodilation. It is a short-acting β2-agonist and represents the first stage of acute and chronic asthma management. If used more than twice a week, or in the presence of nocturnal symptoms, then the next step of treatment should be added (in this case, the second step: inhaled beclomethasone). Thus, the salbutamol should not be stopped.
B	Salbutamol should not be further increased because (1) this would not comply with the British Thoracic Society stepped approach to management, (2) the salbutamol is already causing side effects (i.e. tremor).
C	Prednisolone is an oral corticosteroid. It is the final step in the management of chronic asthma and is also used in the treatment of acute asthma. Note the duration of treatment is also of concern: systemic steroids used for more than 3 weeks create a theoretical risk of adrenal suppression, unmasking addisonian symptoms when treatment is withdrawn (hence a reducing regime is required when prolonged steroids are stopped).
D	This is partially correct, in line with the stepped approach to the management of chronic asthma. A nocturnal cough or use of salbutamol more than twice weekly heralds escalation of treatment.
E	**Correct:** as D above, plus the tremor is a likely consequence of sympathomimetic (β-agonist) overuse, so the patient should be advised of this link.

DECISION OPTIONS

A	STOP SALBUTAMOL 100 MICROGRAMS INHALER	☐
B	INCREASE SALBUTAMOL INHALER TO 2 PUFFS 6-HOURLY	☐
C	ADD PREDNISOLONE 40 MG, DAILY FOR 21 DAYS	☐
D	ADD INHALED BECLOMETHASONE 200 MICROGRAMS, 1 PUFF TWICE DAILY INHALED	☐
E	COUNSEL ABOUT SALBUTAMOL OVERUSE AND ADD INHALED STEROID (BECLOMETHASONE 200 MICROGRAMS, 1 PUFF TWICE DAILY INHALED)	✓

Question 4.3 Planning management item worth 2 marks

CASE PRESENTATION

A 26-year-old carpenter presents to his GP with a 3-day-old cut on his arm from work. On examination there is a superficial, stamp-sized infected wound on his arm. There is some ooze and yellow crusting, and localized erythema. He is otherwise well. He had a tetanus booster 3 months ago.

PAST MEDICAL HISTORY

He has no medical or drug history of note and no known drug allergies.

Question: Select the *most appropriate* treatment option for antibiotic therapy from the list and mark it with a tick.

DECISION OPTIONS

A	METRONIDAZOLE 400 MG, 12-HOURLY FOR 7 DAYS	☐
B	FLUCLOXACILLIN 500 MG, 6-HOURLY FOR 7 DAYS	☐
C	FLUCLOXACILLIN 1 G, IV STAT.	☐
D	AMOXICILLIN 250 MG, 8-HOURLY FOR 7 DAYS	☐
E	CLINDAMYCIN 500 MG, 6-HOURLY FOR 7 DAYS	☐

Question 4.4 Planning management item worth 2 marks

CASE PRESENTATION

A 68-year-old patient is admitted with worsening breathlessness, orthopnoea and leg swelling for the last 3 days. She has no medical history and is taking no regular medications. She has crepitations to both mid-zones with a raised JVP (4 cm) and pitting oedema to the knees. SaO_2 81% (on air). Respiratory rate 30/min. BP: 150/70 mmHg. Blood results (including FBC, CRP, U&E and D-dimer) are normal.

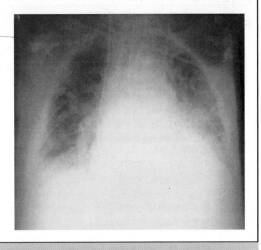

Question: Select the *most appropriate* acute treatment option and mark it with a tick.

DECISION OPTIONS

A	FUROSEMIDE 40 MG ORAL	☐
B	CO-AMOXICLAV 625 MG ORAL	☐
C	BUMETANIDE 1 MG ORAL	☐
D	FUROSEMIDE 40 MG IV	☐
E	BENDROFLUMETHIAZIDE 2.5 MG ORAL	☐

Question 4.3 Answers

A	Metronidazole is typically used for gastrointestinal infections because of its good effects on anaerobes which colonize the gut.
B	**Correct:** the first line antibiotic in skin infections is flucloxacillin.
C	This is the right antibiotic choice but the wrong route. This choice is used for surgical prophylaxis or patients with severe cellulitis and is unlikely to be feasible in a GP surgery.
D	Staphylococci remain susceptible to flucloxacillin but are often resistant to amoxicillin.
E	While effective against gram-positive bacteria such as *Staphylococcus*, it is associated with serious colitis (antibiotic-associated colitis), and is therefore reserved for bone infections.

DECISION OPTIONS

A	METRONIDAZOLE 400 MG, 12-HOURLY FOR 7 DAYS	☐
B	FLUCLOXACILLIN 500 MG, 6-HOURLY FOR 7 DAYS	✓
C	FLUCLOXACILLIN 1 G, IV STAT.	☐
D	AMOXICILLIN 250 MG, 8-HOURLY FOR 7 DAYS	☐
E	CLINDAMYCIN 500 MG, 6-HOURLY FOR 7 DAYS	☐

Question 4.4 Answer

A	There is evidence of right-sided heart failure (peripheral oedema and raised JVP) and left-sided heart failure (bilateral crepitations and breathlessness) collectively giving a diagnosis of congestive cardiac failure (left and right heart failure together). The CXR shows 2 of the 5 signs of pulmonary oedema: cardiomegaly and bilateral pleural effusions. With such a small picture it is difficult to identify upper lobe diversion, bat-wing appearance or Kerley-B lines. Furosemide is the mainstay of treatment in acute heart failure; however, in the acute setting it should be administered intravenously.
B	The normal CRP and WBC make pneumonia unlikely. Unless bilateral, pneumonia usually gives unilateral crepitations.
C	Bumetanide is another loop diuretic, though it is usually reserved for patients resistant to furosemide, and is thus not suitable in this case.
D	**Correct:** see above.
E	Bendroflumethiazide is a thiazide diuretic used in the treatment of hypertension and uncommonly in managing chronic heart failure.

DECISION OPTIONS

A	FUROSEMIDE 40 MG ORAL	☐
B	CO-AMOXICLAV 625 MG ORAL	☐
C	BUMETANIDE 1 MG ORAL	☐
D	FUROSEMIDE 40 MG IV	✓
E	BENDROFLUMETHIAZIDE 2.5 MG ORAL	☐

opioid

Question 4.5 Planning management item worth 2 marks

CASE PRESENTATION

A 66-year-old female patient, recently discharged from hospital after a total hip replacement attends the GP practice where you are working. She explains that her operation went well but now, 3 weeks post-operatively, she is 'seeing double'.

On further questioning, it appears that she is also suffering from a very dry mouth, despite drinking plenty of water, and constipation. You find that she is slightly tachycardic at 104/min.

You wonder if the symptoms could be drug-related. Specifically, you consider whether these are 'anti-muscarinic' side effects.

Question: Which *two* drugs are most likely to be responsible for these anti-muscarinic side effects.
Mark them with ticks in the column provided.

	CURRENT PRESCRIPTIONS				
	Drug name	Dose	Route	Freq.	
A	OMEPRAZOLE	20 MG	ORAL	DAILY	☐
B	CYCLIZINE	50 MG	ORAL	8-HOURLY	☑
C	AMITRIPTYLINE	20 MG	ORAL	NIGHTLY	☑
D	IBUPROFEN	400 MG	ORAL	8-HOURLY	☐
E	ENOXAPARIN	40 MG	S/C	DAILY	☐

Question 4.6 Planning management item worth 2 marks

CASE PRESENTATION

A 55-year-old female patient attends her local GP practice complaining of a sore throat and explains that she has noticed some small, painful ulcers under her tongue.

Past medical history includes osteoarthritis, trigeminal neuralgia, hyperthyroidism (on 'block & replace' regimen), and iron-deficiency anaemia.

A full blood count reveals that she is neutropenic.

Question: From the list of prescribed medications, which drug is *most likely* to have caused neutropenia in this patient? (You should assume that all were commenced around the same time.) Mark it with a tick in the column provided.

	CURRENT PRESCRIPTIONS				
Drug name	Dose	Route	Freq.	
GABAPENTIN	300 MG	ORAL	8-HOURLY	☐
CARBIMAZOLE	20 MG	ORAL	12-HOURLY	☑
LEVOTHYROXINE	75 MICROGRAMS	ORAL	DAILY	☐
FERROUS SULPHATE	200 MG	ORAL	DAILY	☐
CITALOPRAM	20 MG	ORAL	DAILY	☐

Question 4.5 Answer

Correct answers are cyclizine and amitriptyline.

Cyclizine is a sedating antihistamine, mostly used in practice as an antiemetic, and known to have antimuscarinic side effects.

Amitriptyline is a tricyclic antidepressant, used at lower doses in the treatment of neuropathic pain, also known to have antimuscarinic side effects.

CURRENT PRESCRIPTIONS

	Drug name	Dose	Route	Freq.	
A	OMEPRAZOLE	20 MG	ORAL	DAILY	☐
B	CYCLIZINE	50 MG	ORAL	8-HOURLY	✓
C	AMITRIPTYLINE	20 MG	ORAL	NIGHTLY	✓
D	IBUPROFEN	400 MG	ORAL	8-HOURLY	☐
E	ENOXAPARIN	40 MG	S/C	DAILY	☐

Question 4.6 Answer

Correct answer is carbimazole.

Drug-induced neutropenia is a recognized (although rare) side effect of this drug and clinicians are advised to counsel patients on the requirement to report any signs of infection, including sore throat, which might indicate bone marrow suppression.

Carbamazepine, an alternative to gabapentin for treating neuropathic pain, can also cause neutropenia.

CURRENT PRESCRIPTIONS

Drug name	Dose	Route	Freq.	
GABAPENTIN	300 MG	ORAL	8-HOURLY	☐
CARBIMAZOLE	20 MG	ORAL	12-HOURLY	✓
LEVOTHYROXINE	75 MICROGRAMS	ORAL	DAILY	☐
FERROUS SULPHATE	200 MG	ORAL	DAILY	☐
CITALOPRAM	20 MG	ORAL	DAILY	☐

Question 4.7 Planning management item worth 2 marks

CASE PRESENTATION

You review a 78-year-old man at your GP surgery. His daughter reports a stepwise deterioration in his memory and ability to look after himself and is worried he has Alzheimer's disease. His PMH includes a TIA last year and hypertension. He smokes 10 cigarettes per day and is taking no medications. Blood pressure is 180/75 mmHg.

His neurological examination is unremarkable. He scores 8/30 on the mini-mental state examination (MMSE) with relative preservation of short-term memory. A CT head shows small vessel disease only. Routine bloods are normal except a chronically raised potassium (5.2 mmol/L) which has been extensively investigated and no cause found. A blood vitamin B12 level is within normal limits.

Question: Select the *most appropriate* treatment option with regard to his cognitive impairment and mark it with a tick.

	DECISION OPTIONS	
A	ADD DONEPEZIL 5 MG ORAL AT NIGHT	☐
B	ADD MEMANTINE 5 MG ORAL AT NIGHT	☐
C	ADD HYDROXOCOBALAMIN 1 MG IM ALTERNATE DAYS UNTIL NO FURTHER IMPROVEMENT IN COGNITION	☐
D	ADD ASPIRIN 75 MG ORAL DAILY, LISINOPRIL 10 MG ORAL DAILY	☐
E	ADD ASPIRIN 75 MG ORAL DAILY AND AMLODIPINE 5 MG ORAL DAILY	☐

Question 4.8 Planning management item worth 2 marks

CASE PRESENTATION

An 86-year-old female patient, with a history of Parkinson's disease, is admitted to hospital with acute confusion and is diagnosed with a urinary tract infection. She is commenced on a course of antibiotics and haloperidol for agitation, but starts to complain of nausea, so is also commenced on an antiemetic.

Two days into her admission, she develops abnormal movements, which her daughter recognizes as parkinsonian in nature. You are asked to review the patient's drug chart.

Question: From the list of prescribed medication, which one drug is the most likely to have precipitated loss of Parkinson's control in this patient and should thus be stopped? Mark it with a tick in the column provided.

CURRENT PRESCRIPTIONS				
Drug name	Dose	Route	Freq.	
CO-AMOXICLAV	375 MG	ORAL	8-HOURLY	☐
CO-CARELDOPA	125 MG	ORAL	8-HOURLY	☐
DOMPERIDONE	10 MG	ORAL	6-HOURLY	☐
HALOPERIDOL	500 MICROGRAMS	ORAL	AS REQUIRED UP TO 8-HOURLY	☐
OMEPRAZOLE	20 MG	ORAL	DAILY	☐

Question 4.7 Answer

A	Donepezil is licensed for mild to moderate Alzheimer's disease. This patient's MMSE score would not suggest a mild cognitive impairment, and the relative preservation of recent memory would go against a diagnosis of Alzheimer's disease.
B	Memantine is licensed for moderate to severe Alzheimer's disease. As stated above, this patient does not have Alzheimer's disease; certainly the vascular risk factors (smoking and hypertension), previous vascular disease (TIA) and CT results would be in keeping with vascular dementia.
C	When a patient has cognitive impairment a 'confusion screen' should be performed; once the commoner causes of confusion (such as infection) have been excluded, less common (but still reversible) causes should be sought, particularly vitamin B12 deficiency and normal pressure hydrocephalus. Hydroxocobalamin is used to treat vitamin B12 deficiency (and is irrelevant here as there is a normal B12 level).
D	There is little guidance on managing vascular dementia, but given that the only two remaining options are clearly targeting vascular risk factors one can narrow the options quickly. Hypertension management in patients over 55 years old (or black patients of African or Caribbean descent) begins with calcium-channel blockers while that in patients aged under 55 years begins with ACE-inhibitors. The presence of hyperkalaemia should also steer you away from using ACE-inhibitors.
E	**Correct:** as D above, this is the safest of the two options for treating vascular disease (including vascular dementia).

DECISION OPTIONS

A	ADD DONEPEZIL 5 MG ORAL AT NIGHT	☐
B	ADD MEMANTINE 5 MG ORAL AT NIGHT	☐
C	ADD HYDROXOCOBALAMIN 1 MG IM ALTERNATE DAYS UNTIL NO FURTHER IMPROVEMENT IN COGNITION	☐
D	ADD ASPIRIN 75 MG ORAL DAILY, LISINOPRIL 10 MG ORAL DAILY	☐
E	ADD ASPIRIN 75 MG ORAL DAILY AND AMLODIPINE 5 MG ORAL DAILY	✓

Question 4.8 Answer

The correct answer is haloperidol.

Both metoclopramide and haloperidol (a butyrophenone anti-psychotic, licensed for the short-term treatment of acute agitation) are dopamine antagonists and can precipitate parkinsonian symptoms, even in patients who do not have Parkinson's disease.

For this reason, both drugs should be used with extreme caution in patients with a diagnosis of Parkinson's disease and only after discussion with a neurologist.

(It is useful to know that domperidone, another dopamine antagonist licensed for the treatment of nausea, is safe to use for patients with Parkinson's disease as it does not cross the blood-brain barrier).

CURRENT PRESCRIPTIONS

Drug name	Dose	Route	Freq.	
CO-AMOXICLAV	375 MG	ORAL	8-HOURLY	☐
CO-CARELDOPA	125 MG	ORAL	8-HOURLY	☐
DOMPERIDONE	10 MG	ORAL	6-HOURLY	☐
HALOPERIDOL	500 MICROGRAMS	ORAL	AS REQUIRED UP TO 8-HOURLY	✓
OMEPRAZOLE	20 MG	ORAL	DAILY	☐

Question 4.9 Planning management item worth 2 marks

CASE PRESENTATION

A 76-year- old patient with a history of stable angina attends A&E with a 30 minute history of central, crushing chest pain at rest. He is sweaty and has vomited. His examination is unremarkable and his observations are unremarkable.

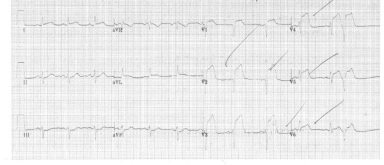

PAST MEDICAL HISTORY

Hypercholesterolaemia and diabetes. He is allergic to opioids.

His ECG is as shown, and a troponin is pending.

You are asked to see him because of severe pain. Until now he has declined analgesia but is now willing to take some.

Question: Select the one most appropriate immediate treatment option for the patient's pain. Mark it with a tick in the column provided.

DECISION OPTIONS

A	PARACETAMOL 1 G ORAL STAT.	☐
B	MORPHINE SULPHATE 10 MG IV STAT.	☐
C	DIAMORPHINE 5 MG IV STAT.	☐
D	GLYCERYL TRINITRATE SPRAY 2 PUFFS SUBLINGUAL	☐
E	GLYCERYL TRINITRATE IV INFUSION 50 MG IN 50 ML 0.9% SALINE AT 2–10 ML/H	☐

Question 4.10 Planning management item worth 2 marks

CASE PRESENTATION

A 70-year-old female was admitted to A&E with acute shortness of breath and left-sided pleuritic chest pain. She has recently been an inpatient under the orthopaedic team having had an elective total right knee replacement. She has a history of chronic obstructive pulmonary disease.

Her respiratory rate is 30/min, oxygen saturations 98% (on air) and heart rate 118/min. Respiratory and cardiovascular examinations are otherwise unremarkable. Her temperature is 36.8°C, she has a swollen left calf and her blood pressure is 162/92 mmHg. She weighs 72 kg.

Chest X-ray shows no focal abnormality. Blood tests (including FBC and CRP) are unremarkable except for an elevated D-dimer (>2000 µg/L).

Question: Select the *most appropriate* management option at this stage and mark it with a tick.

DECISION OPTIONS

A	SUBCUTANEOUS ENOXAPARIN 4,000 UNITS DAILY	☐
B	OXYGEN 60% VIA VENTURI MASK	☐
C	SUBCUTANEOUS DALTEPARIN 15,000 UNITS DAILY	☐
D	FUROSEMIDE 40 MG IV ONCE DAILY	☐
E	AMLODIPINE 5 MG ORAL ONCE DAILY	☐

Question 4.9 Answer

A	While an appropriate first choice analgesic in most situations, this scenario reflects ischaemic heart disease (the ECG shows anterolateral ST elevation indicating a STEMI) and hence the most appropriate immediate treatment option is to give a nitrate to dilate the coronary arteries. The onset of GTN is also much quicker.
B	While opioids often play a part in managing MI, you were told that this patient is allergic to opioids so this is not appropriate.
C	While opioids often play a part in managing MI, this patient is allergic to them so this is not appropriate. Of note, there is little conclusive evidence as to whether diamorphine or morphine confers greater benefit in acute MI despite some preference for the latter. There is a rough equivalency of 5 MG IV diamorphine and 10 MG IV morphine (prefix 'di' means = 2).
D	**Correct:** GTN spray (or tablets) sublingually are rapidly absorbed and give symptomatic benefit. While a failure to respond to GTN spray/tablets may suggest that the current episode of pain is more likely an MI than angina pectoris (which typically responds), it does not preclude using it acutely.
E	When managing acute coronary syndromes, if a patient's chest pain does not subside with GTN spray/tablets an IV infusion of the same drug can be used. It is never used without trying the sublingual route first because (1) this (easier, quicker and cheaper) alternative may give complete resolution; (2) an infusion requires intensive monitoring and risks hypotension.

DECISION OPTIONS

A	PARACETAMOL 1 G ORAL STAT.	☐
B	MORPHINE SULPHATE 10 MG IV STAT.	☐
C	DIAMORPHINE 5 MG IV STAT.	☐
D	GLYCERYL TRINITRATE SPRAY 2 PUFFS SUBLINGUAL	✓
E	GLYCERYL TRINITRATE IV INFUSION 50 MG IN 50 ML 0.9% SALINE AT 2–10 ML/H	☐

Question 4.10 Answer

A	Given the history of recent surgery, an isolated swollen leg (suggesting a DVT) and a raised D-dimer, pulmonary embolism is the most likely diagnosis. This is treated with LMW heparin. However, option A is the prophylactic dose of enoxaparin (not the treatment dose). If in doubt, the BNF will tell you what dose is needed in either situation.
B	Although oxygen is an important part of treating most patients with pulmonary emboli, her saturations are 98% (on air) making 60% oxygen via Venturi mask an inappropriate choice, particularly in a patient at risk of retaining carbon dioxide (COPD).
C	**Correct:** a LMW heparin (enoxaparin, tinzaparin or dalteparin) is appropriate. At her weight (72kg) this is the correct treatment dose of dalteparin.
D	There is no evidence of pulmonary oedema (bilateral crepitations and dullness) so furosemide would not be appropriate.
E	Although the patient is hypertensive this is not the most appropriate treatment as the presumed pulmonary embolism is symptomatic and requires treatment.

DECISION OPTIONS

A	SUBCUTANEOUS ENOXAPARIN 4,000 UNITS DAILY	☐
B	OXYGEN 60% VIA VENTURI MASK	☐
C	SUBCUTANEOUS DALTEPARIN 15,000 UNITS DAILY	✓
D	FUROSEMIDE 40 MG IV ONCE DAILY	☐
E	AMLODIPINE 5 MG ORAL ONCE DAILY	☐

Communicating information

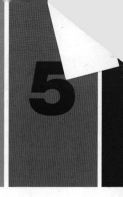

Chapter objectives

- Learn which pieces of information should be communicated to patients when they are started on a particular drug.
- Learn how to select the most appropriate pieces of such information in different clinical scenarios.

STRUCTURE OF THE SECTION WITHIN THE PSA

The 'Communicating information' section will have 6 questions with 2 marks available per question, so a possible total of 12 marks. You will be asked to select one answer from a list of five (i.e. multiple-choice questions).

INTRODUCTION

Patients should always be given adequate information to enable informed decision making about starting a drug, and to ensure its safety and effectiveness. There are no specific guidelines, so this chapter has been divided according to the likely scenarios you will face in the exam. Remember, as in all sections, you have access to the BNF: so if in doubt, use it! We would, however, advocate being familiar with the examples below to avoid running out of time.

QUESTIONS

Question 5.1 Communicating information item worth 2 marks

CASE PRESENTATION
A 27-year-old female is seen in the nephrology clinic.

PAST MEDICAL HISTORY
Chronic kidney disease, focal segmental glomerulosclerosis (FSGS) and hypertension.

DRUG HISTORY
Ramipril 7.5 mg daily for hypertension. She mentions that she is hoping to start a family soon and wonders whether her medication is suitable.

Question: Which one option *best describes* the advice you would give and mark it with a tick.

	DECISION OPTIONS	
A	INCREASE RAMIPRIL TO 10 MG DAILY TO ENSURE BLOOD PRESSURE IS WELL CONTROLLED DURING PREGNANCY	☐
B	STOP RAMIPRIL BECAUSE IT CAN BE TERATOGENIC AND REPLACE WITH LABETALOL BEFORE CONCEPTION	☑
C	STOP RAMIPRIL BECAUSE IT IS TERATOGENIC. NO OTHER MEDICATIONS ARE REQUIRED BECAUSE BLOOD PRESSURE FALLS DURING PREGNANCY	☐
D	REDUCE RAMIPRIL TO 2.5 MG ONCE DAILY AND ADD IN AMLODIPINE 5 MG ONCE DAILY	☐
E	CONTINUE ON RAMIPRIL DURING FIRST TRIMESTER AND CONVERT TO LABETALOL IN THE SECOND TRIMESTER	☐

Question 5.1 Answers

A	Ramipril is teratogenic, particularly in the first trimester. Try not to get bogged down in the unnecessary detail of the question – the key learning point (which is in the BNF) is that ramipril is teratogenic, and should therefore be stopped. You do not need to know detail of FSGS to pass the PSA!
B	**Correct:** ramipril is teratogenic in the first trimester, it is advised to convert to labetalol (first line) before conception.
C	Stopping ramipril although teratogenic would be unsafe given the known history of hypertension. Blood pressure does not fall until the second trimester.
D	Even at low doses ramipril can still be teratogenic. Amlodipine would not be a suitable replacement.
E	Again this would not be suitable due to ramipril's teratogenicity.

DECISION OPTIONS

A	INCREASE RAMIPRIL TO 10 MG DAILY TO ENSURE BLOOD PRESSURE IS WELL CONTROLLED DURING PREGNANCY	☐
B	STOP RAMIPRIL BECAUSE IT CAN BE TERATOGENIC AND REPLACE WITH LABETALOL BEFORE CONCEPTION	✓
C	STOP RAMIPRIL BECAUSE IT IS TERATOGENIC. NO OTHER MEDICATIONS ARE REQUIRED BECAUSE BLOOD PRESSURE FALLS DURING PREGNANCY	☐
D	REDUCE RAMIPRIL TO 2.5 MG ONCE DAILY AND ADD IN AMLODIPINE 5 MG ONCE DAILY	☐
E	CONTINUE ON RAMIPRIL DURING FIRST TRIMESTER AND CONVERT TO LABETALOL IN THE SECOND TRIMESTER	☐

Question 5.2 Communicating information item worth 2 marks

CASE PRESENTATION

A 55-year-old female is seen in the breast clinic following a mastectomy for breast cancer. She is commenced on tamoxifen for positive oestrogen receptors on the tumour.

Question: Select the one *most appropriate* piece of information to communicate to the patient and mark it with a tick.

	DECISION OPTIONS	
A	TAMOXIFEN CONFERS A REDUCED RISK OF ENDOMETRIAL CANCER	☐
B	CAUTION SHOULD BE TAKEN WHEN USING TAMOXIFEN WITH WARFARIN AS IT REDUCES ITS EFFICACY	☐
C	TAKING TAMOXIFEN AT NIGHT WILL REDUCE SYMPTOMS OF 'HOT FLUSHES'	☐
D	SHE SHOULD ATTEND HOSPITAL STRAIGHT AWAY IF SHE NOTICES LEG SWELLING, PAIN OR REDNESS	☐
E	THE TAMOXIFEN DOSE MAY BE DOUBLED AND TAKEN ON ALTERNATE DAYS FOR CONVENIENCE	☐

Question 5.3 Communicating information item worth 2 marks

CASE PRESENTATION

A 75-year-old lady is seen at her GP surgery having had a routine blood test that confirmed an elevated blood sugar. She is commenced on gliclazide 40 mg once daily.

Question: Select the one *most appropriate* piece of information to communicate to the patient and mark it with a tick.

	DECISION OPTIONS	
A	GLICLAZIDE INCREASES THE RISK OF LACTIC ACIDOSIS	☐
B	ADVISE HER TO ENSURE SHE EATS REGULARLY AND AVOIDS MISSING MEALS TO PREVENT HYPOGLYCAEMIA	☑
C	IF A DOSE IS MISSED ENSURE A DOUBLE DOSE IS TAKEN THE NEXT DAY TO AVOID HIGH BLOOD SUGARS	☐
D	MISSING MEALS WILL IMPROVE BLOOD SUGAR CONTROL	☐
E	GLICLAZIDE SHOULD BE TAKEN AT NIGHT IF ON A ONCE-DAILY REGIMEN	☐

Question 5.2 Answers

A	Tamoxifen increases the risk of endometrial carcinoma.
B	Tamoxifen increases the efficacy of warfarin and therefore increases susceptibility to high INR readings.
C	Timing of tamoxifen will not reduce the risk of hot flushes, a common side effect of tamoxifen.
D	**Correct:** tamoxifen increases the risk of venous thromboembolism, and a swollen leg could suggest a deep vein thrombosis which therefore needs urgent medical attention.
E	This is definitely not true!

DECISION OPTIONS

A	TAMOXIFEN CONFERS A REDUCED RISK OF ENDOMETRIAL CANCER	☐
B	CAUTION SHOULD BE TAKEN WHEN USING TAMOXIFEN WITH WARFARIN AS IT REDUCES ITS EFFICACY	☐
C	TAKING TAMOXIFEN AT NIGHT WILL REDUCE SYMPTOMS OF 'HOT FLUSHES'	☐
D	SHE SHOULD ATTEND HOSPITAL STRAIGHT AWAY IF SHE NOTICES LEG SWELLING, PAIN OR REDNESS	✓
E	THE TAMOXIFEN DOSE MAY BE DOUBLED AND TAKEN ON ALTERNATE DAYS FOR CONVENIENCE	☐

Question 5.3 Answers

A	The risk of lactic acidosis is associated with metformin.
B	**Correct:** there is a higher risk of hypoglycaemia associated with sulphonylureas; therefore, patients should not miss meals as this will increase the risk of hypoglycaemia. Note that metformin does not usually cause hypoglycaemia as it works mainly by increasing sensitivity to insulin, and is unlike the sulphonylureas (like gliclazide) which increase insulin production.
C	Under no circumstances should missed doses be doubled up as this will further increase the risk of hypoglycaemia.
D	NO! Missed meals will not improve blood sugar control and will only increase the risk of hypoglycaemia.
E	Gliclazide should be taken in the morning with breakfast. Taking at bedtime will increase the risk of nocturnal hypoglycaemia. If a daily dose of greater than 160 mg is required, then the total daily dose should be divided, but doses should still be given with meals.

DECISION OPTIONS

A	GLICLAZIDE INCREASES THE RISK OF LACTIC ACIDOSIS	☐
B	ADVISE HER TO ENSURE SHE EATS REGULARLY AND AVOIDS MISSING MEALS TO PREVENT HYPOGLYCAEMIA	✓
C	IF A DOSE IS MISSED ENSURE A DOUBLE DOSE IS TAKEN THE NEXT DAY TO AVOID HIGH BLOOD SUGARS	☐
D	MISSING MEALS WILL IMPROVE BLOOD SUGAR CONTROL	☐
E	GLICLAZIDE SHOULD BE TAKEN AT NIGHT IF ON A ONCE-DAILY REGIMEN	☐

Question 5.4 Communicating information item worth 2 marks

CASE PRESENTATION

A 35-year-old man with a history of rheumatoid arthritis is seen in the rheumatology clinic. He is commenced on methotrexate. His baseline chest X-ray and blood tests are satisfactory. You are asked to explain the drug in greater detail following the clinic.

Question: Select the one *most appropriate* piece of information to communicate to the patient and mark it with a tick.

	DECISION OPTIONS	
A	HE WILL REQUIRE 1–2 WEEKLY BLOOD TESTS TO MONITOR FULL BLOOD COUNT	☐
B	METHOTREXATE SHOULD BE TAKEN DAILY	☐
C	THE RISK OF INFECTION IS LOWER WHEN TAKING METHOTREXATE	☐
D	TRIMETHOPRIM SHOULD BE USED AS A FIRST-LINE OPTION FOR URINARY TRACT INFECTIONS	☐
E	FOLIC ACID INCREASES METHOTREXATE TOXICITY	☐

Question 5.5 Communicating information item worth 2 marks

CASE PRESENTATION

A 75-year-old man is admitted to A&E with sudden onset breathlessness and pleuritic chest pain. He has a history of prostate cancer. A CT pulmonary angiogram confirms a sub-segmental pulmonary embolism. He is commenced on LMW heparin and at discharge he is commenced on warfarin and you are asked to discuss this with him.

Question: Select the one *most appropriate* piece of information to communicate to the patient and mark it with a tick.

	DECISION OPTIONS	
A	THE MAJOR ADVERSE EFFECT OF WARFARIN IS BLEEDING	☐
B	NO ADDITIONAL CAUTION NEED BE TAKEN WHEN CONSUMING ALCOHOL	☐
C	ALL 1 MG WARFARIN TABLETS ARE BLUE	☐
D	ALL PATIENTS ON WARFARIN AIM FOR AN INR OF 2.5	☐
E	ONCE WITHIN THE THERAPEUTIC RANGE, WEEKLY BLOODS WILL BE REQUIRED LIFELONG	☐

Question 5.4 Answers

A	**Correct:** regular monitoring of white blood cells is required given the risk of neutropenia.
B	Methotrexate (for non-oncological indications) should ONLY EVER be taken once weekly. More regularly than this increases the risk of neutropenia and other side effects. This is a classic exam trick!
C	Infection risks are much higher given its effect on white blood cells.
D	Folate antagonists, such as trimethoprim and co-trimoxazole, should NEVER be used with methotrexate as they will increase its effect and, therefore, put the patient at risk of severe side effects.
E	Folic acid should be used alongside methotrexate to limit its toxicity to bone marrow.

DECISION OPTIONS

A	HE WILL REQUIRE 1–2 WEEKLY BLOOD TESTS TO MONITOR FULL BLOOD COUNT	✓
B	METHOTREXATE SHOULD BE TAKEN DAILY	☐
C	THE RISK OF INFECTION IS LOWER WHEN TAKING METHOTREXATE	☐
D	TRIMETHOPRIM SHOULD BE USED AS A FIRST-LINE OPTION FOR URINARY TRACT INFECTIONS	☐
E	FOLIC ACID INCREASES METHOTREXATE TOXICITY	☐

Question 5.5 Answers

A	**Correct:** warfarin is an anticoagulant that carries a significant risk of bleeding. This risk is reduced if the INR is regularly monitored.
B	Alcohol affects the metabolism of warfarin and makes monitoring difficult. Acute alcohol intoxication causes enzyme inhibition, while chronic excess causes enzyme induction (see Chapters 1, 2 and 7). If patients wish to drink it should be moderate and spread out over the week as this will have the least impact on INR.
C	Warfarin tablets are colour coded to aid recognition and to allow dose managament. White (0.5 mg), brown (1 mg), blue (3 mg) and pink (5 mg).
D	For most conditions (AF, DVT and PE) an INR of 2.5 is aimed for. For recurrent venous thromboembolism or in patients with mechanical prosthetic valves a higher INR of 3.5 is targeted.
E	Initially, weekly blood tests are required, but once stable these can be performed monthly.

DECISION OPTIONS

A	THE MAJOR ADVERSE EFFECT OF WARFARIN IS BLEEDING	✓
B	NO ADDITIONAL CAUTION NEED BE TAKEN WHEN CONSUMING ALCOHOL	☐
C	ALL 1 MG WARFARIN TABLETS ARE BLUE	☐
D	ALL PATIENTS ON WAFARIN AIM FOR AN INR OF 2.5	☐
E	ONCE WITHIN THE THERAPEUTIC RANGE, WEEKLY BLOODS WILL BE REQUIRED LIFELONG	☐

Question 5.6 Communicating information item worth 2 marks

CASE PRESENTATION

A 50-year-old man with chronic kidney disease, heavy proteinuria and hypertension is seen in the nephrology clinic.

DRUG HISTORY

Amlodipine 10mg once daily. He is commenced on ramipril 2.5mg once daily. You are asked to see him after clinic as the patient wishes to discuss the medication.

Question: Select the one *most appropriate* piece of information to communicate to the patient and mark it with a tick.

	DECISION OPTIONS	
A	RISK OF HYPERKALAEMIA IS LOW WITH RAMIPRIL COMPARED TO OTHER ANTI-HYPERTENSIVES	☐
B	COUGH IS AN UNCOMMON SIDE EFFECT WITH ACE-INHIBITORS	☐
C	PRECAUTIONS NEED TO BE TAKEN IF THE PATIENT DEVELOPS DIARRHOEA OR VOMITING	☐
D	UNLIKE DIURETICS, ACE-INHIBITORS DO NOT CAUSE RENAL FAILURE	☐
E	A REPEAT BLOOD TEST WILL BE REQUIRED IN 6 MONTHS TIME TO MONITOR RENAL FUNCTION	☐

Question 5.7 Communicating information item worth 2 marks

CASE PRESENTATION

An 80-year-old woman presents to her GP with general lethargy and pain around her shoulders and pelvis. Her ESR is elevated at 70 mm/hr and she struggles to lift her arms above her head. A diagnosis of polymyalgia rheumatica is made and she is commenced on prednisolone 30mg once daily. You discuss steroid treatment with her.

Question: Select the one *most appropriate* piece of information to communicate to the patient and mark it with a tick.

	DECISION OPTIONS	
A	STEROIDS DO NOT INCREASE THE RISK OF DIABETES MELLITUS	☐
B	A BISPHOSPHONATE SHOULD BE COMMENCED DUE TO AN INCREASED RISK OF OSTEOPOROSIS	☐
C	GASTRIC PROTECTION IS NOT REQUIRED WHEN ON PREDNISOLONE THERAPY	☐
D	THERE IS NO RISK FROM STOPPING STEROIDS SUDDENLY	☐
E	PATIENTS ARE AT RISK OF HYPOTENSION WITH STEROID THERAPY	☐

Question 5.6 Answers

A	ACE-inhibitors increase the risk of hyperkalaemia.
B	Cough is common with ACE-inhibitors and is thought to be due to the release of bradykinin and is often dose dependent. If patients develop a cough, a trial of an angiotensin-II receptor blocker (e.g. losartan) is an option.
C	**Correct:** caution should be taken, particularly in the elderly who are unwell when on ACE-inhibitors, as it increases the risk of acute kidney injury.
D	Both ACE-inhibitors and diuretics can cause renal failure.
E	It is important to monitor renal function (and potassium) following initiation of ACE-inhibitors, particularly in those with CKD. This should be done 1–2 weeks following initiation.

DECISION OPTIONS

A	RISK OF HYPERKALAEMIA IS LOW WITH RAMIPRIL COMPARED TO OTHER ANTI-HYPERTENSIVES	☐
B	COUGH IS AN UNCOMMON SIDE EFFECT WITH ACE-INHIBITORS	☐
C	PRECAUTIONS NEED TO BE TAKEN IF THE PATIENT DEVELOPS DIARRHOEA OR VOMITING	✓
D	UNLIKE DIURETICS, ACE-INHIBITORS DO NOT CAUSE RENAL FAILURE	☐
E	A REPEAT BLOOD TEST WILL BE REQUIRED IN 6 MONTHS TIME TO MONITOR RENAL FUNCTION	☐

Question 5.7 Answers

A	Long-term steroid therapy increases the risk of diabetes mellitus and blood sugars should be monitored regularly.
B	**Correct:** steroids increase the risk of osteoporosis, particularly in the elderly. If a patient is predicted to take steroid therapy for greater than 3 months (as is typical in polymyalgia rheumatica), prophylactic treatment with a bisphosphonate (e.g. alendronic acid) is an option.
C	There is a small increased risk of gastric irritation and gastric/duodenal ulceration in steroid therapy, thus H2 antagonists (e.g. ranitidine) or proton pump inhibitors (e.g. omeprazole) should be considered for patients considered to be at risk.
D	Those on long courses of steroids should never stop this medication abruptly due to the risk of addisonian crisis.
E	Patients on steroids are at risk of hypertension and should be monitored regularly.

DECISION OPTIONS

A	STEROIDS DO NOT INCREASE THE RISK OF DIABETES MELLITUS	☐
B	A BISPHOSPHONATE SHOULD BE COMMENCED DUE TO AN INCREASED RISK OF OSTEOPOROSIS	✓
C	GASTRIC PROTECTION IS NOT REQUIRED WHEN ON PREDNISOLONE THERAPY	☐
D	THERE IS NO RISK FROM STOPPING STEROIDS SUDDENLY	☐
E	PATIENTS ARE AT RISK OF HYPOTENSION WITH STEROID THERAPY	☐

Question 5.8 Communicating information item worth 2 marks

CASE PRESENTATION

A 30-year-old female with a history of type 1 diabetes mellitus on a basal-bolus insulin regimen attends her GP surgery. She has been low and generally disinterested in life for 5–6 months. She is prescribed citalopram 10mg once daily. You are asked to explain the medication to the patient.

Question: Select the one *most appropriate* piece of information to communicate to the patient and mark it with a tick.

DECISION OPTIONS

A	HER SYMPTOMS ARE LIKELY TO IMPROVE IN 1–2 WEEKS	☐
B	CITALOPRAM MAKES YOU LESS SENSITIVE TO SUNLIGHT	☐
C	TO CONTACT A HEALTH PROFESSIONAL IMMEDIATELY IF SHE HAS THOUGHTS OF SELF HARM OR SUICIDAL IDEATION	☐
D	AGITATION, TEMPERATURES AND HALLUCINATIONS ARE NORMAL SIDE EFFECTS WHEN STARTING CITALOPRAM	☐
E	CITALOPRAM CAN CAUSE EXCESSIVE SALIVATION	☐

Question 5.9 Communicating information item worth 2 marks

CASE PRESENTATION

A 25-year-old male is admitted to hospital with a first presentation of diabetic ketoacidosis and is diagnosed with type 1 diabetes mellitus. He is converted from an insulin sliding scale to a basal-bolus regimen. You are asked to discuss insulin therapy with the patient.

Question: Select the one *most appropriate* piece of information to communicate to the patient and mark it with a tick.

DECISION OPTIONS

A	HYPOGLYCAEMIA SHOULD BE TREATED WITH A BOTTLE OF WATER	☐
B	HbA1c IS A SUITABLE WAY TO MONITOR BLOOD SUGARS FROM DAY-TO-DAY	☐
C	WHEN UNWELL, THE PATIENT'S TOTAL DAILY INSULIN DOSAGE MAY NEED TO BE INCREASED	☐
D	POOR DIABETIC CONTROL IS NOT RELATED TO CARDIOVASCULAR COMPLICATIONS	☐
E	LIPODYSTROPHY IS CAUSED BY REGULARLY ROTATING INJECTION SITES	☐

Question 5.8 Answers

A	It can take up to 6 weeks before there is any improvement in symptoms.
B	Citalopram makes you more photosensitive and precautions should be taken in sunlight.
C	**Correct:** those on anti-depressants can still be suicidal and should seek help immediately. Furthermore, a small proportion of patients will actually feel worse immediately after starting antidepressants before they improve.
D	These symptoms are suggestive of serotonin syndrome which is a life threating complication of selective serotonin reuptake inhibitors (SSRIs). The patient should attend hospital immediately.
E	SSRIs can cause dry mouth.

DECISION OPTIONS

A	HER SYMPTOMS ARE LIKELY TO IMPROVE IN 1–2 WEEKS	☐
B	CITALOPRAM MAKES YOU LESS SENSITIVE TO SUNLIGHT	☐
C	TO CONTACT A HEALTH PROFESSIONAL IMMEDIATELY IF SHE HAS THOUGHTS OF SELF HARM OR SUICIDAL IDEATION	✓
D	AGITATION, TEMPERATURES AND HALLUCINATIONS ARE NORMAL SIDE EFFECTS WHEN STARTING CITALOPRAM	☐
E	CITALOPRAM CAN CAUSE EXCESSIVE SALIVATION	☐

Question 5.9 Answers

A	Depending on consciousness hypoglycaemia should be treated with carbohydrate or glucose tablets/infusions (see Chapter 3).
B	HbA1c gives an average glucose control over a 3-month period. Diabetic patients should target an HbA1c of 48 mmol/mol or less.
C	**Correct:** when unwell, blood glucose increases therefore higher basal doses are required. Failing to do so will increase the risk of diabetic ketoacidosis. Conversely, if patients reduce their oral intake (which many will when ill) there is a risk of hypoglycaemia if the insulin intake is not decreased.
D	Poor glycaemic control significantly increases the risk of microvascular and macrovascular complications.
E	Failure to rotate injection sites can lead to lipodystrophy.

DECISION OPTIONS

A	HYPOGLYCAEMIA SHOULD BE TREATED WITH A BOTTLE OF WATER	☐
B	HbA1c IS A SUITABLE WAY TO MONITOR BLOOD SUGARS FROM DAY-TO-DAY	☐
C	WHEN UNWELL, THE PATIENT'S TOTAL DAILY INSULIN DOSAGE MAY NEED TO BE INCREASED	✓
D	POOR DIABETIC CONTROL IS NOT RELATED TO CARDIOVASCULAR COMPLICATIONS	☐
E	LIPODYSTROPHY IS CAUSED BY REGULARLY ROTATING INJECTION SITES	☐

Question 5.10 Communicating information item worth 2 marks

CASE PRESENTATION

An 80-year-old woman is admitted under the orthopaedic surgeons with a left-side fractured neck of femur. She has had a previous Colles' fracture of her right wrist. She is taking Adcal D3® two tablets once daily and amlodipine 10 mg once daily. She is commenced on alendronic acid. You are asked to explain this medication to the patient.

Question: Select the one *most appropriate* piece of information to communicate to the patient and mark it with a tick.

	DECISION OPTIONS	
A	BISPHOSPHONATES WILL PREVENT ALL FUTURE FRAGILITY FRACTURES	☐
B	ALENDRONIC ACID SHOULD BE TAKEN ON ALTERNATE DAYS	☐
C	BISPHOSPHONATES SHOULD BE TAKEN AT THE SAME TIME AS ADCAL D3®	☐
D	ALENDRONIC ACID IS MOST EFFECTIVE WHEN TAKEN WITH FOOD	☐
E	THE TABLET NEEDS TO BE SWALLOWED WITH A FULL GLASS OF WATER AND SHE SHOULD REMAIN UPRIGHT FOR 30 MIN AFTERWARDS	☑

Question 5.10 Answers

A	They reduce the risk of fractures but certainly do no prevent all fractures.
B	Alendronic acid is a once weekly preparation.
C	Calcium salts reduce the absorption of bisphosphonates and should not be taken at the same time of day.
D	Food should be avoided 2 hours after taking alendronic acid as it reduces its absorption.
E	**Correct:** this is correct and minimizes gastric side effects.

DECISION OPTIONS

A	BISPHOSPHONATES WILL PREVENT ALL FUTURE FRAGILITY FRACTURES	☐
B	ALENDRONIC ACID SHOULD BE TAKEN ON ALTERNATE DAYS	☐
C	BISPHOSPHONATES SHOULD BE TAKEN AT THE SAME TIME AS ADCAL D3®	☐
D	ALENDRONIC ACID IS MOST EFFECTIVE WHEN TAKEN WITH FOOD	☐
E	THE TABLET NEEDS TO BE SWALLOWED WITH A FULL GLASS OF WATER AND REMAIN UPRIGHT FOR 30 MIN AFTERWARDS	✓

Calculation skills

Chapter objectives

- Learn reliable methods for calculating common dosages or administration rates.
- Learn to record this information correctly.
- Learn how to avoid the common traps in the PSA and clinical practice.

STRUCTURE OF THIS SECTION WITHIN THE PSA

The 'Calculation skills' section will have 8 questions with 2 marks available per question, so a possible total of 16 marks. You will be asked to calculate a dose or rate of administration of a medicine.

INTRODUCTION

Calculation assessments can raise anxiety among health care staff, not just because the manipulation of numbers does not always come naturally, even to the most competent practitioner, but also because of the potential implications of a calculation error in 'real life'.

Calculations are, however, a part of almost every aspect of clinical care, from simple multiplication, for example in the case of a drug dosed on a 'milligram per kilogram basis' to complex statistical analysis in the context of clinical research. So it is vital that junior doctors are competent in the interpretation and application of numbers. This is part of the GMC rationale for the PSA.

With this in mind, the 'Calculation skills' section of the PSA will test your ability to make an accurate calculation of drug dosage or rate of administration based on numerical information and to record your answer, using appropriate dosage units.

Fortunately, the vast majority of calculations you will need to perform as a junior doctor are relatively straightforward. This chapter will use examples of calculations common to clinical practice (and hence the PSA) and offer simple strategies for completing them.

While working through these examples, try to keep in mind the following questions:

1. Which pieces of information are relevant? Some questions might include 'distractors', i.e. pieces of information, which might be relevant to the clinical case, but not to your calculation.

2. How can I simplify the information? A handy tip is to pick out and write down the information you select to be relevant in a way that makes it easier for you to manipulate, i.e. accurately completing a calculation question often requires a pencil and a piece of scrap paper!

3. Does my answer look reasonable? When you arrive at your answer, do not just write it down and move on. Compare it with what you already know about drugs and doses and decide if it looks reasonable. This seems an obvious step, but is often missed out.

> **Clinical hint**
>
> 1% means:
> - 1 g in 100 mL (or 10 mg in 1 mL) for weight/volume (w/v) calculations; or
> - 1 g in 100 g for weight/weight (w/w) calculations.

One of the most common calculations in clinical practice involves calculating the volume of a solution that will give the correct dose. For example, what volume of an 80 mg/2 mL solution is required to give a 40 mg dose? (This is an intentionally simple example to illustrate a key equation.) If you have not performed this kind of calculation before and want a quick way of calculating the answer see the following:

1. Write out the information in this format (making sure the units are the same for both numerators and both denominators):

$$\frac{2\,mL}{80\,mg} = \frac{X\,mL}{40\,mg}$$

   Where X is the number you are trying to calculate.

2. Rearrange the equation so that X is on its own:

$$\frac{40 \times 2}{80} = X$$

3. Calculate! (You should get 1 mL as your answer).

4. If you were asked to calculate the dose rather than the volume, use the same equation, but flip the numbers over on both sides so that X is still the numerator. This will make rearranging the equation to solve X much easier.

Now have a go at the example Questions 6.1 and 6.2.

QUESTIONS

> You may use a calculator at any time

Question 6.1 Calculation skills item worth 2 marks

CASE PRESENTATION

You use a bleb of lidocaine (lignocaine) 1% solution to locally anaesthetize an ABG puncture site.

Calculation: How many mg are in 1 mL of a 1% lidocaine solution?

Answer

Question 6.1 Answer

Correct answer and working

By convention, 1% means 1 in 100. In the case of a solution, 1% means 1 g in 100 mL. If there is 1 g in 100 mL, in 1 mL there is 0.01 g or 10 mg.

Learning point

A 1% solution contains 1 g in 100 mL. Memorize this and apply it to similar questions later on.

Clinical point

A 2% solution, which you now know contains 2 g in 100 mL, is double the concentration and perhaps too strong for local anaesthetization for ABG.

Answer | 10 mg

Question 6.2 Calculation skills item worth 2 marks

CASE PRESENTATION

In patients with atrial fibrillation (AF), it might be necessary to administer the cardiac glycoside, digoxin, by the IV route.

Calculation: The IV preparation contains 250 micrograms/mL. Express this as a percentage.

Answer

An alternative way of expressing concentration is demonstrated on adrenaline (epinephrine) preparations in the emergency box on resuscitation trolleys. Different concentrations exist for different indications. A '1 in 1000' (1 g in 1000 mL) preparation is available for the treatment of anaphylaxis. A '1 in 10 000' (1 g in 10 000 mL) preparation is available for use in the setting of cardiopulmonary resuscitation.

Question 6.3 Calculation skills item worth 2 marks

CASE PRESENTATION

An adult male patient is given an intramuscular injection of 0.5 mg of adrenaline 1 in 1000 for the treatment of suspected anaphylaxis after being stung by a bee.

Calculation: What volume of solution was he given?

Answer

Question 6.2 Answer

Correct answer and working

Explanation A (The Long Way Round): You already know that 1% is equivalent to 1 g in 100 mL. So now use it as a reference point:

250 micrograms/mL = 0.25 mg/mL = 2.5 mg/10 mL = 25 mg/100 mL. This is not a 25% solution. Do not be caught out. Note the units.

25 mg/100 mL = 0.025 g/100 mL. This is a 0.025% solution.

Explanation B (the quick way):

250 micrograms/mL = 0.25 mg/mL = 0.00025 g/mL
0.00025 g × 100 (mL) = 0.025%

Learning point

Get your units right! Some of you may have jumped to '25%' as the answer using explanation A. Errors like this can and do happen, particularly when doctors are tired on long night shifts. Avoid this by always thinking about the units you are working with and convert all volumes or masses into the same unit.

You should also know that micrograms are always written out in full in drug charts. This protects patients from drug errors. You should spot (and underline) micrograms in this question, and be drawn to thinking about the units and that they indicate a small expected size of a dose – this is consistent with 0.025% and not 25%.

Answer	0.025%

Question 6.3 Answer

Correct answer and working

Explanation A: 1 in 1000 = 1 g in 1000 mL = 1000 mg/1000 mL = 1 mg/mL = 0.5 mg/0.5 mL
Explanation B: 0.5 mg = 0.0005 g × (1000 mL ÷ 1 g)

Clinical point

Why 1 in 1000? Adrenaline (epinephrine) is available as an easy-to-administer intramuscular injection (EpiPen®) for the treatment of anaphylaxis outside of the hospital (i.e. in the community setting). A 1 in 1000 concentration allows a substantial dose (0.3 mg) to be given in just 0.3 mL of solution. A 1 in 10000 solution would require 3 mL to be administered intramuscularly: a painful and avoidable alternative.

Answer	0.5 mL

The next few sample questions move away from concentrations of solutions. For some, the calculations involved in these questions will seem more intuitive as the answers are proportions of vials or fixed volumes, which are easier to visualize.

We have included some 'distracting' information so that our examples resemble those that might be used in the PSA and indeed present in real-life.

You may use a calculator at any time

Question 6.4 Calculation skills item worth 2 marks

CASE PRESENTATION

A 57-year-old male patient, weighing 80 kg, is given 4 mL of furosemide 50 mg in 5 mL solution by slow IV injection.

Calculation: What dose (in milligrams) of furosemide was given?

Answer   40

You may use a calculator at any time

Question 6.5 Calculation skills item worth 2 marks

CASE PRESENTATION

Later on, you decide to give the same patient a further 75 mg of furosemide.

Calculation: How many millilitres of 50 mg/5 mL solution do you need to give?

Answer   7.4

You may use a calculator at any time

Question 6.6 Calculation skills item worth 2 marks

CASE PRESENTATION

While working on a paediatric ward, you are asked by a staff nurse to double-check a dose calculation. An 11-year-old girl, weighing 30 kg, requires a 2 mg/kg slow IV bolus dose of antibiotic X. The ampoule contains 80 mg in 2 mL.

Calculation: What volume of solution is required?

Answer   1.5

Question 6.4 Answer

Correct answer and working

Remember to get your units right!
50 mg/5 mL = 10 mg/1 mL – this is the dose in 1 mL
4 (mL) × 10 (mg/mL) = 40 mg

Clinical point

If in doubt, work out the dose in 1 mL then multiply by the volume given. Using distracting information, like age and weight, is a useful tip when writing questions to test yourself. It reflects real-life clinical practice.

Answer | 40 mg

Question 6.5 Answer

Correct answer and working

50 mg/5 mL = 10 mg/mL
75 (mg) × (1 (mL) ÷ 10 (mg)) = 7.5 mL

Answer | 7.5 mL

Question 6.6 Answer

Correct answer and working

- This is a perfect opportunity to ask yourself the three questions discussed in the introduction to this chapter:
  o Which pieces of information are relevant? 30 kg, 2 mg/kg and 80 mg/2 mL.
  o How can I simplify the information? Write the relevant bits down and discard the rest.
  o Does my answer look reasonable? If you have calculated a volume of 15 mL, this is highly unlikely to be appropriate for slow IV bolus administration in a paediatric patient.
- 30 (kg) × 2 (mg/kg) = 60 mg (dose required).
- Either:
  o 60 (mg)/80 (mg) = 0.75 (i.e. three-quarters of the ampoule) = 1.5 mL, or
  o 60 (mg) × (2 (mL) ÷ 80 (mg)) = 1.5 mL.

Answer | 1.5 mL

You may use a
calculator at any time

Question 6.7 Calculation skills item worth 2 marks

CASE PRESENTATION

Baby Leon weighs 3 kg and requires a daily maintenance dose of IV digoxin of 25 micrograms. Digoxin is available as 500 micrograms/2 mL ampoules.

Calculation: What volume do you need to give?

Answer

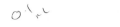 0.1 mL

You may use a
calculator at any time

Question 6.8 Calculation skills item worth 2 marks

CASE PRESENTATION

Mary Bett, a 50 kg, 62-year-old patient, has a swollen left calf. Investigations reveal the following:

- D-dimer – positive
- Wells' score – 6
- Serum creatinine – 64 µmol/L (creatinine clearance >30 mL/min).

You decide to initiate treatment dose enoxaparin (LMW heparin) at a dose of 1.5 mg/kg (or 150 units/kg).

Calculation: What dose do you give? Express the dose in both 'mg' and 'units'

Answer

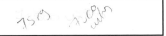 75 mg 7500 units

You may use a
calculator at any time

Question 6.9 Calculation skills item worth 2 marks

CASE PRESENTATION

Elsevier Hospital

Enoxaparin Prescription

Qualitative and quantitative composition

Prefilled syringes

20 mg injection	Equivalent to 2000 units anti-Xa activity in 0.2 mL water for injection
40 mg injection	Equivalent to 4000 units anti-Xa activity in 0.4 mL water for injection
60 mg injection	Equivalent to 6000 units anti-Xa activity in 0.6 mL water for injection
80 mg injection	Equivalent to 8000 units anti-Xa activity in 0.8 mL water for injection

Calculation: Which syringe size will you choose for Mrs Bett? Note that you can discard any excess. (If you are extra keen, you can express as a volume how much you would need to discard.)

Answer

Question 6.7 Answer

Correct answer and working

Use the equation and calculate $(2 \div 500) \times 25$.

Answer 0.1 mL

Question 6.8 Answer

Correct answer and working

The calculation for this question requires little explanation. It is a simple multiplication. The key thing here is the amount of 'distracting' information and you should get used to spotting the relevant information. All of the information is clinically relevant, but not for your calculation.

Clinical point

Doctors often try to 'save time' by using the abbreviation 'IU' or 'U' instead of the word 'units'. This can **and has** led to doses being misread and inadvertently increased by a factor of 10, for example '150 U' can be misread as '1500'. This has occurred on several occasions with insulin, leading to catastrophic results. Protect your patients and always take the time to write out the word 'units' in full. You might think your writing is easy to read, but others may not and it is, after all, only 3 or 4 more letters.
Remember too, you must write out the word 'micrograms' in full for a similar reason to that above.

Answer 75 mg or 7500 units

Question 6.9 Answer

Correct answer and working

If this is not immediately obvious, work out how many units are in 1 mL:
8000 units/0.8 mL = 10 000 units/1 mL.
Then calculate how many millilitres contain 500 units. Use the equation to calculate that if:
10 000 units = 1 mL *then* 500 units = 0.05 mL.
Again, this question requires little explanation. Choose the syringe size from which you can give the whole dose. Your patients will not thank you for giving them two injections when they could have one!

Clinical point

Most hospitals now use drug charts that make LMW heparin syringe size selection easier. If not, there is nothing to stop you from making it clear on the drug chart. The more information you can give to the nursing staff administering the drugs, the safer your prescription will be.

Answer 80 mg (8000 units) (discard 500 units, i.e. 0.05 mL)

In the PSA, you may be asked to interpret more complex data. This may involve interpreting information in the form of charts or graphs in order to find an answer. Do not be intimidated by this kind of question. They are often no more difficult to answer.

> You may use a calculator at any time

Question 6.10 Calculation skills item worth 2 marks

CASE PRESENTATION

You are asked to re-prescribe gentamicin for a 65 kg patient. Blood results are as follows:

- Creatinine clearance = 63 mL/min
- Gentamicin serum concentration = 6.2 micrograms/mL
- Time since last dose (h) = 10.

You are using a 'once-daily' regimen of 7 mg/kg/day.

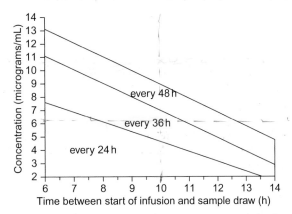

Data from Nicolau DP, et al. Experience with a once-daily aminoglycoside program administered to 2,184 adult patients. *Antimicrobial Agents and Chemotherapy* 1995;39: 650–655.

Calculation: Use the nomogram above to select a suitable dose and dosing interval.

Answer

> You may use a calculator at any time

Question 6.11 Calculation skills item worth 2 marks

CASE PRESENTATION

A 30-weeks pregnant patient is sent to the obstetrics department by her GP. Her blood pressure is 145/100 mmHg. She has proteinuria and brisk reflexes. You treat her as an emergency for pre-eclampsia. The nurse puts equipment on the bedside as shown in the Figure.

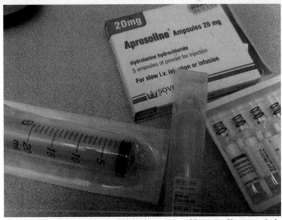

With kind permission of Sovereign Pharmaceuticals.

Calculation: 1. How much sodium chloride (NaCl) 0.9% would you need to add to an ampoule of hydralazine 20 mg/2 mL to make a 1 mg/mL dilution?

2. How much of the 1 mg/mL solution would you need to administer 5 mg?

Answer

Question 6.10 Answer

Correct answer and working

Recall that gentamicin is a nephrotoxic and ototoxic antibiotic so dosing is carefully calculated using renal function and the patient's weight (see Chapter 3). Abnormal monitoring results stimulate changes in the dosing interval (frequency) rather than the dose. The Hartford nomogram above can be used to adjust the dosing interval in response to plasma level monitoring for 7 mg/kg dosing (the Urban and Craig nomogram is used for 5 mg/kg regimens).
For this question:

- Establish that gentamicin is safe to prescribe. 'High-dose' regimens of gentamicin, such as this one, are not recommended for patients whose creatinine clearance is <20 mL/min.

- Interval: plot the serum concentration (6.2 micrograms/mL) against the time since the last dose (10 hours). The area of the graph into which this point falls dictates the next dosing interval (in this case 36 hours between doses (i.e. every 36 hours)). Note that if the point falls on the boundary between two areas, choose the longer dosage interval.

- Dose: 7 (mg) x 65 (kg) = 455 mg.

Answer | 455 mg every 36 hours

Question 6.11 Answer

Correct answer and working

Hydralazine is presented as a 20 mg/2 mL ampoule. Adding 18 mL of NaCl 0.9% would therefore result in a concentration of 1 mg/mL.

1 mg/mL = 5 mg/5mL

Answer 1 | 18 mL

Answer 2 | 5 mL

Question 6.12 Calculation skills item worth 2 marks

CASE PRESENTATION

A neurosurgical patient is prescribed phenytoin 300 mg daily, which she is being given in capsule form. A few days after her operation, she complains of difficulty swallowing the capsules and the nurse asks you if you can re-prescribe phenytoin in liquid form.

Phenytoin is available as a liquid, but it contains phenytoin base rather than the sodium salt of phenytoin (as is in the capsules) such that 100 mg administered as a capsule is equivalent in therapeutic effect to approximately 92 mg administered as liquid.

Calculation: What dose of liquid phenytoin should you prescribe?

Answer	

Question 6.12 Answer

Correct answer and working

It is possible to use our equation to answer this type of question: $(92 \div 100) \times 300$.

Clinical point

Phenytoin is an example of a drug with a narrow therapeutic index. This concept is explained in Chapter 8, so we will only reinforce here the fact that small dose changes for this type of drug can result in either sub-therapeutic or toxic levels. For drugs with a wide therapeutic index, a dose amendment of <10% is unlikely to have any clinical significance. Other drugs for which formulations may differ in terms of the so-called 'salt-factor' are digoxin and sodium fusidate. Use caution when switching patients from one formulation to another.

Answer

276 mg

Prescribing: doing it yourself

Chapter objectives

- Revisit the PReSCRIBER routine described in Chapter 2.
- Practise writing prescriptions with worked answers to reinforce the principles.

STRUCTURE OF THIS SECTION WITHIN THE PSA

The 'Prescribing' section will have 8 questions with 10 marks available per question, so there is a possible total of 80 marks. You will be asked to write a single prescription in each question.

PRESCRIBING PITFALLS

To highlight the common prescribing pitfalls, please complete the scenario in Question 7.1.

Question 7.1 Prescribing item: example scenario

CASE PRESENTATION

Diane Stubbings, 83, is admitted with diarrhoea. Two other residents from her care home also have diarrhoea. Her medical history includes hypertension, asthma, osteoarthritis and a haemorrhagic stroke 3 weeks ago. She has constant pain from her arthritis. She reports an allergy to penicillin (develops anaphylaxis).

ON EXAMINATION

BP 150/110 mmHg, HR 126 b.p.m., UO 100 mL/24 h, SaO$_2$ 100% (on air), chest clear, no oedema, JVP not raised.

INVESTIGATIONS

	Value	Normal range		Value	Normal range
Ur	37.1 mmol/L	(3–7 mmol/L)	K	5.3 mmol/L	(3.5–5.0 mmol/L)
Cr	230 µmol/L	(60–125 µmol/L)	Hb	122 g/L	(120–150 g/L (female))
Na	152 mmol/L	(135–145 mmol/L)			

Pharmacy Stamp *Please do not stamp over age box*	Name: STUBBINGS, DIANE Age: 83 years D.o.B: 01/02/1930	Address: 1 The Close The Ivies Care Home Small City AB1 2PQ Hospital Number: 038942
	CO-CODAMOL 30/500. 2 TABLETS 6-HOURLY ORAL ASPIRIN 75 MG DAILY ORAL LISINOPRIL 10 MG DAILY ORAL PARACETAMOL 1 G 'AS REQUIRED' UP TO 6-HOURLY ORAL IBUPROFEN 200 MG 'AS REQUIRED' UP TO 8-HOURLY ORAL	
Signature of Prescriber Dr B. Smith		Date 01/02/2013
For Dispenser No. of Prescns. on form	Small City Health Authority Dr B. Smith 1 The Lane Small City CA1 3JQ Tel: 01234 567839	
	FP10NC0109	

Prescribing request: Please complete the prescription chart including old drugs and treatment for this episode.

Inpatient Prescription Chart

Weight (kg)	Height (cm)	Surface Area (m²)

Admission Date	Ward	Consultant(s)

Name

Hospital no.

Date of Birth

Address

Use label

Oral medication in surgical pre-op patients

Give ALL oral medication apart from hypoglycaemics even if 'nil by mouth'

Allergies & sensitivities

If none, state '*None*'. Record source of information, e.g. '*patient*', '*notes*', etc

Latex Allergy	☐ Yes		☐ No
☐ Patient	☐ Medical notes		☐ GP
☐ Dr	☐ Nurse		☐ Pharmacist
Signed		Name	Date

Non-administration of drugs

Reasons for non-administration of drugs must be recorded:

1. Nil by mouth	5. Medical instruction
2. Off ward	6. No IV canula in situ
3. Vomiting/nausea	7. Contraindicated
4. Refused	8. Drug not available

Thromboprophylaxis risk assessment
Complete for ALL ADULT PATIENTS, excluding OBSTETRIC patients. REVIEW EVERY 3 DAYS

STEP ONE: ASSESS THROMBOSIS RISK FACTORS - Tick all boxes that apply or tick here if NO thrombosis risk factor ☐

Procedure related factors	Patient related factors
LMWH indicated according to guideline for procedure ☐	Active cancer or cancer treatment ☐
Surgical procedures lasting >30 minutes ☐	Acute surgical admission with inflammatory or abdominal condition ☐
Bilateral uni-compartmental knee replacements ☐	Age >60 years ☐
Critical Care admission ☐	Dehydration ☐
Hip replacement/hip fracture ☐	Known thrombophilia ☐
Major trauma ☐	Medical morbidity (heart failure; respiratory disease; infection; inflammatory conditions; metabolic, diabetic/endocrine crisis) ☐
Major abdominal/pelvic/gynaecological surgery ☐	Obesity (BMI >30 kg/m²) ☐
Plaster cast immobilization of lower limb ☐	On HRT or oestrogen-containing contraceptive pill ☐
Total knee replacement ☐	Personal history or first degree relative with PE or DVT ☐
	Reduced mobility ☐
	Varicose veins with phlebitis ☐

STEP TWO: REVIEW RISK OF ANTICOAGULATION – Tick all boxes that apply or tick here if NO anticoagulation risk factor ☐

Procedure related factors	Patient related factors
Neurosurgery, spinal surgery or eye surgery ☐	Acute stroke in previous month (infarct or haemorrhage) ☐
Other procedure with high bleeding risk ☐	Already on anticoagulant (e.g. warfarin) therapy ☐
	Bleeding from any source/major bleeding risk, e.g. active peptic ulcer ☐
	Blood pressure >230 systolic or >120 diastolic ☐
	Haemophilia, other bleeding disorder, platelet count <75 ☐
	Heparin allergy or heparin-induced thrombocytopenia (seek advice) ☐
	Mobile and high fall risk ☐
	Possible intracranial haemorrhage, e.g. chronic sub-dural haematoma ☐
	Severe liver disease (INR >1.3 or known varices) ☐

STEP THREE: If any box ticked in STEP ONE, consider prescribing drug thromboprophylaxis.
If any box ticked in STEP TWO, consider if anticoagulation risk contraindicates the prescribing of drug thromboprophylaxis.
If prescribing enoxaparin reduce standard dose of 40 mg to 20 mg od if eGFR <30 mL/minute/1.73m².

Drug thromboprophylaxis indicated LMWH ☐ **Other** ☐ | **Drug thromboprophylaxis not indicated** ☐
(Prescribe drug in 'Thromboprophylaxis' section of drug chart)

STEP FOUR: ANTI-EMBOLISM STOCKINGS – indicated in all surgical patients with any box ticked in STEP ONE, unless the following contraindications are present: lower limb dermatitis, ulceration, gangrene, risk of compartment syndrome, peripheral vascular disease, leg deformity preventing proper application, recent skin graft, severe leg oedema **Tick box to prescribe** ☐

Name:	Signature:	Date:

Signature Record

All prescribers MUST complete the Signature Record (including signature as used on the prescription chart)

Date	Name (BLOCK CAPITALS)	Status	Signature	Date	Name (BLOCK CAPITALS)	Status	Signature
	1.				2.		
	3.				4.		
	5.				6.		

Once-only drugs

Name:

Hospital no.:

Date to be given	Time to be given		Drug (approved name)	Dose	Route	Prescriber's signature & bleep number	Given by	Time given	Pharmacy
		1.							
		2.							
		3.							
		4.							
		5.							
		6.							
		7.							
		8.							

Noticeboard

This section is used by healthcare professionals to record useful information relevant to this prescription chart

Antibiotic prescriptions

Indication and stop or review date MUST be completed by prescriber

Name:

Hospital no.:

Date ▶
Circle times or enter other times ▼

1. Antibiotic (approved name)		Start date													
		06													
Dose	Route	12													
		14													
Frequency/Other Instructions	Pharmacy	18													
		22													
Indication(s)		24													
Prescriber's Signature	Bleep no.	Initial stop/review date		Revised stop/review date		Revised stop/review date		Stop/review date must be updated if course continues beyond initial stop/review date							

2. Antibiotic (approved name)		Start date													
		06													
Dose	Route	12													
		14													
Frequency/other instructions	Pharmacy	18													
		22													
Indication(s)		24													
Prescriber's Signature	Bleep no.	Initial stop/review date		Revised stop/review date		Revised stop/review date		Stop/review date must be updated if course continues beyond initial stop/review date							

3. Antibiotic (approved name)		Start date													
		06													
Dose	Route	12													
		14													
Frequency/other instructions	Pharmacy	18													
		22													
Indication(s)		24													
Prescriber's Signature	Bleep no.	Initial stop /review date		Revised stop/review date		Revised stop/review date		Stop/review date must be updated if course continues beyond initial stop/review date							

Oxygen therapy

	Name							Hospital no.			

Date ▸											
Guide times for checking oxygen administration ▾											

1. Target SpO$_2$(%)   Start date

88–92% ☐   94–98% ☐   **OR**   Min.........% Max..........%
(if at risk of CO$_2$ retention)

Nursing staff to sign chart at each drug round to confirm that the specified target oxygen saturation is being achieved.
The method & rate of oxygen delivery should be adjusted by nursing staff to achieve the target oxygen saturation.

Is controlled(Venturi) delivery essential? Yes ☐ No ☐

Continuous ☐   or   PRN ☐

Humidified? ☐

Additional instructions: ....

Prescriber's signature	Bleep no.

	06										
	12										
	18										
	22										

2. Target SpO$_2$(%)   Start date

88–92% ☐   94–98% ☐   **OR** Min.........% Max..........%
(if at risk of CO$_2$ retention)

Nursing staff to sign chart at each drug round to confirm that the specified target oxygen saturation is being achieved.
The method & rate of oxygen delivery should be adjusted by nursing staff to achieve the target oxygen saturation.

Is controlled(Venturi) delivery essential?   Yes ☐ No ☐

Continuous ☐   or   PRN ☐

Humidified? ☐

Additional instructions: ....

Prescriber's signature	Bleep no.

	06										
	12										
	18										
	22										

Regular prescriptions

Date ▸											
Circle times or enter other times ▾											

4. Drug (approved name)		Start date	06									
			08									
Dose	Route	Stop date	12									
			14									
Frequency	Pharmacy	DH ☐ New ☐	18									
			22									
Prescriber's signature		Bleep no.	24									

5. Drug (approved name)		Start date	06									
			08									
Dose	Route	Stop date	12									
			14									
Frequency	Pharmacy	DH ☐ New ☐	18									
			22									
Prescriber's signature		Bleep no.	24									

6. Drug (approved name)		Start date	06									
			08									
Dose	Route	Stop date	12									
			14									
Frequency	Pharmacy	DH ☐ New ☐	18									
			22									
Prescriber's signature		Bleep no.	24									

7. Drug (approved name)		Start date	06									
			08									
Dose	Route	Stop date	12									
			14									
Frequency	Pharmacy	DH ☐ New ☐	18									
			22									
Prescriber's signature		Bleep no.	24									

As required prescriptions

| Name | | | Hospital no. | |

1. Drug (approved name)		Start date	Date/time	/	/	/	/	/	/	/	/	/	/
Dose	Route	Frequency	Route										
Indication/other instructions	Pharmacy		Dose										
Prescriber's Signature		Bleep no.	Given by	/	/	/	/	/	/	/	/	/	/

2. Drug (approved name)		Start date	Date/time	/	/	/	/	/	/	/	/	/	/
Dose	Route	Frequency	Route										
Indication/other instructions	Pharmacy		Dose										
Prescriber's Signature		Bleep no.	Given by	/	/	/	/	/	/	/	/	/	/

3. Drug (approved name)		Start date	Date/time	/	/	/	/	/	/	/	/	/	/
Dose	Route	Frequency	Route										
Indication/other instructions	Pharmacy		Dose										
Prescriber's Signature		Bleep no.	Given by	/	/	/	/	/	/	/	/	/	/

4. Drug (approved name)		Start date	Date/time	/	/	/	/	/	/	/	/	/	/
Dose	Route	Frequency	Route										
Indication/other instructions	Pharmacy		Dose										
Prescriber's Signature		Bleep no.	Given by	/	/	/	/	/	/	/	/	/	/

5. Drug (approved name)		Start date	Date/time	/	/	/	/	/	/	/	/	/	/
Dose	Route	Frequency	Route										
Indication/other instructions	Pharmacy		Dose										
Prescriber's Signature		Bleep no.	Given by	/	/	/	/	/	/	/	/	/	/

Intravenous fluids

| Name | | | | | | Hospital no. | | | |

Date	Fluid	Volume	Additive & dose	Duration (hrs) or rate (mL/hr)	Prescriber's signature and bleep no.	Given by	Start time	End time
	1.					/		
	2.					/		
	3.					/		
	4.					/		
	5.					/		
	6.					/		
	7.					/		
	8.					/		

Question 7.1 Answer

Inpatient Prescription Chart

Weight (kg)	Height (cm)	Surface Area (m²)

Admission Date	Ward	Consultant(s)

Name DIANE STUBBINGS   *Hospital no.* **038942**

Date of Birth **01/02/1930**

Address **The Ivies Care Home, Small City, AB1 2PQ**

Use label

Oral medication in surgical pre-op patients

Give ALL oral medication apart from hypoglycaemics even if 'nil by mouth'

Non-administration of drugs

Reasons for non-administration of drugs must be recorded:
1. Nil by mouth   5. Medical instruction
2. Off ward   6. No IV canula in situ
3. Vomiting/nausea   7. Contraindicated
4. Refused   8. Drug not available

Allergies & sensitivities

If none, state 'None'. Record source of information, e.g. 'patient', 'notes', etc

PENICILLIN – ANAPHYLAXIS

Latex Allergy ☐ Yes   ☐ No

☐ Patient   ☐ Medical notes   ☐ GP
☐ Dr   ☐ Nurse   ☐ Pharmacist

Signed	Name	Date
Will Brown	**WILL BROWN**	01/02/2013

Thromboprophylaxis risk assessment
Complete for ALL ADULT PATIENTS, excluding OBSTETRIC patients. REVIEW EVERY 3 DAYS

STEP ONE: ASSESS THROMBOSIS RISK FACTORS - Tick all boxes that apply or tick here if NO thrombosis risk factor   ☐

Procedure related factors		Patient related factors	
LMWH indicated according to guideline for procedure	☐	Active cancer or cancer treatment	☐
Surgical procedures lasting >30 minutes	☐	Acute surgical admission with inflammatory or abdominal condition	☐
Bilateral uni-compartmental knee replacements	☐	Age >60 years	☑
Critical Care admission	☐	Dehydration	☐
Hip replacement/hip fracture	☐	Known thrombophilia	☐
Major trauma	☐	Medical morbidity (heart failure; respiratory disease; infection;	☑
Major abdominal/pelvic/gynaecological surgery	☐	inflammatory conditions; metabolic, diabetic/endocrine crisis)	
Plaster cast immobilization of lower limb	☐	Obesity (BMI >30 kg/m²)	☐
Total knee replacement	☐	On HRT or oestrogen-containing contraceptive pill	☐
		Personal history or first degree relative with PE or DVT	☐
		Reduced mobility	☐
		Varicose veins with phlebitis	☐

STEP TWO: REVIEW RISK OF ANTICOAGULATION – Tick all boxes that apply or tick here if NO anticoagulation risk factor   ☐

Procedure related factors		Patient related factors	
Neurosurgery, spinal surgery or eye surgery	☐	Acute stroke in previous month (infarct or haemorrhage)	☑
Other procedure with high bleeding risk	☐	Already on anticoagulant (e.g. warfarin) therapy	☐
		Bleeding from any source/major bleeding risk, e.g. active peptic ulcer	☐
		Blood pressure >230 systolic or >120 diastolic	☐
		Haemophilia, other bleeding disorder, platelet count <75	☐
		Heparin allergy or heparin induced thrombocytopenia (seek advice)	☐
		Mobile and high fall risk	☐
		Possible intracranial haemorrhage, e.g. chronic sub-dural haematoma	☐
		Severe liver disease (INR >1.3 or known varices)	☐

STEP THREE: If any box ticked in STEP ONE, consider prescribing drug thromboprophylaxis.
If any box ticked in STEP TWO, consider if anticoagulation risk contraindicates the prescribing of drug thromboprophylaxis.
If prescribing enoxaparin reduce standard dose of 40 mg to 20 mg od if eGFR <30 mL/minute/1.73m².

Drug thromboprophylaxis indicated LMWH ☐   **Other** ☐   **Drug thromboprophylaxis not indicated** ☑
(Prescribe drug in 'Thromboprophylaxis' section of drug chart)

STEP FOUR: ANTI-EMBOLISM STOCKINGS – indicated in all surgical patients with any box ticked in STEP ONE, unless the following contraindications are present: lower limb dermatitis, ulceration, gangrene, risk of compartment syndrome, peripheral vascular disease, leg deformity preventing proper application, recent skin graft, severe leg oedema   **Tick box to prescribe**   ☑

Name: WILL BROWN	Signature: *Will Brown*	Date: 01/02/2013

Signature Record

All prescribers MUST complete the Signature Record (including signature as used on the prescription chart)

Date	Name (BLOCK CAPITALS)	Status	Signature	Date	Name (BLOCK CAPITALS)	Status	Signature
01/02/13	1. **WILL BROWN**	CT2	*Will Brown*		2.		
	3.				4.		
	5.				6.		

Regular prescriptions

4. Drug (approved name) **COCODAMOL 30/500**		Start date **01/02/13**	Date ▶ 01/02/13 Circle times or enter other times ▼											
			⑥											
			08											
Dose **TWO TABLETS**	Route **ORAL**	Stop date	⑫											
			14											
Frequency **6-HRLY**	Pharmacy	DH ☐ New ☐	⑱											
			22											
Prescriber's signature *Will Brown*		Bleep no. **1234**	㉔											
5. Drug (approved name)		Start date	06											
			08											
Dose	Route	Stop date	12											
			14											
Frequency	Pharmacy	DH ☐ New ☐	18											
			22											
Prescriber's signature		Bleep no.	24											

As required prescriptions

Name: Hospital no.

1. Drug (approved name) **CYCLIZINE**		Start date **01/02/13**	Date/time									
Dose **50 MG**	Route **IV**	Frequency **8-HRLY**	Route									
Indication/other instructions **NAUSEA OR VOMITING**	Pharmacy		Dose									
Prescriber's Signature *Will Brown*		Bleep no. **1234**	Given by									
2. Drug (approved name) **MORPHINE SULPHATE (10 MG/5 ML)**		Start date **01/02/13**	Date/time									
Dose **5 mg**	Route **ORAL**	Frequency **4-HRLY**	Route									
Indication/other instructions **PAIN**	Pharmacy		Dose									
Prescriber's signature *Will Brown*		Bleep no. **1234**	Given by									

Intravenous fluids

Name: Hospital no.

Date	Fluid	Volume	Additive & dose	Duration (hrs) or rate (mL/hr)	Prescriber's signature and bleep no.	Given by	Start time	End time
01/02/13	1. **5% DEXTROSE**	**1 L**	**NIL**	**1 HOUR**	*Will Brown* **1234**			
	2.							
	3.							
	4.							
	5.							
	6.							
	7.							
	8.							

This scenario highlights both how complicated prescribing can be, but also how dangerous it is when done incorrectly. You **MUST** follow a routine when prescribing to ensure you do not fall foul of the common pitfalls encountered in clinical practice and the Prescribing Safety Assessment (PSA), e.g. the PReSCRIBER routine (see Chapter 2 for more details).

Note that in this section of the PSA you will, in fact, only be required to write one prescription (i.e. one prescription for one drug), and the scenarios below reflect this; however, the above scenario (Question 7.1) is much more representative of real life!

This chapter (and section in the PSA) uses the same theory learned in previous chapters but changes the format of questioning. However, note the wealth of marks to be gained from this section of the PSA (80/200 in total): this is a section to master!

REMEMBER PReSCRIBER

- **P** – **p**atient details
- **Re** – **re**action (allergy plus the reaction)
- **S** – **s**ign the front of the chart
- **C** – check **c**ontraindications to each drug
- **R** – check **r**oute for each drug
- **I** – prescribe **i**ntravenous fluids if needed
- **B** – prescribe **b**lood clot prophylaxis if needed
- **E** – prescribe anti**e**metic if needed
- **R** – prescribe pain **r**elief if needed.

REMEMBER THE BASIC PRINCIPLES FOR ALL PRESCRIBING

Always remember that every drug prescription must be:

- Legible
- Unambiguous (e.g. not a range of doses such as 30–60 mg of codeine, which is a common error and entirely your fault if the patient is overdosed within your prescribed dosage range)
- Approved (generic) name: e.g. salbutamol not Ventolin®
- In capitals
- Instructional if drug is to be used 'as required', i.e. provide: (1) indication and (2) a maximum frequency
- Without abbreviations
- Signed (even when practising or in an exam it is advisable to sign and make up a bleep number in order to get into this routine)
- Inclusive of the indication and the stop/review date if an antibiotic is being prescribed
- Inclusive of treatment duration if the treatment is not long-term (e.g. antibiotics) or if it is in a GP setting (e.g. 7 or 28 days).

Note that the duration of an antibiotic course is given in the *British National Formulary* under each indication. However, as a general rule, most courses are for 5 days; with the following notable exceptions of uncomplicated urinary tract infections in women requiring a course for 3 days, while bone infections (septic arthritis or osteomyelitis) and endocarditis require a course for many weeks. Another general rule is that once a patient is clinically improving, intravenous antibiotics should be converted to the oral route where possible.

SEVEN

Prescribing: Doing It Yourself

Question 7.2 Prescribing item worth 10 marks

CASE PRESENTATION

A 26-year-old woman attends A&E following sudden onset breathlessness and haemoptysis. She has complained of a tender and swollen left calf for the last three days. She has no past medical history. She has a family history of Factor V Leiden though has never been tested herself.

ON EXAMINATION

RR 22/min, Sa0$_2$ 91% (on air) and afebrile. BP 118/72 mmHg and HR 108 b.p.m. Her chest examination is unremarkable. Her left calf is swollen. She weighs 80 kg.

INVESTIGATIONS

Hb and MCV normal. Renal function is normal. A CT pulmonary angiogram has been arranged for tomorrow.

Prescribing request: Write a prescription for ONE drug that is indicated immediately in the treatment of the presumed pulmonary embolus. (*Use the 'once only medicines' prescription chart provided.*)

ONCE ONLY MEDICINES

Date	Time	Medicine (approved name)	Dose	Route	Prescriber – sign + print	Time given	Given by

Question 7.2 Answer

A. Drug choice	Score	Feedback/justification	B. Dose, route, frequency	Score	Feedback/justification
1. DALTEPARIN	4	LMW heparin is needed to prevent the clot enlarging while the body breaks it down; it does not thrombolyse the clot itself. Factor V Leiden is the most common inherited thrombophilia (i.e. increased likelihood of thromboembolism).	15 000 UNITS S/C ONCE DAILY	4	This is the treatment dose (remember LMW heparin may be used for treatment or prophylaxis). It should be continued until warfarin has achieved a therapeutic INR (i.e >2). Use the BNF to calculate the dose according to weight.
2. ENOXAPARIN	4	As above	120 MG OR 12 000 UNITS S/C ONCE DAILY (can be prescribed either way)	4	As above (it does not matter which of the three LMW heparins you use: in real life it reflects hospital policy and dalteparin is cheapest at present!)
3. TINZAPARIN	4	As above	14 000 UNITS S/C ONCE DAILY	4	As above
4. ALTEPLASE	1	Thrombolytics activate plasminogen to form plasmin, which degrades fibrin and so breaks up thrombi. Thrombolysis in PE is definitely not warranted here: it is reserved for patients with PE in cardiac arrest or cardiogenic shock (BP < 90 mmHg) resistant to IV fluid and inotropes.	10 MG IV OVER 1–2 MIN	4	Correct dose for initial therapy; then requires infusion.
5. ASPIRIN	0	Aspirin is an antiplatelet and has no role in the treatment of PE or deep DVT.	N/A		300 mg is the 'treatment dose' for acute coronary syndrome or stroke; 75 mg is the prophylactic dose for IHD, stroke, peripheral vascular disease and thromboembolism from AF.
6. WARFARIN	2	Warfarin is the oral anticoagulant of choice. It inhibits the synthesis of vitamin K, preventing formation of the vitamin K-dependent clotting factors (II, VII, IX and X) hence prolonging the PT/INR. Its anticoagulant effects occur after 48–72 h, so concomitant heparin must be given. This question specifically asked for a drug that is indicated immediately in the treatment of this PE, i.e. LMW heparin, although warfarin will probably be started concomitantly.	10 MG ORAL	4	Follow local policy, but most hospitals give patients 10 mg on the first day, then check the INR to direct following days. (Most patients will require 2–3 days of 10 mg before the INR increases from 1).

A and B. Marking Guide for Questions 7.2–7.10
4 marks: optimal answer that cannot be improved.
3 marks: good answer but minor problem (e.g. cost-effectiveness, likely adherence).
2 marks: answer likely to provide benefit but is suboptimal for more than one reason.
1 mark: answer that has some justification and deserves some credit.

C. Timing. 1 mark for correctly dating (and timing) the prescription.

D. Signature. 1 mark for signing the prescription.

Question 7.2 Answer *(Cont'd)*

For example, the prescription should appear as:

ONCE ONLY MEDICINES

Date	Time	Medicine (approved name)	Dose	Route	Prescriber – sign + print	Time given	Given by
01/01/13	18 00	DALTEPARIN	15 000 UNITS	S/C	*YOUR SIGNATURE AND PRINTED NAME*		

You may use the BNF at any time

www.bnf.org

Question 7.3 Prescribing item worth 10 marks

CASE PRESENTATION

A 78-year-old man attends his GP complaining of a 6-month history of mild breathlessness on exertion. He has also noticed that he has to sleep with three pillows as he is breathless when he lies flat. He has a history of asthma for which he occasionally needs a salbutamol inhaler; the inhaler has not helped his recent breathlessness. He is currently taking furosemide 20 mg once daily.

ON EXAMINATION

RR 16/min, SaO_2 93% (on air) and afebrile. BP 140/72 mmHg and HR 68 b.p.m. His chest examination is unremarkable and his JVP is not elevated. Mild pitting oedema is present. His peak flow is 100% of its usual value.

INVESTIGATIONS

His serum biochemistry is normal. An echocardiogram has also been requested.

He admits that he has only come at his wife's request and does not find the breathlessness too troublesome.

Prescribing request: Write a prescription for ONE drug for long-term treatment of his condition. (*Use the 'regular medication' prescription chart provided.*)

REGULAR MEDICATION		Date						
		Time						
Drug (Approved name)		6						
		8						
Dose	Route	12						
Prescriber – sign + print	Start date	14						
		18						
Notes	Frequency	22						

Question 7.3 Answer

A. Drug choice	Score	Feedback/justification	B. Dose, route, frequency	Score	Feedback/justification
1. ENALAPRIL	4	Enalapril is an ACE-inhibitor which in combination with a beta-blocker is a first-line therapy for management of chronic heart failure. Selection of an ACE-inhibitor over a beta-blocker in this scenario reflects the presence of asthma which contraindicates a beta-blocker.	2.5 MG ORAL NIGHTLY	4	2.5 mg is the starting dose for heart failure. NOTE: ACE-inhibitors can cause postural hypotension so they are best given in the evening. There are marks for giving the correct timing of the drug: if in doubt, look it up!
2. LISINOPRIL	4	Lisinopril is also an ACE-inhibitor.	2.5 MG ORAL NIGHTLY	4	2.5 mg is the starting dose for heart failure.
3. PERINDOPRIL ERBUMINE	4	Perindopril is also an ACE-inhibitor. NOTE: there are two forms of perindopril with different doses (perindopril erbumine and perindopril arginine); both are licensed in heart failure but the differing doses stress the need to write full names.	2.0 MG ORAL DAILY	4	2.0 mg is the starting dose for heart failure. The BNF recommends giving perindopril in the morning: the only ACE-inhibitor with this advice.
4. RAMIPRIL	4	Ramipril is also an ACE-inhibitor.	1.25 MG ORAL NIGHTLY	4	1.25 mg is the starting dose for heart failure.
5. ANY OTHER ACE-INHIBITOR AT THE CORRECT DOSE	4		CORRECT DOSE ACCORDING TO BNF	4	
6. ANY BETA-BLOCKER	0	While beta-blockers are given in combination with ACE-inhibitors in the management of chronic heart failure, this patient has asthma so they are contraindicated. Be wary of the question asking for one prescription for a condition usually requiring two drugs – there will be a catch!			
7. FUROSEMIDE	1	Furosemide is used in the treatment of acute heart failure but has no role in the management of chronic heart failure (although often patients remain on furosemide from acute exacerbations). It has no effect on mortality while ACE-inhibitors and beta-blockers do.	20 MG ORAL DAILY (in the morning) OR 40 MG ORAL DAILY (in the morning)	4	Should be given in the morning due to subsequent diuresis. (i.e. not at night.)
8. SPIRONOLACTONE	2	Spironolactone is used as an adjunct in moderate-to-severe heart failure when ACE-inhibitors and beta-blockers are inadequate (i.e. should have picked ACE-inhibitors first as this is neither a moderate nor a severe case).	25 MG ORAL DAILY	4	Should be given in the morning (potassium-sparing diuretic).

Question 7.3 Answer *(Cont'd)*

A. Drug choice	Score	Feedback/ justification	B. Dose, route, frequency	Score	Feedback/justification
9. ANY ASTHMA TREATMENT	0	This patient has chronic congestive cardiac failure. Further, the peak flow (a measure of severity of bronchoconstriction and hence asthma) is at his baseline.			

For example, the prescription should appear as:

REGULAR MEDICATION		Date						
		Time						
Drug (Approved name)		**6**						
ENALAPRIL		**8**						
Dose 2.5 MG	Route ORAL	**12**						
Prescriber – sign + print *YOUR SIGNATURE AND NAME*	Start date *TODAY'S DATE*	**14**						
		(18)						
Notes	Frequency AT NIGHT	**22**						

You may use the BNF at any time

BNF

www.bnf.org

Question 7.4 Prescribing item worth 10 marks

CASE PRESENTATION

A 48-year-old Caucasian male requires treatment for hypertension after home monitoring has recorded a mean blood pressure of 160/102 mmHg. He denies any medical history.

ON EXAMINATION

HR 82 b.p.m. Chest clear, JVP not raised, no peripheral oedema.

INVESTIGATIONS

His serum biochemistry is found below:

	Value	Normal range		Value	Normal range
WCC	7.3×10^9/L	(4–11×10^9/L)	Ur	3 mmol/L	(3–7 mmol/L)
Neut.	6.1×10^9/L	(2–8×10^9/L)	Cr	72 μmol/L	(60–125 μmol/L)
Lymph.	1.2×10^9/L	(1–4.8×10^9/L)	Na	136 mmol/L	(135–145 mmol/L)
Hb	$140 \times$ g/L	(135–175 g/L (male))	K	3.4 mmol/L	(3.5–5.0 mmol/L)
MCV	82 fL	(76–99 fL)			

Prescribing request: Write a prescription for ONE drug for long-term treatment of his condition. (*Use the 'regular medication' prescription chart provided.*)

REGULAR MEDICATION		Date						
		Time						
Drug (Approved name)		**6**						
		8						
Dose	Route	**12**						
Prescriber – sign + print	Start date	**14**						
		18						
Notes	Frequency	**22**						

Question 7.4 Answer

A. Drug choice	Score	Feedback/justification	B. Dose, route, frequency	Score	Feedback/justification
1. ENALAPRIL	4	Enalapril is an ACE-inhibitor. ACE-inhibitors are first-line therapy for hypertension in those under 55 years. The British Hypertension Society suggests offering angiotensin receptor blocker (ARB) as an alternative first-line of treatment, but the BNF suggests this only if ACE-inhibitors are not tolerated. His mild hypokalaemia may actually be helped by an ACE-inhibitor (which can cause hyperkalaemia); it should obviously be investigated and monitored but that is not the focus of this question.	5 MG ORAL NIGHTLY	4	NOTE: ACE-inhibitors can cause postural hypotension so generally they are best given in the evening.
2. LISINOPRIL	4	See above	10 MG ORAL NIGHTLY	4	As above
3. PERINDOPRIL ERBUMINE	4	See above. Note there are two forms of perindopril with different doses (perindopril erbumine and perindopril arginine); both are licensed in hypertension but the differing doses stress the need to write full names.	4 MG ORAL DAILY	4	The BNF recommends giving perindopril in the morning: the only ACE-inhibitor with this advice.
4. RAMIPRIL	4	See above	1.25 MG ORAL NIGHTLY OR 2.5 MG ORAL NIGHTLY	4	NOTE: ACE-inhibitors can cause postural hypotension so they are best given in the evening.
5. ANY OTHER ACE-INHIBITOR AT THE CORRECT DOSE	4	See above	CORRECT DOSE ACCORDING TO BNF	4	
6. ANY ARB	2	See above	CORRECT DOSE ACCORDING TO BNF	4	
7. ANY CALCIUM-CHANNEL BLOCKER	1	Patients under 55 years should be treated with ACE-inhibitors (or if not tolerated an ARB; calcium-channel blockers are reserved for first-line treatment of those aged over 55, or black patients of African or Caribbean family origin of any age).	CORRECT DOSE ACCORDING TO BNF	4	
8. ANY THIAZIDE DIURETIC	1	Thiazide diuretics (e.g. bendroflumethiazide, chlortalidone or indapamide) are indicated in patients over the age of 55 (or black patients of African or Caribbean family origin of any age) who don't tolerate calcium channel blockers, or who have/are at high risk of heart failure.	CORRECT DOSE ACCORDING TO BNF	4	

Question 7.4 Answer *(Cont'd)*

For example, the prescription should appear as:

REGULAR MEDICATION

		Date							
		Time							
Drug (Approved name) ENALAPRIL		**6**							
		8							
Dose 5MG	Route ORAL	**12**							
Prescriber – sign + print YOUR SIGNATURE AND NAME	Start date TODAY'S DATE	**14**							
		⑱							
Notes	Frequency AT NIGHT	**22**							

You may use the BNF at any time BNF

www.bnf.org

Question 7.5 Prescribing item worth 10 marks

CASE PRESENTATION

A 19-year-old patient is admitted with 6 hours of severe breathlessness. She has a background of asthma and has just started smoking. She is getting little benefit from her salbutamol inhaler (her only medication). Her expiratory peak flow is 230 L/min (best 540 L/min).

ON EXAMINATION

There is widespread polyphonic expiratory wheeze throughout the chest. RR 32/min; SaO_2 82% (on air); the nurses are just applying an oxygen mask with high-flow oxygen.

INVESTIGATIONS

Results are pending.

Prescribing request: You are the first doctor to see the patient. Write a prescription for THE FIRST drug to rapidly improve the dyspnoea. *(Please use the 'once only' prescription chart.)*

ONCE ONLY MEDICINES

Date	Time	Medicine (approved name)	Dose	Route	Prescriber – sign + print	Time given	Given by

Question 7.5 Answer

A. Drug choice	Score	Feedback/justification	B. Dose, route, frequency	Score	Feedback/justification
1. SALBUTAMOL	4	This patient has an acute exacerbation of asthma. The PEF is 43% of normal (i.e. a severe exacerbation). After oxygen (which you are told is being arranged), the treatment includes salbutamol and ipratropium nebulizers, oral or intravenous steroids and potentially theophylline; much later magnesium may be considered. As the question asked for the first drug for relief of breathlessness, salbutamol should be first.	5 MG NEBULIZED stat.	4	As this is severe, inhaler salbutamol would not be helpful; nebulized is much more effective and does not rely on inhaler technique (as it is delivered through a mask). Further, she is not benefitting from inhaled salbutamol.
2. TERBUTALINE	4	Terbutaline is another less commonly used short-acting β2 agonist.	10 MG NEBULIZED stat.	4	This is the correct dose and route in acute asthma.
3. IPRATROPIUM	2	Ipratropium is a muscarinic antagonist. While a core part of managing an exacerbation of asthma, its onset of action is slower than salbutamol, hence salbutamol is a more appropriate answer.	250– 500 MICROGRAMS NEBULIZED stat.	4	Note that unlike salbutamol which may be given back-to-back and whose total dose is only limited by side effects (usually tachycardia and tremor), ipratropium should only be given x4-6/day.
4. PREDNISOLONE	0	While prednisolone has an important part to play in managing exacerbations, its effects are not noted for 2–3 days through reduction of bronchial inflammation. It therefore has no effect on acute breathlessness.	N/A		
5. HYDROCORTISONE	0	See above; generally use prednisolone (oral) for moderate exacerbations and hydrocortisone (IV) for severe or life-threatening exacerbations.	N/A		

For example, the prescription should appear as:

ONCE ONLY MEDICINES

Date	Time	Medicine (approved name)	Dose	Route	Prescriber – sign + print	Time given	Given by
01/01/13	18 00	SALBUTAMOL	5 MG	NEBULIZED	YOUR SIGNATURE AND PRINTED NAME		

Question 7.6 Prescribing Item

CASE PRESENTATION

An 81-year-old lady is an inpatient on the vascular ward awaiting a femoral-popliteal bypass graft for peripheral vascular disease. She also had a transient ischaemic attack last year and has controlled hypertension. You are asked to see her because of central crushing chest pain which came on when she walked to the toilet two minutes ago. It is starting to improve but she still rates the pain as 5/10.

ON EXAMINATION

Her chest and heart examination are unremarkable. Observations are normal.

INVESTIGATIONS

An ECG is shown below and the nurse has just sent off some bloods.

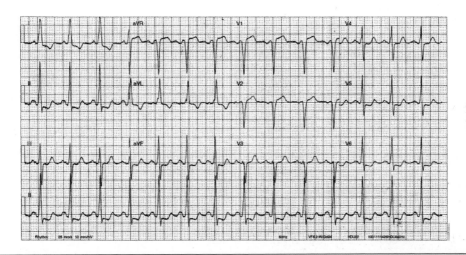

Prescribing request: Write a prescription for THE FIRST drug to give relief of chest pain. *(Please use the 'once only' prescription chart.)*

ONCE ONLY MEDICINES

Date	Time	Medicine (approved name)	Dose	Route	Prescriber – sign + print	Time given	Given by

Question 7.6 Answer

A. Drug choice	Score	Feedback/justification	B. Dose, route, frequency	Score	Feedback/justification
1. GTN SPRAY (GLYCERYL TRINITRATE)	4	GTN is one of the few therapies you could abbreviate – if in doubt always write out the full drug name.	2 SPRAYS (or symbol for two) SUBLINGUAL	4	This is the correct dose. As there is only one strength (concentration) of spray available one typically does not write the 400 micrograms/metered dose, but if you wish to it should go with the drug name, i.e. GTN spray (400 micrograms/metered dose) then 2 sprays in dose box.
2. GTN TABLET (GLYCERYL TRINITRATE)	4	As above	0.3–1 MG SUBLINGUAL	4	This is the correct dose. Note you must actually pick a dose you should never prescribe a range for any drug as it is your responsibility, not the nurses, to ensure a specific, safe dose. There will be a local policy for the management of chest pain, which will give you some guidance.
3. ASPIRIN	0	This patient's history is very suggestive of stable angina (which she is certainly at risk of given other vascular disease) and the ECG shows infero-lateral ST depression. Aspirin, while important in the treatment of ACS (and sometimes given pre-emptively before the diagnosis is confirmed) may improve outcomes, but would provide little symptomatic benefit beyond its (unintentional in this case) anti-inflammatory properties.	300 MG ORAL stat.	4	This is the correct treatment dose. (75 mg oral is a prophylactic dose and therefore incorrect.)
4. CLOPIDOGREL	0	As above: acute ACS treatment (except STEMI) comprises ABC, symptomatic therapy (GTN ± morphine) and aspirin/clopidogrel/heparin to improve outcome, ± beta-blockade afterwards.	N/A		
5. MORPHINE	1	While useful and likely to improve her pain, morphine is reserved for severe pain in ACS. Therefore, its side effect profile should prevent its use in stable angina.	2–10 MG SLOW INTRAVENOUS INJECTION	4	The dose of morphine required by different patients varies considerably. Again note that a specific dose (not a range) must be specified.
6. DIAMORPHINE	1	As above	1–5 MG SLOW INTRAVENOUS INJECTION	4	As above

For example, the prescription should appear as:

ONCE ONLY MEDICINES

Date	Time	Medicine (approved name)	Dose	Route	Prescriber – sign + print	Time given	Given by
01/01/13	1800	GTN SPRAY (GLYCERYL TRINITRATE)	2 SPRAYS (OR SYMBOL FOR TWO)	SUBLINGUAL	*YOUR SIGNATURE AND PRINTED NAME*		

You may use the
BNF at any time

BNF

www.bnf.org

Question 7.7 Prescribing item worth 10 marks

CASE PRESENTATION

An 77-year-old man is admitted with two weeks of mild breathlessness. Beyond asthma for which he uses a beclomethasone inhaler, twice daily, he has no medical history of note.

ON EXAMINATION

HR 135 b.p.m, BP 132/88 mmHg, RR 18/min, SaO_2 94% (on air). Afebrile.

His chest is clear and there are no murmurs on auscultation of the heart.

INVESTIGATIONS

An ECG is shown below; electrolytes, TSH and troponin are normal.

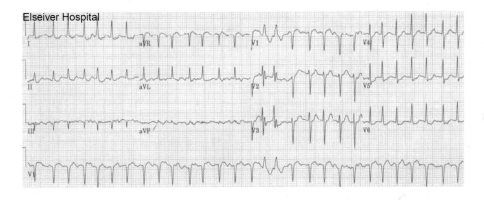

Prescribing request: Write a prescription for ONE drug to treat the underlying cause of his breathlessness. *(Please use the 'regular medication' prescription chart.)*

REGULAR MEDICATION		Date							
		Time							
Drug (Approved name)		6							
		8							
Dose	Route	12							
Prescriber – sign + print	Start date	14							
		18							
Notes	Frequency	22							

Question 7.7 Answer

A. Drug choice	Score	Feedback/justification	B. Dose, route, frequency	Score	Feedback/justification
1. DILTIAZEM	4	This patient has AF. His age, lack of a precipitant or adverse features make rate control preferable to rhythm control (he would also require formal anticoagulation if cardioversion were to be attempted as onset was over 48 hours ago). First-line therapy for rate control is either a rate-limiting calcium-channel blocker (e.g. diltiazem or verapamil) or beta-blockers. Beta-blockers are contraindicated in asthma.	120 MG ORAL DAILY USING A MODIFIED-RELEASE PREPARATION	4	NOTE: although the most commonly given calcium-channel blocker for AF, diltiazem is not actually licensed for AF and, if given the choice, we suggest opting for verapamil despite its risk of profound bradycardia in the presence of beta-blockers (clearly not relevant here).
2. VERAPAMIL	4	As above	40–120 MG ORAL 8-HOURLY	4	It would be most appropriate to start at low dose (i.e. 40 mg 8-hourly then work up), but the BNF does not specify this so up to 120 mg should be given full marks.
3. DIGOXIN	2	Digoxin should be used in patients in whom beta or calcium-channel blockade is inadequate (as poly-therapy) or contraindicated (as mono-therapy).	125–250 MICROGRAMS ORAL DAILY	4	Digoxin requires oral (or intravenous when more sick) loading, usually in the form of 250–500 micrograms oral 12-hourly for the first 24 h before starting this regular dose.
4. ANY BETA-BLOCKER	0	Beta-blockers are contraindicated in asthma.	N/A		
5. ASPIRIN OR WARFARIN	0	While aspirin or warfarin will likely be needed for thromboprophylaxis, the question specifically asks for treatment of his underlying cause of breathlessness.	N/A		

For example, the prescription should appear as:

REGULAR MEDICATION

		Date				
		Time				
Drug (Approved name) VERAPAMIL		⑥ 8				
Dose 40 MG	Route ORAL	12				
Prescriber – sign + print *YOUR SIGNATURE AND NAME*	Start date *TODAY'S DATE*	⑭ 18				
Notes	Frequency 8-HOURLY	㉒				

You may use the
BNF at any time

BNF

www.bnf.org

SEVEN

Prescribing: Doing It Yourself

Question 7.8 Prescribing item worth 10 marks

CASE PRESENTATION

A 68-year-old patient with benign prostatic hyperplasia is admitted with lethargy. He says he has not passed urine for five days and reports painful abdominal distension.

ON EXAMINATION

HR 115 b.p.m, BP 132/88 mmHg, RR 18/min, Sa0$_2$ 99% (on air). Examination reveals a palpable bladder with over a litre of urine visible on bladder scan.

INVESTIGATIONS

	Value	Normal range		Value	Normal range
WCC	8.3×10^9/L	(4–11×10^9/L)	Ur	18 mmol/L	(3–7 mmol/L)
Neut.	6.1×10^9/L	(2–8×10^9/L)	Cr	346 µmol/L	(60–125 µmol/L)
Lymph.	1.2×10^9/L	(1–4.8×10^9/L)	Na	136 mmol/L	(135–145 mmol/L)
Hb	160 g/L	(135–175 g/L (male))	K	7.1 mmol/L	(3.5–5.0 mmol/L)
MCV	82 fL	(76–99 fL)	Glucose	7.2 mmol/L	

An ECG shows tall T-waves throughout and sinus tachycardia.

Prescribing request: Write a prescription for the FIRST DRUG to lower the patient's potassium. *(Please use the 'once only' section.)*

ONCE ONLY MEDICINES

Date	Time	Medicine (approved name)	Dose	Route	Prescriber – sign + print	Time given	Given by

Question 7.8 Answer

A. Drug choice	Score	Feedback/justification	B. Dose, route, frequency	Score	Feedback/justification
1. SHORT-ACTING INSULIN (E.G. ACTRAPID® OR NOVORAPID®) WITH GLUCOSE	4	The hyperkalaemia here is secondary to renal failure (remember the mnemonic DREAD). The first potassium-lowering therapy is insulin and dextrose; insulin causes cellular uptake of potassium, and the dextrose is given to prevent subsequent hypoglycaemia.	10 UNITS OF ACTRAPID® (or NOVORAPID®) IN 100 ML OF 20% DEXTROSE OVER 30 MIN IV	4	See below
2. SHORT-ACTING INSULIN (E.G. ACTRAPID® OR NOVORAPID®) WITH GLUCOSE	4	As above	5–10 UNITS OF ACTRAPID® (or NOVORAPID®) IN 50 ML OF 50% DEXTROSE OVER 5–15 MIN IV	3	This is the standard (and easily memorable) prescription; however, it can irritate veins so some elect lower concentrations of dextrose.
3. SALBUTAMOL	2	Salbutamol is a second-line therapy for hyperkalaemia.	2.5–5 MG NEBULIZED stat.	4	This is an appropriate dose.
4. POLYSTYRENE SULFONATE RESIN (E.G. CALCIUM RESONIUM)	2	Also an effective treatment for hyperkalaemia but not first-line.	15 G ORAL OR 30 G PR	4	These are appropriate doses.
5. CALCIUM GLUCONATE	0	While the first treatment for hyperkalaemia (given to protect the myocardium from the effects of hyperkalaemia, preventing arrhythmias) it has no effect on potassium level which the question requested.	N/A		

For example, the prescription should appear as:

ONCE ONLY MEDICINES

Date	Time	Medicine (approved name)	Dose	Route	Prescriber – sign + print	Time given	Given by
01/02/13	13 00	ACTRAPID®	10 UNITS IN 100 ML OF 20% DEXTROSE, OVER 30 MINS	IV	*YOUR SIGNATURE AND PRINTED NAME*		

Question 7.9 Prescribing item worth 10 marks

CASE PRESENTATION

An 32-year-old woman who is trying for a baby has just been diagnosed with epilepsy following multiple complex partial seizures; an MRI of her head has revealed a small temporal meningioma which currently does not require surgery. Her sodium is low but stable (128 mmol/L) which the endocrinology registrar suspects is due to syndrome of inappropriate ADH secretion (SIADH) caused by tumour.

Prescribing request: Write a prescription for a drug to prevent seizures. *(Please use the 'regular medication' prescription chart.)*

REGULAR MEDICATION		Date						
		Time						
Drug (Approved name)		6						
		8						
Dose	Route	12						
Prescriber – sign + print	Start date	14						
		18						
Notes	Frequency	22						

Question 7.9 Answer

A. Drug choice	Score	Feedback/justification	B. Dose, route, frequency	Score	Feedback/justification
1. LAMOTRIGINE	4	Focal epilepsy is best managed with lamotrigine or carbamazepine (see Chapter 4). Carbamazepine, however, also causes SIADH and is therefore not appropriate here as the sodium would likely drop further which itself may provoke more seizures. Furthermore, lamotrigine has the best safety profile in pregnancy of all antiepileptic drugs.	25 MG ORAL DAILY	4	In reality, as an F1 you are unlikely to be prescribing in this situation, but the question is designed to test your knowledge of antiepileptic drugs and their side effects.
2. CARBAMAZEPINE	1	See above.	100 MG ORAL DAILY *OR* 200 MG ORAL DAILY *OR* 100 MG ORAL 12-HOURLY *OR* 200 MG ORAL 12-HOURLY	4	
3. SODIUM VALPROATE	1	Not only is valproate highly teratogenic, NICE do not recommend it as a first-line drug for focal seizures.	600 MG ORAL DAILY (or in divided doses)	4	
4. PHENYTOIN	1	As above; because of its narrow therapeutic index, phenytoin is avoided unless the patient is in status epilepticus or cannot swallow (as can be given IV).	150–300 MG ORAL DAILY (or in divided dose)	4	

For example, the prescription should appear as:

REGULAR MEDICATION

		Date						
		Time						
Drug (Approved name)		6						
LAMOTRIGINE		⑧						
Dose 25 MG DAILY	Route ORAL	12						
Prescriber – sign + print *YOUR SIGNATURE AND PRINTED NAME*	Start date *TODAY'S DATE*	14						
		18						
Notes	Frequency DAILY	22						

Question 7.10 Prescribing item worth 10 marks

CASE PRESENTATION

An 42-year-old woman reports polyuria and polydipsia for the last 2 months. She has a BMI of 18 and no other medical history.

A fasting blood glucose was 8.8 mmol/L so the GP started dietary and exercise management for type 2 diabetes. She returns to your clinic four months later with an HbA1C of 58 mmol/mol (target <48 mmol/mol) and still reporting her old symptoms. Her random blood glucose today is 14 mmol/L. Her creatinine is 172 µmol/L.

Prescribing request: Write a prescription for a drug to improve her diabetic control. (*Please use the 'regular medication' prescription chart.*)

REGULAR MEDICATION		Date							
		Time							
Drug (Approved name)		6							
		8							
Dose	Route	12							
Prescriber – sign + print	Start date	14							
		18							
Notes	Frequency	22							

Question 7.10 Answer

A. Drug choice	Score	Feedback/justification	B. Dose, route, frequency	Score	Feedback/justification
1. GLICLAZIDE	4	Gliclazide, tolbutamide, glipizide and glibenclamide are sulphonylureas. When selecting the first oral hypoglycaemic drug for diabetic patients, generally pick metformin if overweight or a sulphonylurea if normal/underweight; a creatinine of >150 µmol/L should also preclude using metformin (see Chapter 4).	40 MG ORAL DAILY WITH FIRST MEAL *OR* 80 MG ORAL DAILY WITH FIRST MEAL	4	
2. TOLBUTAMIDE	4	As above	0.5 G ORAL DAILY WITH/IMMEDIATELY AFTER FIRST MEAL *OR* 1 G ORAL DAILY WITH/IMMEDIATELY AFTER FIRST MEAL *OR* 1.5 G ORAL DAILY WITH/IMMEDIATELY AFTER FIRST MEAL	4	
3. GLIPIZIDE	4	As above	2.5 MG ORAL DAILY WITH/IMMEDIATELY AFTER FIRST MEAL *OR* 5 MG ORAL DAILY WITH/IMMEDIATELY AFTER FIRST MEAL	4	
4. GLIMEPIRIDE	4	As above	1 MG ORAL DAILY BEFORE/WITH FIRST MEAL	4	
5. GLIBENCLAMIDE	3	Glipenclamide is a longer-acting sulphonylurea and is hence a less appropriate starting drug.	5 MG ORAL DAILY WITH/IMMEDIATELY AFTER FIRST MEAL	4	
6. METFORMIN	0	Metformin should be used first-line in overweight patients (as it causes appetite suppression), but also avoided in those with a creatinine >150 µmol/L due to the risk of lactic acidosis. Therefore it is inappropriate and unsafe here.	N/A		
7. ANY INSULIN	0	Insulin is not generally used first-line in type 2 diabetes unless all other agents are contraindicated (or an acute sliding scale of insulin is required).	N/A		

For example, the prescription should appear as:

REGULAR MEDICATION		Date						
		Time						
Drug (Approved name)		**6**						
GLICLAZIDE		**⑧**						
Dose 40 MG	Route ORAL	**12**						
Prescriber – sign + print *YOUR SIGNATURE AND PRINTED NAME*	Start date *TODAY'S DATE*	**14**						
		18						
Notes	Frequency DAILY WITH FIRST MEAL	**22**						

Drug monitoring

Chapter objectives

- Learn how to monitor the beneficial and harmful effects of commonly used drugs.
- Practise identifying the most appropriate course of action for managing different clinical scenarios.

STRUCTURE OF THIS SECTION WITHIN THE PSA

The 'Drug monitoring' section will have 8 questions with 2 marks available per question and a possible total of 16 marks. You will be asked to identify the most appropriate option from a list of five for each scenario (see Fig. 8.1).

INTRODUCTION

The 'Drug monitoring' section will test your ability to effectively monitor the beneficial and harmful effects of drugs. Unlike previous sections, this section predominantly assesses your ability to plan monitoring for particular drugs (rather than respond to their results). Effective drug monitoring utilizes history and clinical examination as well as investigations.

You will be asked to plan an appropriate monitoring strategy by choosing the most suitable option from a list of five for a given scenario. The emphasis here is the most suitable option: multiple options may have a role in monitoring, but as in clinical practice the scenario should help you select the most applicable to the patient in hand. For example, statins are associated with a risk of myopathy in those with risk factors for it, i.e. a personal or family history of muscular disorders, previous history of muscular toxicity, a high alcohol intake, renal impairment, hypothyroidism and in the elderly. When prescribing simvastatin, a creatine kinase level should be checked at baseline in these patients. However, if the clinical situation reveals no such risk factors then a baseline check of creatine kinase is not the most suitable option and alternatives, e.g. serum alanine transaminase should be sought.

Rather than presenting a dry list of parameters to check for each drug, this chapter uses clinical scenarios (as in the exam) to work through the drugs that commonly require monitoring. Much of this chapter is revision of previous ones.

QUESTIONS

Question 8.1 Drug monitoring item worth 2 points – vancomycin

CASE PRESENTATION

A 67-year-old male patient with a diagnosis of epidural abscess is referred to the microbiologists for selection of a suitable antibiotic regimen. The microbiologist contacts you to advise commencement of IV vancomycin of which the patient is likely to require a prolonged course.

Question: Before prescribing vancomycin, which *one* of the following parameters would be the most important for you to check? Mark it with a tick in the column provided.

DECISION OPTIONS

A	SERUM CREATININE	☐
B	SERUM ALT	☐
C	CRP	☐
D	NEUTROPHIL COUNT	☐
E	PLATELET COUNT	☐

Question 8.1 Answers

A	**Correct:** clearance of vancomycin is reduced in patients with renal dysfunction. Renal function must be taken into account when choosing a dosing regimen for vancomycin. For your own learning, the two classic side effects of vancomycin are nephrotoxicity and ototoxicity. Look out for these in similar questions about vancomycin.
B	Vancomycin is renally eliminated and is not known to be hepatotoxic. A measure of ALT would not be necessary at this stage.
C	CRP is an acute phase protein used to check for the presence of inflammation (and thus infection); while helpful in identifying infection (and thus likely to already be available in this patient), it is not required at baseline for monitoring of therapy with vancomycin. It would help in monitoring the inflammatory response (and thus presence of infection), but clinical markers of response would be more helpful. (Generally in such questions, the clinical response (history/examination/observations) correlates better with improvement or deterioration than data.)
D	Vancomycin may uncommonly cause neutropenia, but this would normally occur after at least a week of therapy. Neutrophil count is not required for baseline monitoring.
E	Thrombocytopenia is a rare side effect of therapy with vancomycin. Platelet count is not required for baseline monitoring.

DECISION OPTIONS

A	SERUM CREATININE	✓
B	SERUM ALT	☐
C	CRP	☐
D	NEUTROPHIL COUNT	☐
E	PLATELET COUNT	☐

Question 8.2 Drug monitoring item worth 2 points – simvastatin

CASE PRESENTATION

During a routine check-up with the GP a 60-year-old female patient is found to have a 10-year cardiovascular disease risk of 26.6%. Following a discussion between the patient and the GP a decision is made to start her on the cholesterol-lowering agent simvastatin.

Question: Before prescribing simvastatin, which *one* of the following parameters would be the most important to check? Mark it with a tick in the column provided.

	DECISION OPTIONS	
A	SERUM ALT	☐
B	BLOOD PRESSURE	☐
C	CREATINE KINASE	☐
D	SERUM ALBUMIN	☐
E	WEIGHT	☐

Question 8.3 Drug monitoring item worth 2 points – phenytoin

CASE PRESENTATION

A 36-year-old male patient is prescribed phenytoin for the treatment of seizures related to a severe head injury sustained after falling off a pushbike. He is given an initial 'loading dose' of 1200 mg (20 mg/kg) by IV infusion followed by a maintenance dose of 300 mg orally daily. At day 14 of treatment a pre-dose 'trough' phenytoin level is requested in order to ensure that it is within the normal reference range. The reported level is 54 µmol/L (reference range: 40–80 µmol/L). (Note that this represents a 'total phenytoin' level.)

Question: Which *one* of the following statements is true regarding this patient's phenytoin therapy? Mark it with a tick in the column provided.

	DECISION OPTIONS	
A	300 MG DAILY IS A SUITABLE MAINTENANCE DOSE FOR THIS PATIENT	☐
B	300 MG DAILY IS TOO HIGH A MAINTENANCE DOSE AND SHOULD BE REDUCED	☐
C	300 MG DAILY IS TOO LOW A MAINTENANCE DOSE AND SHOULD BE INCREASED	☐
D	A POST-DOSE LEVEL IS REQUIRED IN ORDER TO ASCERTAIN THE SUITABILITY OF THIS DOSE FOR THIS PATIENT	☐
E	THE REPORTED LEVEL CAN BE CONSIDERED ALONE, WITHOUT INFORMATION ABOUT SEIZURE CONTROL	☐

Question 8.2 Answers

A	**Correct:** statins should be used with caution in patients with a history of liver disease, as they are metabolized by the liver, so hepatic impairment will increase their levels and thus the risk of myopathy. If active liver disease or transaminases (ALT or AST) are raised more than three times the normal range then statins are contraindicated (or if already being taken should be stopped). Note that transaminases (i.e. ALT or AST) should be checked 3 and 12 months after starting treatment (by requesting LFTs).
B	A measurement of blood pressure might be useful in assessing cardiovascular risk in this patient, but is not specifically relevant to therapy with simvastatin.
C	Creatine kinase need only be checked at baseline in patients who are considered to be at increased risk of the rare side effect of myopathy. There is no indication that this patient is at increased risk.
D	Serum albumin is a measure of the (synthetic) function of the liver (see Chapter 3). Statins should be used with caution in patients with a history of liver disease. However, NICE guidance only requires a measure of transaminases before commencing statins. Thus, this is not the most appropriate answer.
E	The dose of simvastatin is not weight based.

DECISION OPTIONS

A	SERUM ALT	✓
B	BLOOD PRESSURE	☐
C	CREATINE KINASE	☐
D	SERUM ALBUMIN	☐
E	WEIGHT	☐

Question 8.3 Answers

A	**Correct:** the reported level is within the normal reference range (40–80 µmol/L) which is available in the BNF. (Be careful as there are two normal ranges presented with different units.) Based on the information you have, it would be reasonable to assume that no dose change is required.
B	See justification for Option A.
C	See justification for Option A.
D	Post-dose phenytoin levels are not routinely required. The average half-life of phenytoin (approximately 24 hours) is such that after 14 days of therapy there is unlikely to be significant diurnal variation in the plasma level.
E	The normal range quoted (40–80 µmol/L) is a reference range only and based on population data. One should consider the level in the context of the patient: if there are no seizures (i.e. a therapeutic effect), the dose (of this potentially toxic drug) should not be increased. Conversely, if there are side effects despite a 'normal' trough level, then the dose should be decreased (if seizure control is adequate) or an alternative sought (see Chapter 3 for more detail).

DECISION OPTIONS

A	300 MG DAILY IS A SUITABLE MAINTENANCE DOSE FOR THIS PATIENT	✓
B	300 MG DAILY IS TOO HIGH A MAINTENANCE DOSE AND SHOULD BE REDUCED	☐
C	300 MG DAILY IS TOO LOW A MAINTENANCE DOSE AND SHOULD BE INCREASED	☐
D	A POST-DOSE LEVEL IS REQUIRED IN ORDER TO ASCERTAIN THE SUITABILITY OF THIS DOSE FOR THIS PATIENT	☐
E	THE REPORTED LEVEL CAN BE CONSIDERED ALONE, WITHOUT INFORMATION ABOUT SEIZURE CONTROL	☐

Question 8.4 Drug monitoring item worth 2 points – lithium

CASE PRESENTATION

Following psychiatric evaluation a 40-year-old female patient is prescribed lithium for the prophylaxis of acute mania. She is told that she will be required to attend her GP surgery for regular blood tests, which will be more frequent during the first few months of therapy.

Question: Which *one* of the following statements regarding monitoring therapy with lithium is true? Mark it with a tick in the column provided.

	DECISION OPTIONS	
A	SERUM CONCENTRATION OF LITHIUM SHOULD BE MEASURED ON A SAMPLE TAKEN 2–4 HOURS FOLLOWING THE LAST DOSE	☐
B	SERUM CONCENTRATIONS OF LITHIUM WHICH ARE ABOVE 1.5 MMOL/L ARE LIKELY TO MANIFEST WITH TOXIC EFFECTS	☑
C	FULL BLOOD COUNTS SHOULD BE CHECKED REGULARLY IN PATIENTS WHO ARE PRESCRIBED LITHIUM	☑
D	FOR PATIENTS STABILIZED ON LONG-TERM TREATMENT WITH LITHIUM, SERUM CONCENTRATIONS OF LITHIUM NEED ONLY BE CHECKED IF THERE IS CLINICAL SUSPICION OF TOXICITY	☐
E	SERUM LITHIUM LEVELS ARE UNAFFECTED BY SODIUM INTAKE	☐

Question 8.5 Drug monitoring item worth 2 points – methotrexate

CASE PRESENTATION

Following a discussion regarding risks and benefits, a 60-year-old woman is commenced on methotrexate by a consultant rheumatologist for the treatment of rheumatoid arthritis. She is prescribed a low dose initially of 7.5 mg to be taken once a week, and on the same day each week.

Question: Concerning the appropriate monitoring of methotrexate therapy, which *one* of the following statements is true? Mark it with a tick in the column provided.

	DECISION OPTIONS	
A	A FULL BLOOD COUNT SHOULD BE CHECKED AT BASELINE AND REPEATED EVERY 1–2 WEEKS THROUGHOUT THE DURATION OF THERAPY	☐
B	A BASELINE CHEST X-RAY SHOULD BE CHECKED PRIOR TO COMMENCING TREATMENT	☐
C	TREATMENT WITH METHOTREXATE SHOULD NOT BE STARTED IF LIVER FUNCTION TESTS ARE ABNORMAL	☐
D	IN THE EVENT OF A CLINICALLY SIGNIFICANT DROP IN WHITE CELL OR PLATELET COUNT, THE DOSE OF METHOTREXATE SHOULD BE REDUCED	☐
E	REGULAR MONITORING OF RENAL FUNCTION IS NOT REQUIRED DURING THERAPY WITH METHOTREXATE AS IT IS NOT CLEARED RENALLY	☐

Question 8.4 Answers

A	The recommended sampling time for lithium is 12 hours after the last dose.
B	**Correct:** the normal reference range for lithium is 0.4–0.8 mmol/L and toxic effects are likely to manifest at serum concentrations above 1.5 mmol/L.
C	Full blood counts are not routinely required in patients on lithium.
D	Routine serum lithium monitoring should be performed weekly after initiation and after each dose change until concentrations are stable, and then every 3 months thereafter.
E	Sodium depletion is known to increase the risk of lithium toxicity and patients are advised to avoid making changes in their diet that would lead to increased or decreased sodium intake.

DECISION OPTIONS

A	SERUM CONCENTRATION OF LITHIUM SHOULD BE MEASURED ON A SAMPLE TAKEN 2–4 HOURS FOLLOWING THE LAST DOSE	☐
B	SERUM CONCENTRATIONS OF LITHIUM WHICH ARE ABOVE 1.5 MMOL/L ARE LIKELY TO MANIFEST WITH TOXIC EFFECTS	✓
C	FULL BLOOD COUNTS SHOULD BE CHECKED REGULARLY IN PATIENTS WHO ARE PRESCRIBED LITHIUM	☐
D	FOR PATIENTS STABILIZED ON LONG-TERM TREATMENT WITH LITHIUM, SERUM CONCENTRATIONS OF LITHIUM NEED ONLY BE CHECKED IF THERE IS CLINICAL SUSPICION OF TOXICITY	☐
E	SERUM LITHIUM LEVELS ARE UNAFFECTED BY SODIUM INTAKE	☐

Question 8.5 Answers

A	Methotrexate has been known to cause fatal blood dyscrasias. Monitoring of full blood count at regular intervals is imperative, but once therapy has been stabilized, full blood count can be monitored every 2–3 months.
B	According to the BNF, a CXR is not required at baseline (although the British Society of Rheumatology recommend one); however, it may be required later on if pulmonary toxicity is suspected.
C	**Correct:** owing to the risk of liver cirrhosis, treatment with methotrexate should not be started if liver function tests are abnormal.
D	No! Methotrexate must be stopped immediately under these circumstances.
E	Methotrexate is predominantly renally excreted and toxicity is more likely in the presence of renal dysfunction.

DECISION OPTIONS

A	A FULL BLOOD COUNT SHOULD BE CHECKED AT BASELINE AND REPEATED EVERY 1–2 WEEKS THROUGHOUT THE DURATION OF THERAPY	☐
B	A BASELINE CHEST X-RAY SHOULD BE CHECKED PRIOR TO COMMENCING TREATMENT	☐
C	TREATMENT WITH METHOTREXATE SHOULD NOT BE STARTED IF LIVER FUNCTION TESTS ARE ABNORMAL	✓
D	IN THE EVENT OF A CLINICALLY SIGNIFICANT DROP IN WHITE CELL OR PLATELET COUNT, THE DOSE OF METHOTREXATE SHOULD BE REDUCED	☐
E	REGULAR MONITORING OF RENAL FUNCTION IS NOT REQUIRED DURING THERAPY WITH METHOTREXATE AS IT IS NOT CLEARED RENALLY	☐

Question 8.6 Drug monitoring item worth 2 points – olanzapine

CASE PRESENTATION

Following psychiatric evaluation, a 55-year-old male patient is prescribed olanzapine for the treatment of symptoms of schizophrenia. He has no other significant past medical history.

Question: Which *one* of the following parameters is important to check and record before commencing treatment? Mark it with a tick in the column provided.

	DECISION OPTIONS	
A	CHEST X-RAY	☐
B	FASTING BLOOD GLUCOSE	☑
C	HEART RATE	☐
D	TEMPERATURE	☐
E	ECG	☐

Question 8.7 Drug monitoring item worth 2 points – oral contraceptive pill

CASE PRESENTATION

A 34-year-old female patient attends an annual review appointment at her GP surgery. She has no significant past medical history but has been taking a combined oral contraceptive pill containing ethinylestradiol and levonorgestrel for the last 2 years. She requests a prescription for a further supply of her pill.

Question: Before responding to her request, which *one* of the following parameters would it be most important to check? Mark it with a tick in the column provided.

	DECISION OPTIONS	
A	SERUM CREATININE	☐
B	RESTING HEART RATE	☐
C	BLOOD PRESSURE	☑
D	SERUM AST	☐
E	HAEMOGLOBIN	☐

Question 8.6 Answers

A	Not required at baseline.
B	**Correct:** hyperglycaemia and diabetes can occur in patients prescribed antipsychotic drugs, particularly olanzapine. Fasting blood glucose must be tested at baseline and at regular intervals thereafter.
C	Not routinely required at baseline.
D	Not required at baseline.
E	Baseline ECG prior to commencing an antipsychotic drug is only usually indicated in patients with cardiovascular disease or associated risk factors. We are told that this patient has no significant past medical history, so this is not the most appropriate choice in this case.

DECISION OPTIONS

A	CHEST X-RAY	☐
B	FASTING BLOOD GLUCOSE	✓
C	HEART RATE	☐
D	TEMPERATURE	☐
E	ECG	☐

Question 8.7 Answers

A	Routine monitoring of renal function is not required for patients on a combined oral contraceptive pill.
B	Not required.
C	**Correct:** hypertension is known to increase the risk of arterial disease associated with contraceptive medication.
D	Not required.
E	Not specifically required for patients on contraceptive medication unless anaemia is suspected.

DECISION OPTIONS

A	SERUM CREATININE	☐
B	RESTING HEART RATE	☐
C	BLOOD PRESSURE	✓
D	SERUM AST	☐
E	HAEMOGLOBIN	☐

Question 8.8 Drug monitoring item worth 2 points – amiodarone

CASE PRESENTATION

While on a cardiology ward, a 56-year-old female patient is prescribed oral amiodarone for the treatment of an arrhythmia. She is to be 'loaded' with amiodarone, starting on a dose of 200 mg 3 times daily for 1 week, and reduced to 200 mg twice daily for a further week, and then reduced again to 200 mg once daily as a maintenance dose.

Question: Which *one* of the following statements is true regarding appropriate monitoring of amiodarone? Mark it with a tick in the column provided.

	DECISION OPTIONS	
A	SERUM THYROXINE (T4) ALONE IS A SUFFICIENT MEASURE OF THYROID FUNCTION IN PATIENTS TAKING AMIODARONE	☐
B	A BASELINE CHEST X-RAY SHOULD BE CHECKED BEFORE COMMENCING TREATMENT	☑
C	LIVER FUNCTION SHOULD BE CHECKED AT BASELINE AND REPEATED DURING THERAPY IF HEPATOTOXICITY SUSPECTED	☐
D	SERUM CREATININE SHOULD BE MEASURED BEFORE COMMENCING TREATMENT	☐
E	AMIODARONE SHOULD BE COMMENCED WITH CAUTION IN PATIENTS WITH HYPERKALAEMIA	☐

Question 8.9 Drug monitoring item worth 2 points – carbimazole

CASE PRESENTATION

A 44-year-old female patient is prescribed carbimazole by her GP as part of a 'block and replace' regimen for the treatment of thyrotoxicosis. The GP advises her to report any sore throat immediately.

Question: Which *one* of the following should be checked first in a patient presenting with a sore throat who is prescribed carbimazole? Mark it with a tick in the column provided.

	DECISION OPTIONS	
A	NEUTROPHIL COUNT	☑
B	THROAT SWAB	☐
C	BLOOD CULTURES	☐
D	SERUM ALT	☐
E	TFTs	☐

Question 8.8 Answers

A	T3, TSH *and* T4 must all be included in a measurement of thyroid function in patients taking amiodarone. T4 may be raised in the absence of hyperthyroidism.
B	**Correct:** a baseline chest X-ray should be carried out owing to the risk of pulmonary toxicity with amiodarone.
C	Raised serum transaminases and acute liver dysfunction are recognized side effects of amiodarone. It is important to monitor liver function at regular intervals throughout the duration of therapy, and not only in the case of suspected hepatotoxicity.
D	The dose of amiodarone is chosen independently of renal function, and renal failure is not a recognised side effect.
E	Amiodarone should be commenced with caution in patients with hypokalaemia owing to an increased risk of arrhythmias.

DECISION OPTIONS

A	SERUM THYROXINE (T4) ALONE IS A SUFFICIENT MEASURE OF THYROID FUNCTION IN PATIENTS TAKING AMIODARONE	☐
B	A BASELINE CHEST X-RAY SHOULD BE CHECKED BEFORE COMMENCING TREATMENT	✓
C	LIVER FUNCTION SHOULD BE CHECKED AT BASELINE AND REPEATED DURING THERAPY IF HEPATOTOXICITY SUSPECTED	☐
D	SERUM CREATININE SHOULD BE MEASURED BEFORE COMMENCING TREATMENT	☐
E	AMIODARONE SHOULD BE COMMENCED WITH CAUTION IN PATIENTS WITH HYPERKALAEMIA	☐

Question 8.9 Answers

A	**Correct:** sore throat may be an indication of infection, which could be a result of carbimazole-induced bone marrow suppression and thus agranulocytosis. A full blood count, including neutrophil count, is imperative.
B	It is more important in the first instance to rule out bone marrow suppression. A throat swab will not reveal bone-marrow suppression and is not indicated at this point.
C	Blood cultures are not indicated at this point without other features of infection, and would (like throat swabs) take much longer to deliver a result (e.g. infection), which is non-specific (i.e. a patient could have a throat infection without neutropenia). They may be indicated later.
D	Carbimazole is known to be associated with hepatic disorders, but this is not the priority in the first instance.
E	Thyroid function tests at this stage would not allow bone marrow suppression to be confirmed nor ruled out and are, therefore, not the most appropriate 'first' parameter to check. The priority at this stage is to assess for bone marrow suppression.

DECISION OPTIONS

A	NEUTROPHIL COUNT	✓
B	THROAT SWAB	☐
C	BLOOD CULTURES	☐
D	SERUM ALT	☐
E	TFTs	☐

Question 8.10 Drug monitoring item worth 2 points – gentamicin: multiple daily dose regimen

CASE PRESENTATION

A 56-year-old male patient with a diagnosis of endocarditis, caused by viridans streptococci, is commenced on benzylpenicillin and gentamicin on the recommendation of microbiology. The dose of gentamicin is 60 mg, by IV infusion, 3 times daily.

Question: Concerning the monitoring of gentamicin therapy in infective endocarditis, which *one* of the following statements is true? Mark it with a tick in the column provided.

	DECISION OPTIONS	
A	ONE-HOUR (PEAK) SERUM CONCENTRATION SHOULD BE 5–10 MG/L	☑
B	ONE-HOUR (PEAK) SERUM CONCENTRATION SHOULD BE 3–5 MG/L	☐
C	PRE-DOSE (TROUGH) SERUM CONCENTRATION SHOULD BE LESS THAN 2 MG/L	☐
D	ONLY PRE-DOSE (TROUGH) LEVELS ARE REQUIRED FOR THE MONITORING OF A MULTIPLE DAILY DOSE REGIMEN FOR GENTAMICIN	☐
E	MONITORING OF RENAL FUNCTION IS NOT ROUTINELY REQUIRED WITH GENTAMICIN AS IT IS NOT SIGNIFICANTLY RENALLY CLEARED	☐

Question 8.11 Drug monitoring item worth 2 points – ramipril

CASE PRESENTATION

A 63-year-old female patient with a history of acute myocardial infarction is diagnosed with mild heart failure and commenced on ramipril.

Question: Which *one* of the following parameters would be the most important for you to monitor at regular intervals in the primary care setting? Mark it with a tick in the column provided.

	DECISION OPTIONS	
A	HEART RATE	☐
B	URINARY SODIUM	☐
C	URINE OUTPUT	☐
D	SERUM UREA AND ELECTROLYTES	☑
E	SERUM ACE LEVEL	☐

Question 8.10 Answers

A	For a multiple daily dose regimen, 1 hour (peak) serum concentration should be 3–5 mg/L for the treatment of endocarditis (see Chapter 3).
B	**Correct:** for a multiple daily dose regimen, 1 hour (peak) serum concentration should be 3–5 mg/L for the treatment of endocarditis.
C	For a multiple daily dose regimen, pre-dose (trough) serum concentration should be less than 1 mg/L for the treatment of endocarditis.
D	For a multiple daily dose regimen, both pre- and post-dose levels must be checked at regular intervals.
E	Gentamicin is principally renally excreted from the body. Patients with renal dysfunction are at increased risk of toxicity, thus monitoring of renal function is required at regular intervals in patients on gentamicin.

DECISION OPTIONS

A	ONE-HOUR (PEAK) SERUM CONCENTRATION SHOULD BE 5–10 MG/L	☐
B	ONE-HOUR (PEAK) SERUM CONCENTRATION SHOULD BE 3–5 MG/L	✓
C	PRE-DOSE (TROUGH) SERUM CONCENTRATION SHOULD BE LESS THAN 2 MG/L	☐
D	ONLY PRE-DOSE (TROUGH) LEVELS ARE REQUIRED FOR THE MONITORING OF A MULTIPLE DAILY DOSE REGIMEN FOR GENTAMICIN	☐
E	MONITORING OF RENAL FUNCTION IS NOT ROUTINELY REQUIRED WITH GENTAMICIN AS IT IS NOT SIGNIFICANTLY RENALLY CLEARED	☐

Question 8.11 Answers

A	ACE inhibitors do not affect heart rate and therefore this would not be the appropriate answer. It is possible that the patient may have been concomitantly started on a beta blocker but this is not mentioned.
B	While ramipril may cause hyponatraemia, urinary sodium would not be a suitable method for detecting this.
C	Serum creatinine is a sufficient measure of renal function. Measuring urine output would not be practical in a primary care setting.
D	**Correct:** ACE-inhibitors are known to cause hyperkalaemia, hyponatraemia and, in some cases, acute kidney injury. U&Es should be checked at baseline and after every dose change.
E	It is possible to measure serum levels of ACE, but it is not a relevant measurement in the monitoring of either ACE-inhibitor therapy or of heart failure. Serum ACE is characteristically raised in active sarcoidosis.

DECISION OPTIONS

A	HEART RATE	☐
B	URINARY SODIUM	☐
C	URINE OUTPUT	☐
D	SERUM UREA AND ELECTROLYTES	✓
E	SERUM ACE LEVEL	☐

Question 8.12 Drug monitoring item worth 2 points – digoxin

CASE PRESENTATION

A 72-year-old sedentary male with a new diagnosis of AF is commenced on aspirin for stroke prophylaxis and digoxin 62.5 micrograms daily for rate control.

Question: Which *one* of the following parameters would be the most important to monitor during treatment with digoxin? Mark it with a tick in the column provided.

	DECISION OPTIONS	
A	PLASMA DIGOXIN CONCENTRATION	☑
B	SERUM CREATININE	☐
C	BLOOD PRESSURE	☐
D	CHEST X-RAY	☐
E	SERUM SODIUM	☐

Question 8.13 Drug monitoring item worth 2 points – sodium valproate

CASE PRESENTATION

A 72-year-old male patient with no significant medical history is commenced on sodium valproate for the management of generalized seizures.

Question: Before starting treatment, which *one* of the following parameters would be the most important for you to check? Mark it with a tick in the column provided.

	DECISION OPTIONS	
A	PANCREATIC AMYLASE	☐
B	SERUM VITAMIN D LEVEL	☐
C	SERUM POTASSIUM	☐
D	ALT	☑
E	SERUM CREATININE	☐

Question 8.12 Answers

A	Plasma digoxin concentration is not measured unless toxicity, non-compliance or inadequate effect are suspected.
B	**Correct:** digoxin is predominantly renally excreted and patients with renal dysfunction are at increased risk of toxicity.
C	Not required for patients on digoxin. It does not cause hypotension (unlike calcium-channel blockers and beta-blockers) which makes it a good choice for patients with arrhythmias and hypotension needing treatment.
D	Not required for patients on digoxin.
E	Serum sodium is not specifically required in the monitoring of digoxin therapy (although it would likely be checked as part of U&Es). Serum potassium is a more relevant parameter as hypokalaemia increases the risk of digoxin toxicity.

DECISION OPTIONS

A	PLASMA DIGOXIN CONCENTRATION	☐
B	SERUM CREATININE	✓
C	BLOOD PRESSURE	☐
D	CHEST X-RAY	☐
E	SERUM SODIUM	☐

Question 8.13 Answers

A	Pancreatitis is a known side effect of sodium valproate, but a measurement of pancreatic amylase would only be required if a patient were to report symptoms of pancreatitis whilst on therapy.
B	Vitamin D supplementation should be considered for patients on sodium valproate at risk of osteoporosis; however, a vitamin D level would not be routinely checked at baseline.
C	Not required.
D	**Correct:** sodium valproate therapy is associated with hepatotoxicity and liver function should be measured at baseline as well as at regular intervals throughout the duration of therapy.
E	A measure of renal function is not routinely required prior to commencing treatment with sodium valproate. It is neither significantly renally cleared nor nephrotoxic. In patients with severe renal impairment, it might be necessary to adjust the dose based on careful monitoring, but we are not given any indication that this patient has severe renal impairment.

DECISION OPTIONS

A	PANCREATIC AMYLASE	☐
B	SERUM VITAMIN D LEVEL	☐
C	SERUM POTASSIUM	☐
D	ALT	✓
E	SERUM CREATININE	☐

Question 8.14 Drug monitoring item worth 2 points – clozapine

CASE PRESENTATION

A patient is commenced on clozapine for the treatment of schizophrenia, having failed to respond to two other antipsychotic drugs.

The psychiatrist asks you to ensure that appropriate monitoring is carried out so that therapy can continue.

Question: Regarding the appropriate monitoring of therapy with clozapine, which *one* of the following statements is correct? Mark it with a tick in the column provided.

	DECISION OPTIONS	
A	FULL BLOOD COUNT MUST BE CHECKED WEEKLY FOR THE FIRST 18 WEEKS	☑
B	REGISTRATION WITH A CLOZAPINE MONITORING SERVICE IS RESERVED FOR PATIENTS WITH A BASELINE NEUTROPENIA	☐
C	SERUM CREATININE SHOULD BE CHECKED AT REGULAR INTERVALS THROUGHOUT THE DURATION OF THERAPY	☐
D	IF LEUKOCYTE COUNT DROPS TO BELOW 3000/MM^3, THE DOSE SHOULD BE REDUCED	☐
E	IF NEUTROPHIL COUNT DROPS TO BELOW 1500/MM^3, THE DOSE SHOULD BE REDUCED	☐

Question 8.14 Answers

A	**Correct:** owing to the risk of neutropenia and potentially fatal agranulocytosis, routine monitoring of full blood count is required at regular intervals as dictated by the product license throughout the duration of treatment.
B	Registration with a clozapine monitoring service is required for all patients.
C	Not routinely required in patients on clozapine.
D	No! Clozapine must be immediately stopped under these circumstances.
E	No! Clozapine must be immediately stopped under these circumstances.

DECISION OPTIONS

A	FULL BLOOD COUNT MUST BE CHECKED WEEKLY FOR THE FIRST 18 WEEKS	✓
B	REGISTRATION WITH A CLOZAPINE MONITORING SERVICE IS RESERVED FOR PATIENTS WITH A BASELINE NEUTROPENIA	☐
C	SERUM CREATININE SHOULD BE CHECKED AT REGULAR INTERVALS THROUGHOUT THE DURATION OF THERAPY	☐
D	IF LEUKOCYTE COUNT DROPS TO BELOW 3000/MM^3, THE DOSE SHOULD BE REDUCED	☐
E	IF NEUTROPHIL COUNT DROPS TO BELOW 1500/MM^3, THE DOSE SHOULD BE REDUCED	☐

Adverse drug reactions

Chapter objectives

- Learn to identify and predict adverse reactions for specific drugs.
- Learn to identify likely drug interactions.
- Know how best to prevent or manage these reactions.

STRUCTURE OF THIS SECTION WITHIN THE PSA

The 'Adverse drug reactions' section will have 8 questions with 2 marks available per question, so a possible total of 16 marks. You will be asked to identify the most appropriate option from a list of five for each scenario.

INTRODUCTION

Around 5% of NHS admissions are related to adverse drug reactions (ADRs). This places a considerable burden on the NHS in terms of morbidity, mortality and cost. Evidence suggests that a significant proportion of ADRs are avoidable (see Pirmohamed M, et al. Adverse drug reactions as a cause of admission to hospital: Prospective analysis of 18820 patients. *BMJ* 2004:329;15–19P).

The 'Adverse drug reaction' section of the PSA will test your ability to detect, respond to and prevent potential ADRs and drug interactions. There are four different types of question you might be asked in this section and it is likely you will be asked one of each type. Much of this chapter will be revision of earlier concepts.

TYPE 1: ADVERSE EFFECTS OF COMMON DRUGS

This question will ask you to identify adverse effects associated with a specific drug. (See Chapter 2 for theory).

> **Handy tip**
>
> The emphasis here is on common and/or serious side effects of commonly used drugs. While we have listed the side effects of the most common drug groups in Chapter 2 and extended this in Table 9.1 (and in doing so covered all examples in the PSA blueprint), you can reassure yourself by listing the five most common drugs for each body system and learning the common side effects.

TYPE 2: RECOGNIZING THE COMMON REACTIONS

This question will ask you to identify the most likely drug to have caused a specific presentation. (See Chapter 2 for theory).

> **Handy tip**
>
> It is advisable to know the difference between a common reaction and a dangerous one. For example, a common reaction to statins is myalgia and a dangerous one is rhabdomyolysis. Common reactions covered might include new renal impairment, hypokalaemia, hepatic dysfunction and urinary retention. This type of reaction is sometimes referred to as a Type A reaction – common, predictable and dose related. Type B reactions (sometimes called idiosyncratic) are bizarre and unexpected reactions related to gene/host/environmental interactions. Type A and B reactions are comprehensively discussed in pharmacology texts, but this summary should suffice for the PSA.

Table 9.1: Drugs and their common ADRs (see Chapter 2)

Type	Examples	Adverse Drug Reactions
Antibiotics	Gentamicin Vancomycin	Nephrotoxicity, ototoxicity
	Any antibiotic (but most commonly the broad-spectrum antibiotics like cephalosporins or ciprofloxacin)	*Clostridium difficile* colitis
Antihypertensives	ACE-inhibitors, e.g. lisinopril	Hypotension, electrolyte abnormalities, acute kidney injury, dry cough
	Beta-blockers, e.g. bisoprolol	Hypotension, bradycardia, wheeze in asthmatics, worsens acute heart failure (but helps chronic heart failure)
	Calcium-channel blockers, e.g. diltiazem	Hypotension, bradycardia, peripheral oedema, flushing
	Diuretics, e.g. furosemide, bendroflumethiazide, spironolactone	Hypotension, electrolyte abnormalities, acute kidney injury, subclass-dependent effects
Anticoagulants/ antiplatelets	Heparins	Haemorrhage (especially if renal failure or <50 kg), heparin-induced thrombocytopaenia
	Warfarin	Haemorrhage (note that ironically warfarin has a pro-coagulant effect initially as well as taking a few days to become an anti-coagulant; thus heparin should be prescribed alongside warfarin and continued until the INR exceeds 2.
		(WARFarin (Wisconsin Alumni Research Foundation) is a vitamin K reductase inhibitor. Vitamin K was named by German biochemists 'koagulation vitamin')
	Aspirin	Haemorrhage, peptic ulcers and gastritis, tinnitus in large doses
Other antiarrhythmics	Digoxin	Nausea, vomiting and diarrhoea, blurred vision, confusion and drowsiness, xanthopsia (disturbed yellow/green visual perception including 'halo' vision)
		Digoxin competes with potassium at the myocyte Na^+/K^+ ATPase, limiting Na^+ influx. Since Ca^{2+} outflow relies on Na^+ influx, Ca^{2+} accumulates in the cell. This lengthens the action potential and slows the heart rate. This summary is important because changes in serum K^+ at the receptor can compete with digoxin; low K^+ augments digoxin effect. High levels limit the effect
	Amiodarone	Interstitial lung disease (pulmonary fibrosis), thyroid disease (both hypo- and hyperthyroidism are reported; it is structurally related to iodine, hence its name amIODarone), skin greying, corneal deposits
Mood stabilizers	Lithium	Early – tremor
		Intermediate – tiredness
		Late – arrhythmias, seizures, coma, renal failure, diabetes insipidus
Antipsychotics	Haloperidol	Dyskinesias, e.g. acute dystonic reactions, drowsiness
	Clozapine	Agranulocytosis (requires intensive monitoring of full blood count)
Corticosteroids	Dexamethasone and prednisolone	STEROIDS: **S**tomach ulcers, **T**hin skin, **E**dema, **R**ight and left heart failure, **O**steoporosis, **I**nfection (including *Candida*), **D**iabetes (commonly causes hyperglycaemia; uncommonly progresses to diabetes); and Cushing's **S**yndrome
	Fludrocortisone	Hypertension/sodium and water retention
NSAIDs	Ibuprofen	NSAID: **N**o urine (renal failure), **S**ystolic dysfunction (heart failure), **A**sthma, **I**ndigestion (any cause), **D**yscrasia (clotting abnormality)
Statins	Simvastatin	Myalgia, abdominal pain, increased ALT/AST (can be mild), rhabdomyolysis (can be just mildly increased creatine kinase though)

TYPE 3: CLINICALLY IMPORTANT DRUG INTERACTIONS

To answer this question type, you will need to identify potential interactions between prescribed drugs and state those that are of clinical importance. Table 9.2 summarizes the information below.

Handy tips

A useful approach to this type of question is to 'spot' the drugs on the list that are known to interact. Drugs that are known to interact usually fall into one of three categories:

1. **Drugs with a narrow therapeutic index**, such as warfarin, digoxin and phenytoin. Interactions resulting in increased or decreased levels of these drugs can result in subtherapeutic or toxic levels. Try to spot these drugs in the questions.
2. **Drugs that require careful titration of dose according to effect**, such as antihypertensives and antidiabetic drugs (where over-treatment can lead to clinically significant consequences – hypotension or hypoglycaemia respectively). Furthermore, the body's handling of these drugs may be affected by the addition of other drugs. For example, iodinated contrast media can cause renal impairment, which increases the risk of metformin-induced lactic acidosis or ACE-inhibitor associated acute kidney injury. This might seem quite complicated, but will become clearer as you start to practise some questions of this type. A useful hint is that if the scenario presented refers to symptoms of low GCS or acidotic behaviour, look for metformin in the question!
3. **Drugs that affect (or are affected by) the cytochrome P450 enzyme system** (i.e. enzyme inducers/enzyme inhibitors/substrates – see Box 9.1). Knowing the types of drugs in these categories will guide and focus your revision and aid 'drug spotting' during the assessment.

Table 9.2: Common interacting drugs

Drugs with a narrow therapeutic index: warfarin, digoxin, phenytoin, theophylline	*Drugs which require careful dosage control:* antihypertensives, antidiabetic drugs
Enzyme inducers:	*Enzyme inhibitors* (most common): ketoconazole, ciprofloxacin and erythromycin. Do not forget grapefruit juice (not included below)!
PC BRAS:	**AODEVICES:**
Phenytoin	**A**llopurinol
Carbamazepine	**O**meprazole
Barbiturates	**D**isulfiram
Rifampicin	**E**rythromycin
Alcohol (chronic)	**V**alproate
Sulphonylureas	**I**soniazid
Synergistic effects: β-blockers and verapamil together may cause profound hypotension and asystole and the combination is therefore avoided (and strictly contraindicated if IV verapamil)	**C**iprofloxacin
	Ethanol (acute intoxication)
	Sulphonamides

Box 9.1   A fresh look at enzyme induction/inhibition

The cytochrome P450 isoenzyme system is involved in the metabolism of toxins (e.g. drugs). This short summary aims to add some depth to the understanding of this family of enzymes.

- Cytochromes are a family of membrane-bound ring structures that provide energy for reactions. They have functional iron components that contribute to their role as energy sources for reactions. They are active in oxidative phosphorylation and the electron transport chain.
- P stands for pigment because local iron, complexed as haem groups, makes these enzymes red.
- 450 represents the maximum absorption wavelength in the presence of carbon monoxide (a consequence of early measuring systems).

The cytochrome P450 enzymes are termed isoenzymes, which means that they are each different molecules, (with different amino acid sequences) but perform the same function (i.e. catalyse the same reaction). A good example of another group of isoenzymes is the lactate dehydrogenase isoenzymes. Different configurations optimize their work in different tissues.

The liver is not the only site of cytochrome P450 enzyme activity. The duodenum also has a role. It acts almost as a 'backstop' for the stomach, modifying toxic foodstuffs/poisons before further absorption in the gut. Drug companies are aware of this and modify their doses accordingly, sometimes doubling the physiological requirement to combat losses sustained in the duodenum. One problem is that everyday foodstuffs can interfere with their action. For example a single glass of grapefruit juice can inhibit the duodenal cytochrome P450 system for approximately 24 hours. This means excessive drug doses can pass through the duodenum, a particular problem for drugs with a narrow therapeutic index and others that require careful dosage control.

Enzyme induction takes days–weeks to establish but inhibition only takes hours–days. Keeping in mind that foodstuffs can also affect enzyme activity, doctors need to remain vigilant for ADRs because they can present weeks after medication changes or anytime patients change eating habits.

(Alcohol deserves a special mention because of its common use, under-reported misuse and widespread interaction with prescription drugs. For example, drinking alcohol while on metronidazole can cause fulminant nausea and vomiting, see Table 9.3).

Table 9.3: Drugs with potent interactions with alcohol

Gastrointestinal bleeding caused by: nonsteroidal anti-inflammatory drugs, including aspirin and ibuprofen	**Lactic acidosis caused by**: metformin
Increased anticoagulation caused by: warfarin (with acute alcohol due to enzyme inhibition); chronic alcohol causes enzyme induction and thus reduces anticoagulant effect	**Hypertensive crisis caused by**: monoamine oxidase inhibitors
Sweating, flushing, nausea and vomiting caused by: metronidazole and disulfiram	**Sedation caused by**: barbiturates, opioids and benzodiazepines

TYPE 4: RECOGNIZING AND MANAGING AN ADR

This type of question will ask you to determine the most appropriate action following an ADR. This might include acute anaphylaxis, excessive anticoagulation, drug-induced hyperglycaemia or diuretic-induced dehydration. Essentially, this type of question is asking you to put the theory you have acquired into practice in a proposed clinical scenario in order to answer type 1, 2 and 3 questions. The management of an ADR involves assessment of the reaction, selection of an appropriate treatment plan/course of action and symptom management and you should consider all of these aspects when reading the scenario you are presented with.

Question 9.1 Adverse drug reactions item worth 2 marks

CASE PRESENTATION

A 58-year-old man is attending a routine follow-up appointment after starting lisinopril for the treatment of hypertension 3 months earlier.

On questioning, you establish that he has been compliant with his medicine and has had no significant problems. You decide to titrate his dose up but carry out a blood test before proceeding.

Question: Based on the known adverse effect profile of lisinopril, select the *one parameter* you are most interested in checking when you carry out the blood test. Mark it with a tick in the column provided.

DECISION OPTIONS

A	WHITE CELL COUNT	☐
B	NEUTROPHIL COUNT	☐
C	SERUM SODIUM	☐
D	SERUM ALBUMIN	☐
E	SERUM POTASSIUM	☑

Question 9.2 Adverse drug reactions item worth 2 marks

CASE PRESENTATION

You wish to start a 62-year-old female on propranolol for migraine prophylaxis. She is quite an anxious lady and is keen to avoid taking medication if she possibly can.
She asks you for advice about the common side effects so that she can make an informed decision as to whether she would like to start treatment.

Question: Which *one* of the following is a common side effect of propranolol that you might discuss with your patient? Mark it with a tick in the column provided.

DECISION OPTIONS

A	HEAT INTOLERANCE	☐
B	TREMOR	☐
C	HYPERTENSION	☐
D	FATIGUE	☑
E	TACHYCARDIA	☐

Question 9.1 Answer

ACE-inhibitors are known to cause renal impairment, so a measure of serum creatinine is necessary before any dose titration (but this is not given as an option). Additionally, ACE-inhibitors can accumulate in renal impairment.

ACE-inhibitors are known to cause hyperkalaemia (either directly due to inhibition of the renin-angiotensin-aldosterone system, or indirectly through renal impairment).

ACE-inhibitors can cause hyponatraemia, but checking the potassium is more important as abnormalities can cause fatal arrhythmias.

DECISION OPTIONS

A	WHITE CELL COUNT	☐
B	NEUTROPHIL COUNT	☐
C	SERUM SODIUM	☐
D	SERUM ALBUMIN	☐
E	SERUM POTASSIUM	✓

Question 9.2 Answers

A	Beta-blockers are not associated with heat intolerance. In fact, a common side effect of beta-blockers is cold extremities.
B	Beta-blockers do not cause tremor, and in fact are used to treat essential tremor and anxiety-related tremor. Conversely beta-agonists (such as salbutamol) can cause tremor.
C	Beta-blockers are used in the treatment of hypertension and are more likely to cause hypotension as a side effect.
D	**Correct:** this option is a less-recognized side effect, but a quick look in the BNF (which is available at all times during your exam) would reveal this.
E	Beta-blockers block adrenoceptors in the heart and slow the heart rate causing bradycardia.

DECISION OPTIONS

A	HEAT INTOLERANCE	☐
B	TREMOR	☐
C	HYPERTENSION	☐
D	FATIGUE	✓
E	TACHYCARDIA	☐

Question 9.3 Adverse drug reactions item worth 2 marks

CASE PRESENTATION

A 48-year-old man, with a history of polymyalgia rheumatica, attends the A&E department, complaining of abdominal pain and having noticed some blood in his stool. Amongst your differential diagnoses is peptic ulcer disease. His current medication is listed.

Question: Select the *one* drug from the list which would be the most likely to have caused peptic ulcer disease. Mark it with a tick in the column provided.

CURRENT PRESCRIPTIONS

Drug name	Dose	Route	Freq.	
LISINOPRIL	10 MG	ORAL	DAILY	☐
AMLODIPINE	5 MG	ORAL	DAILY	☐
BENDROFLUMETHIAZIDE	2.5 MG	ORAL	DAILY	☐
NAPROXEN	500 MG	ORAL	12-HOURLY	☑
CODEINE PHOSPHATE	30 MG	ORAL	6-HOURLY	☐

Question 9.4 Adverse drug reactions item worth 2 marks

CASE PRESENTATION

A 78-year-old man is being treated as an inpatient for a severe urinary tract infection. His baseline creatinine, on admission, was recorded as 98 µmol/L, however, on day 4 of his admission it is reported to be 178 µmol/L.

He has been adequately hydrated throughout his admission and has no history of renal impairment. You are asked to review his medication chart (see current prescriptions).

Question: Select *one* drug that is most likely to have caused the deterioration in this patient's renal function. Mark it with a tick in the column provided.

CURRENT PRESCRIPTIONS

Drug name	Dose	Route	Freq.	
PARACETAMOL	1 G	IV	8-HOURLY	☐
CO-BENELDOPA 100/25	2 TABLETS	ORAL	6-HOURLY	☐
DOMPERIDONE	10 MG	ORAL	6-HOURLY	☐
SELEGILINE	5 MG	ORAL	DAILY	☐
DICLOFENAC	50 MG	ORAL	8-HOURLY	☐

Question 9.3 Answer

The correct answer is naproxen.

Naproxen is an NSAID, which inhibits prostaglandin synthesis needed for gastric mucosal protection from acid. It therefore increases the risk of gastric inflammation and ulceration.

Another group of drugs which may cause peptic ulcers (which are not offered in this question) are corticosteroids (e.g. prednisolone), which inhibit gastric epithelial renewal thus predisposing to ulceration.

CURRENT PRESCRIPTIONS

Drug name	Dose	Route	Freq.	
LISINOPRIL	10 MG	ORAL	DAILY	☐
AMLODIPINE	5 MG	ORAL	DAILY	☐
BENDROFLUMETHIAZIDE	2.5 MG	ORAL	DAILY	☐
NAPROXEN	500 MG	ORAL	12-HOURLY	✓
CODEINE PHOSPHATE	30 MG	S/C	6-HOURLY	☐

Question 9.4 Answer

The correct answer is diclofenac.

Diclofenac (and the other NSAIDs) can cause acute kidney injury, usually by affecting renal haemodynamics or in a condition known as acute interstitial nephritis. Again, NSAID-induced nephrotoxicity is more likely to occur in patients with pre-existing renal impairment.

Learning point: ACE-inhibitors and NSAIDs should not be co-prescribed.

- ACE-inhibitors relax vessels leaving the kidney (i.e. efferent blood flow and often remembered as '(e)F off', as in go away). This decreases renal hydraulic pressure, and protects the fine friable vascular network of the kidney from the damaging effects of hypertension. As a consequence this reduces pressures, but also costs a few mL/h in filtration rate (GFR).

- NSAIDs inhibit prostaglandins. This class of drugs modify the afferent vessels (recalled as 'a'fferent/'a'pproaching). In normal physiology prostaglandins dilate the afferent renal vessels, promoting flow into the kidney and, therefore, renal perfusion. So it follows that NSAIDs diminish the inward flow. This also lowers renal hydraulic pressure. If the vessel inwards constricts and the vessel out dilates, the pressure in the kidney falls away too much and GFR tails off. The kidney relies on good perfusion, like any organ. Low flow indicates ischaemia.

Avoid prescribing ACE inhibitors and NSAIDs together, particularly in elderly patients, who already have a degree of renal impairment.

CURRENT PRESCRIPTIONS

Drug name	Dose	Route	Freq.	
PARACETAMOL	1 G	IV	8-HOURLY	☐
CO-BENELDOPA 100/25	2 TABLETS	ORAL	6-HOURLY	☐
DOMPERIDONE	10 MG	ORAL	6-HOURLY	☐
SELEGILINE	5 MG	ORAL	DAILY	☐
DICLOFENAC	50 MG	ORAL	8-HOURLY	✓

Question 9.5 Adverse drug reactions item worth 2 marks

CASE PRESENTATION

A 55-year-old woman with a history of rheumatoid arthritis, for which she currently takes methotrexate, is admitted to hospital for a total hip replacement, having sustained a hip fracture. During her admission she develops a urinary tract infection and is treated with antibiotics.

Over the following 2 weeks, routine blood tests reveal that her neutrophil count appears to be gradually declining and you are asked to review the patient. A list of her newly prescribed medication is provided (see current prescriptions).

Question: Select the *one* drug that is most likely to have caused the decline in neutrophil count. Mark it with a tick in the column provided.

CURRENT PRESCRIPTIONS

Drug name	Dose	Route	Freq.	
GABAPENTIN	300 MG	ORAL	8-HOURLY	☐
BENDROFLUMETHIAZIDE	2.5 MG	ORAL	DAILY	☐
AMLODIPINE	5 MG	ORAL	DAILY	☐
TRIMETHOPRIM	200 MG	ORAL	12-HOURLY	☑
CYCLIZINE	50 MG	ORAL	AS REQUIRED	☐

Question 9.6 Adverse drug reactions item worth 2 marks

CASE PRESENTATION

A 67-year-old woman is admitted to the CCU with a diagnosis of worsening congestive cardiac failure. On day 5 of her admission, she is stable enough to be transferred to a general ward.

The nurse asks you to review her blood results prior to transferring her as one of her electrolytes is outside of the reference range:

	Value	Normal range		Value	Normal range
Na	140 mmol/L	(135–145 mmol/L)	Ur	3.2 mmol/L	(3–7 mmol/L)
K	6.2 mmol/L	(3.5–5.0 mmol/L)	Cr	78 µmol/L	(60–125 µmol/L)

Question: Select the *one* drug that is most likely to have caused this patient's hyperkalaemia. Mark it with a tick in the column provided.

CURRENT PRESCRIPTIONS

Drug name	Dose	Route	Freq.	
CODEINE	30 MG	ORAL	DAILY	☐
CYCLIZINE	50 MG	ORAL	8-HOURLY	☐
AMILORIDE	5 MG	ORAL	DAILY	☑
ASPIRIN	75 MG	ORAL	DAILY	☐
CARVEDILOL	6.25 MG	ORAL	DAILY	☐

Question 9.5 Answer

The correct answer is trimethoprim.

Trimethoprim is a folate antagonist, as is methotrexate. Taking both together can lead to additive toxicity in the form of bone marrow suppression, pancytopenia and neutropenic sepsis. In fact, taking trimethoprim is strictly contraindicated in patients taking methotrexate.

CURRENT PRESCRIPTIONS

Drug name	Dose	Route	Freq.	
GABAPENTIN	300 MG	ORAL	8-HOURLY	☐
BENDROFLUMETHIAZIDE	2.5 MG	ORAL	DAILY	☐
AMLODIPINE	5 MG	ORAL	DAILY	☐
TRIMETHOPRIM	200 MG	ORAL	12-HOURLY	✓
CYCLIZINE	50 MG	ORAL	AS REQUIRED	☐

Question 9.6 Answer

The correct answer is amiloride.

Amiloride is a potassium-sparing diuretic, which is known to cause hyperkalaemia. The other group of drugs which commonly cause hyperkalaemia are ACE-inhibitors (due to their inhibition of the renin-angiotensin-aldosterone system).

It is worth noting that the combination of a potassium-sparing diuretic and an ACE-inhibitor should always alert you to the potential for developing hyperkalaemia. Patients on this combination should have their electrolytes monitored regularly, and particularly following dose changes.

CURRENT PRESCRIPTIONS

Drug name	Dose	Route	Freq.	
CODEINE	30 MG	ORAL	DAILY	☐
CYCLIZINE	50 MG	ORAL	8-HOURLY	☐
AMILORIDE	5 MG	ORAL	DAILY	✓
ASPIRIN	75 MG	ORAL	DAILY	☐
CARVEDILOL	6.25 MG	ORAL	DAILY	☐

Question 9.7 Adverse drug reactions item worth 2 marks

CASE PRESENTATION

A 76-year-old man with a history of AF, for which he is prescribed warfarin (target INR 2.0–3.0), presents at his local A&E department describing an episode of haematuria. An INR is reported as 7.2.

A week earlier, he had been commenced on a course of oral antibiotics for the treatment of a LRTI, by his general practitioner.

Question: On the basis that this is likely to be the result of a drug interaction, which *one* of the following antibiotics do you suspect that the patient is most likely to have been prescribed for the treatment of his LRTI? Mark it with a tick in the column provided.

DECISION OPTIONS

	Drug name	
A	AMOXICILLIN	☐
B	ERYTHROMYCIN	☑
C	AUGMENTIN®	☐
D	CO-AMOXICLAV	☐
E	TRIMETHOPRIM	☐

Question 9.8 Adverse drug reactions item worth 2 marks

CASE PRESENTATION

An 80-year-old man is brought to the accident and emergency department by his daughter (who is his carer). She explains to you that she noticed a small amount of blood in his urine (haematuria) earlier in the day which is confirmed on urine dipstick. His blood pressure is normal and he feels well.

He is currently taking warfarin for thromboprophylaxis as he has a diagnosis of AF. His target INR is 2.0 to 3.0 and he had his most recent INR check a month ago, which was reported to be 2.7.

You request an emergency INR, which is reported as 8.2.

Question: Which *one* of the following would be the most appropriate immediate course of action? Mark it with a tick in the column provided.

DECISION OPTIONS

A	GIVE WARFARIN AT LOWER DOSE	☐
B	GIVE VITAMIN K BY MOUTH	☐
C	GIVE VITAMIN K BY SLOW IV INJECTION	☑
D	WITHHOLD 1–2 DOSES OF WARFARIN AND RESTART AT LOWER DOSE	☐
E	GIVE PROTAMINE BY SLOW IV INJECTION	☐

Question 9.7 Answer

The correct answer is erythromycin.

You will find that all of the above options are listed in the BNF as potentially interacting with warfarin. The trick is to find the 'potentially serious' interactions, as indicated in the BNF by a black dot. Note that Augmentin® is a brand name for co-amoxiclav.

The mechanism of the potentially serious interaction between warfarin and erythromycin is, at least in part, due to inhibition of the cytochrome P-450 enzyme system by erythromycin (see Chapter 2).

The mechanism of the interaction between warfarin and ciprofloxacin (not offered as an option here, but well known for its enzyme-inhibiting properties) is less clear.

DECISION OPTIONS

	Drug name	
A	AMOXICILLIN	☐
B	ERYTHROMYCIN	✓
C	AUGMENTIN®	☐
D	CO-AMOXICLAV	☐
E	TRIMETHOPRIM	☐

Question 9.8 Answers

A	This would only be appropriate if the INR was less than 6 without bleeding (see Chapter 2).
B	Vitamin K should be given via the IV route in this scenario. It could be given by mouth if there was no bleeding.
C	**Correct:** as INR is over 8.
D	This course of action would only be appropriate if there was no bleeding and the INR was between 6 and 8.
E	Protamine is used to reverse the anticoagulant effects of heparin.

DECISION OPTIONS

A	GIVE WARFARIN AT LOWER DOSE	☐
B	GIVE VITAMIN K BY MOUTH	☐
C	GIVE VITAMIN K BY SLOW IV INJECTION	✓
D	WITHHOLD 1–2 DOSES OF WARFARIN AND RESTART AT LOWER DOSE	☐
E	GIVE PROTAMINE BY SLOW IV INJECTION	☐

Question 9.9 Adverse drug reactions item worth 2 marks

CASE PRESENTATION

You are called urgently to a ward to review an 18-year-old girl who appears to be suffering from an allergic reaction after receiving co-amoxiclav for a urinary tract infection.

She was not previously known to be allergic to penicillin.

Her symptoms include throat swelling and hypotension and she appears very unwell.

Question: Which _one_ of the following would be the most appropriate immediate course of action? Mark it with a tick in the column provided.

	DECISION OPTIONS	
A	SWITCH TO AN ALTERNATIVE ANTIBIOTIC	☐
B	ATTEMPT TO INDUCE EMESIS	☐
C	SECURE AIRWAY	☐
D	ADMINISTER IV HYDROCORTISONE	☐
E	ADMINISTER INTRAMUSCULAR ADRENALINE	☐

Question 9.10 Adverse drug reactions item worth 2 marks

CASE PRESENTATION

A 78-year-old male patient on your ward is prescribed oral gliclazide 120 mg 12-hourly for the treatment of type 2 diabetes.

You are interrupted by one of the nurses during your morning ward round to be told that the patient's blood glucose has been reported as 2.9 mmol/L and, although conscious, he is drowsy and seems agitated.

You immediately review the patient.

Question: Which _one_ of the following statements is true concerning the treatment of drug-induced hypoglycaemia? Mark it with a tick in the column provided.

	DECISION OPTIONS	
A	A CONSCIOUS PATIENT SHOULD BE GIVEN 10–20 G OF GLUCOSE BY MOUTH	☑
B	AN UNCONSCIOUS PATIENT SHOULD BE GIVEN AN IV INFUSION OF 50% GLUCOSE	☐
C	DRUG-INDUCED HYPOGLYCAEMIA CAN BE MANAGED WITHOUT HOSPITAL ADMISSION	☐
D	IM/IV/SC GLUCAGON SHOULD BE FIRST LINE IN A CONSCIOUS PATIENT WITH HYPOGLYCAEMIA	☐
E	DRUG-INDUCED HYPOGLYCAEMIA IS LESS LIKELY TO OCCUR IN PATIENTS ON SULPHONYLUREAS THAN IN PATIENTS ON METFORMIN	☐

Question 9.9 Answers

A	The co-amoxiclav should indeed by stopped and switched to an alternative antibiotic; however, the question asks you specifically for your immediate course of action.
B	Promoting emesis will not alleviate the symptoms in this scenario.
C	**Correct:** this patient has throat swelling which may compromise her airway (the most worrying consequence of an anaphylactic reaction). When severe this causes stridor then (without intervention) total occlusion and death. Whether through a head-tilt-chin-lift, a simple airway adjunct (such as a nasopharyngeal airway) or simply calling an anaesthetist, securing the airway is the priority here.
D	Hydrocortisone may be given, but its onset of action is delayed for several hours, thus it has a role in preventing further deterioration. Again, remember that the question asks you for your immediate actions.
E	Whilst intramuscular adrenaline is the first drug in the management of anaphylaxis, the patient will not gain much benefit from it without a patent airway. Always begin with ABCs when asked for acute management.

DECISION OPTIONS

A	SWITCH TO AN ALTERNATIVE ANTIBIOTIC	☐
B	ATTEMPT TO INDUCE EMESIS	☐
C	SECURE AIRWAY	✓
D	ADMINISTER IV HYDROCORTISONE	☐
E	ADMINISTER INTRAMUSCULAR ADRENALINE	☐

Question 9.10 Answers

A	**Correct:** if the patient is conscious (with little subsequent risk of aspiration) a sugar-rich snack is recommended.
B	Glucose 50% is not recommended due to the high risk of extravasation injury and because administration is difficult (due to viscosity).
C	Drug-induced hypoglycaemia should be managed in hospital as the hypoglycaemic effects of these drugs can persist for many hours.
D	Glucagon is usually used in an unconscious patient (or one who is too drowsy to safely swallow) when there is no IV access to enable IV dextrose administration.
E	Metformin is less likely to cause hypoglycaemia than the sulphonylureas. Learning point: metformin is a biguanide, it acts by limiting hepatic gluconeogenesis (creation of new sugar by the liver). Lactate is usually taken up in this process, and without new sugar production in the liver it can build up leading to lactic acidosis. Sulphonylureas, in simple terms, act by chemically squeezing insulins out of the pancreas. This is achieved by indirectly modifying calcium levels in beta cells. This calcium shift changes the cell membrane potential and makes insulin granules bind to it and exocytose more readily. Sulphonylureas are more dangerous (see answer E) because they act directly on insulin levels, rather than indirectly by sugar production (e.g. metformin).

DECISION OPTIONS

A	A CONSCIOUS PATIENT SHOULD BE GIVEN 10–20 G OF GLUCOSE BY MOUTH	✓
B	AN UNCONSCIOUS PATIENT SHOULD BE GIVEN AN IV INFUSION OF 50% GLUCOSE	☐
C	DRUG-INDUCED HYPOGLYCAEMIA CAN BE MANAGED WITHOUT HOSPITAL ADMISSION	☐
D	IM/IV/SC GLUCAGON SHOULD BE FIRST LINE IN A CONSCIOUS PATIENT WITH HYPOGLYCAEMIA	☐
E	DRUG-INDUCED HYPOGLYCAEMIA IS LESS LIKELY TO OCCUR IN PATIENTS ON SULPHONYLUREAS THAN IN PATIENTS ON METFORMIN	☐

EXAM 1

Question 10.1 Prescription review item worth 4 marks

CASE PRESENTATION

A 43-year-old woman is admitted with cholecystitis and your consultant has asked you to designate her 'nil by mouth' and prepare her for emergency surgery tomorrow morning.

Question: Please identify which *three* drugs you would stop before surgery with ticks in column A and which *two* you would stop and instigate an alternative therapy for with ticks in column B.

CURRENT PRESCRIPTIONS

Drug name	Dose	Route	Freq.	A	B
METFORMIN	1 G	ORAL	12-HOURLY	☑	☐
MICROGYNON 30 ED®	ONE	ORAL	DAILY	☑	☐
ENOXAPARIN	40 MG	S/C	DAILY	☐	☑
ASPIRIN	75 MG	ORAL	DAILY	☐	☐
BISOPROLOL	5 MG	ORAL	DAILY	☐	☐
NOVOMIX 30®	15 UNITS	S/C	12-HOURLY	☑	☑
PARACETAMOL	1 G	ORAL	6-HOURLY	☐	☐
LANSOPRAZOLE	30 MG	ORAL	DAILY	☐	☐

Question 10.2 Prescription review item worth 4 marks

CASE PRESENTATION

A 47-year-old man has been admitted with pneumonia and is improving with medical management (i.e. antibiotics and IV fluids). He has a background of hypertension, hypercholesterolaemia and arthritis; he has some knee pain. He denies any allergies.

Question: Please identify the *four* drug errors to address in this patient with ticks in column A.

CURRENT PRESCRIPTIONS

Drug name	Dose	Route	Freq.	A
BENDROFLUMETHIAZIDE	2.5 MG	ORAL	DAILY	☐
PARACETAMOL	500 MG	ORAL	AS REQUIRED UP TO 6-HOURLY	☑
SIMVASTATIN	20 G	ORAL	NIGHTLY	☑
TAMOXIFEN	20 MG	ORAL	DAILY	☐
AMOXICILLIN (FOR 7 DAYS)	500 MG	ORAL	8-HOURLY	☐
LISINOPRIL	10 MG	ORAL	NIGHTLY	☐
CO-CODAMOL 30/500	2 TABLETS	ORAL	6-HOURLY	☑
ALENDRONIC ACID	70 MG	ORAL	DAILY	☑

Question 10.3 Prescription review item worth 4 marks

CASE PRESENTATION

A 63-year-old presents with dizziness and a dry cough. His PMH includes depression, hypertension, stable angina and a TIA two months ago. He has not used his GTN spray for years.
His examination is unremarkable except BP 98/72 mmHg.

Question: Please identify which *two* drugs should be stopped with ticks in column A.

CURRENT PRESCRIPTIONS

Drug name	Dose	Route	Freq.	A
ASPIRIN	375 MG	ORAL	DAILY	☐
LISINOPRIL	20 MG	ORAL	NIGHTLY	☑
GTN SPRAY	1 SPRAY	SUBLINGUAL	AS REQUIRED UP TO 1-HOURLY	☐
CLOPIDOGREL	75 MG	ORAL	DAILY	☐
ST JOHN'S WORT	5 MG	ORAL	DAILY	☐
PRAVASTATIN	10 MG	ORAL	NIGHTLY	☑
PARACETAMOL	1 G	ORAL	6-HOURLY	☐

Question 10.4 Prescription review item worth 4 marks

CASE PRESENTATION

A 47-year-old with arthritis, hypertension and angina comes into your GP surgery for routine review. He has no new complaints and admits he is just here for a chat! You take the opportunity to review his prescription which he has handwritten for you.

Question: Please identify the *two* major drug errors with ticks in column A.

CURRENT PRESCRIPTIONS

Drug name	Dose	Route	Freq.	A
CO-CODAMOL 8/500	2 TABLETS	ORAL	4-HOURLY	☑
AMLODIPINE	5 MG	ORAL	DAILY	☐
ASPIRIN	75 MG	ORAL	DAILY	☐
ENALAPRIL	10 MG	ORAL	DAILY	☐
PROPRANOLOL	40 MG	ORAL	8-HOURLY	☐
QLAIRA®	1 TABLET	ORAL	DAILY	☐
IBUPROFEN	200 MG	ORAL	AS REQUIRED UP TO 8-HOURLY	☐

Question 10.5 Prescription review item worth 4 marks

CASE PRESENTATION

A 72-year-old female is admitted with confusion and agitation. Her PMH is notable for arthritis and hypertension. Her urine smells offensive and a dipstick supports the diagnosis of a urinary tract infection. She is treated with trimethoprim and diazepam to control her aggression on the ward. She requests ibuprofen for her joint pain. The next day she is much better, but on the second day she is very drowsy and only rouses to pain. You note her respiratory rate is also quite slow. You perform some blood tests.

	On admission	Now	Normal range		On admission	Now	Normal range
Na	138 mmol/L	146 mmol/L ↑	(135–145 mmol/L)	Cr	87 µmol/L	327 µmol/L ↑	(60–125 µmol/L)
K	4.2 mmol/L	5.2 mmol/L ↑	(3.5–5.0 mmol/L)	WCC	14.7 × 10⁹/L	14.1 × 10⁹/L	(4–11 × 10⁹/L)
Ur	7.1 mmol/L	11 mmol/L ↑	(3–7 mmol/L)			AKI	

Question: Please identify which *four* drugs to stop in this patient with ticks in column A.

CURRENT PRESCRIPTIONS

Drug name	Dose	Route	Freq.	A
COCODAMOL 8/500	2 TABLETS	ORAL	6-HOURLY	☑
DIAZEPAM	2 MG	ORAL	12-HOURLY	☑
LISINOPRIL	10 MG	ORAL	NIGHTLY	☑
ASPIRIN	75 MG	ORAL	DAILY	☐
IBUPROFEN	400 MG	ORAL	8-HOURLY	☑
TRIMETHOPRIM	200 MG	ORAL	12-HOURLY	☐

Question 10.6 Prescription review item worth 4 marks

CASE PRESENTATION

A 71-year-old patient with a PMH of diabetes, COPD, atrial fibrillation and hypertension presents to the emergency department complaining of polydipsia and indigestion. His regular medications are listed (see current prescriptions chart). Today he finishes courses of erythromycin and prednisolone prescribed for an exacerbation of COPD; there have otherwise been no recent changes to his medications. Examination reveals epigastric tenderness. His blood results are as follows:

	Value	Normal range		Value	Normal range
Na	142 mmol/L	(135–145 mmol/L)	Hb	82 g/L	(135–175 g/L (male))
K	5.4 mmol/L	(3.5–5.0 mmol/L)	INR	8.2	(Target 2–3)
Ur	14 mmol/L	(3–7 mmol/L)	Glucose	26 mmol/L	
Cr	274 µmol/L	(60–125 µmol/L)			

A: Select the *two* prescriptions that are most likely to be contributing to the indigestion. Mark with ticks in column A.

B: Select the *one* prescription most likely to be contributing to the hyperglycaemia. Mark with a tick in column B.

C: Select the *one* prescription most likely to be contributing to the acute deterioration in the coagulation profile. Mark with a tick in column C.

CURRENT PRESCRIPTIONS

Drug name	Dose	Route	Freq.	A	B	C
PARACETAMOL	1 G	ORAL	6-HOURLY	☐	☐	☐
NAPROXEN	500 MG	ORAL	12-HOURLY	☑	☐	☐
WARFARIN	2 MG	ORAL	DAILY	☐	☐	☐
PREDNISOLONE	30 MG	ORAL	DAILY	☑	☑	☐
RAMIPRIL	2.5 MG	ORAL	NIGHTLY	☐	☐	☐
ALLOPURINOL	100 MG	ORAL	DAILY	☐	☐	☐
ERYTHROMYCIN	500 MG	ORAL	6-HOURLY	☐	☐	☑

Question 10.7 Prescription review item worth 4 marks

CASE PRESENTATION

A 72-year-old attends preoperative assessment clinic before elective inguinal hernia repair which is scheduled for 2 weeks' time. His medical history includes hypertension, polymyalgia rheumatica, bipolar disorder and gout. His respiratory examination is normal, and he has no murmurs. His BP is 103/62 mmHg and HR 92/min. He feels very well with no postural dizziness.

Question: Please identify which *four* drugs you will amend (increase, supplement, withhold or stop) before his surgery and mark with ticks in column A.

CURRENT PRESCRIPTIONS

Drug name	Dose	Route	Freq.	A
ALLOPURINOL	100 MG	ORAL	DAILY	☐
BENDROFLUMETHIAZIDE	5 MG	ORAL	DAILY	☑
LITHIUM CARBONATE MR	600 MG	ORAL	12-HOURLY	☑
ASPIRIN	75 MG	ORAL	DAILY	☑
BISOPROLOL	5 MG	ORAL	DAILY	☐
PREDNISOLONE	5 MG	ORAL	DAILY	☑
PARACETAMOL	1 G	ORAL	6-HOURLY	☐
LANSOPRAZOLE	30 MG	ORAL	DAILY	☐

Question 10.8 Prescription review item worth 4 marks

CASE PRESENTATION

You are performing medicines reconciliation with a pharmacist for all new inpatients. A 28-year-old woman has been admitted with deep vein thrombosis and is being treated with enoxaparin (LMW heparin). Beyond migraine (with aura), she has no medical history. The patient has not passed urine since she was admitted over 24 hours ago. On examination she has no palpable bladder or hydronephrosis. She weighs 60 kg. You request some routine blood tests and your registrar asks you to review the drug chart while the results are pending.

Question: Please identify the *four* drugs that should be withheld or amended with ticks in column A.

CURRENT PRESCRIPTIONS

Drug name	Dose	Route	Freq.	A
ENOXAPARIN	40 MG	S/C	DAILY	☐
PARACETAMOL	1 MG	ORAL	6-HOURLY	☑
YASMIN®	1 TABLET	ORAL	DAILY	☑
IBUPROFEN	200 MG	ORAL	8-HOURLY	☑
PROPRANOLOL	40 MG	ORAL	12-HOURLY	☐
CYCLIZINE	50 MG	ORAL	AS REQUIRED UP TO 8-HOURLY	☑

Question 10.9 Data interpretation item worth 2 marks

CASE PRESENTATION

A 42-year-old woman with bipolar disorder is admitted with increasing lethargy, an episode of palpitations and her first-ever seizure. Her mood has achieved excellent control with lithium, and she has had no recent dose changes. She has recently started bendroflumethiazide and lisinopril for hypertension.

HR 90 b.p.m. BP 112/72 mmHg. SaO$_2$ 100% (on air). RR 16/min.

	Value	Normal range		Value	Normal range
WCC	7 × 10^9/L	(4–11 × 10^9/L)	Ur	6 mmol/L	(3–7 mmol/L)
Neut.	5 × 10^9/L	(2–8 × 10^9/L)	Cr	142 µmol/L ↑	(60–125 µmol/L)
Lymph.	1.3 × 10^9/L	(1–4.8 × 10^9/L)	Na	139 mmol/L	(135–145 mmol/L)
Hb	123 g/L	(120–150 g/L (female))	K	4.5 mmol/L	(3.5–5.0 mmol/L)
MCV	82 fL	(76–99 fL)	Li	2.3 mmol/L ↑	(0.4–0.8 mmol/L)

Your registrar has inserted a central line and is arranging dialysis. She asks you to prescribe routine medications.

Question: Select the *most appropriate* acute treatment option and mark it with a tick.

DECISION OPTIONS

A	REDUCE LITHIUM	☐
B	STOP LITHIUM	☐
C	REDUCE LITHIUM, STOP BENDROFLUMETHIAZIDE	☑
D	STOP LITHIUM, STOP BENDROFLUMETHIAZIDE	☐
E	STOP LITHIUM, STOP BENDROFLUMETHIAZIDE, STOP LISINOPRIL	☐

Question 10.10 Data interpretation item worth 2 marks

CASE PRESENTATION

A 29-year-old with hypothyroidism due to Hashimoto's thyroiditis attends your surgery for her most recent thyroid function test results. These were pre-empted by increasing anxiety, difficulty sleeping and loose stools. A stool culture was negative. Current medications are as follows:

LORAZEPAM 500 MICROGRAMS SUBLINGUAL AS REQUIRED
LOPERAMIDE 8 MG ORAL 12-HOURLY
LEVOTHYROXINE 200 MICROGRAMS ORAL DAILY

	Value	Normal range		Value	Normal range
WCC	6×10^9/L	(4–11×10^9/L)	Ur	6 mmol/L	(3–7 mmol/L)
Neut.	5×10^9/L	(2–8×10^9/L)	Cr	72 µmol/L	(60–125 µmol/L)
Lymph.	1.3×10^9/L	(1–4.8×10^9/L)	Na	139 mmol/L	(135–145 mmol/L)
Hb	130 g/L	(120–150 g/L (female))	K	4.5 mmol/L	(3.5–5.0 mmol/L)
MCV	88 fL	(76–99 fL)	TSH	0.2 µIU/L	(0.5–5.0 µIU/L)
			CRP	6 mg/L	(<10 mg/L)

Your colleague, who requested the blood tests, has forgotten to request a T4 level, but the patient is going on holiday tomorrow and requests treatment before the results are available.

Question: Select the *most appropriate* treatment option and mark it with a tick.

DECISION OPTIONS

A	INCREASE LOPERAMIDE	☐
B	INCREASE LEVOTHYROXINE TO 250 MICROGRAMS DAILY	☐
C	INCREASE LEVOTHYROXINE TO 300 MICROGRAMS DAILY	☐
D	DECREASE LEVOTHYROXINE TO 150 MICROGRAMS DAILY	☑
E	DECREASE LEVOTHYROXINE TO 100 MICROGRAMS DAILY	☐

Question 10.11 Data interpretation item worth 2 marks

CASE PRESENTATION

A 65-year-old patient with no medical history except arthritis was admitted 4 days ago with acute renal failure due to ibuprofen taken for his arthritis. The ibuprofen has since been stopped. He was catheterised and given aggressive IV fluid therapy for 3 days and his blood results improved (see below). He is starting to tolerate a little oral intake (about 500 mL over the last 24 hours).

	On admission	Yesterday	Normal range		On admission	Yesterday	Normal range
Na	138 mmol/L	145 mmol/L	(135–145 mmol/L)	Ur	23 mmol/L	2.0 mmol/L	(3–7 mmol/L)
K	6.2 mmol/L	3.3 mmol/L	(3.5–5.0 mmol/L)	Cr	792 µmol/L	142 µmol/L	(60–125 µmol/L)

His total fluid balance since admission is shown below:

	Input	Output	Balance		Input	Output	Balance
Day 1	6 L	1 L	5 L positive	Day 3	4 L	4 L	0
Day 2	5 L	3 L	2 L positive	Today	3 L	6 L	3 L negative

The nurses have spotted his improving blood results and (just before midnight) ask you if they can stop IV fluids and encourage oral intake alone.

Question: Select the *most appropriate* treatment option and mark it with a tick.

DECISION OPTIONS

A	ENCOURAGE ORAL FLUIDS	☐
B	GIVE 1 L 0.9% SALINE WITH 20 MMOL KCL OVER 12 HOURS	☐
C	GIVE 1 L 5% DEXTROSE WITH 20 MMOL KCL OVER 12 HOURS	☐
D	GIVE 1 L 5% DEXTROSE WITH 20 MMOL KCL OVER 4 HOURS	☐
E	GIVE 1 L 5% DEXTROSE WITH 40 MMOL KCL OVER 1 HOURS	☐

Question 10.12 Data interpretation item worth 2 marks

CASE PRESENTATION

A 49-year-old has been on regular phenytoin monotherapy for epilepsy. He attends your epilepsy clinic reporting two seizures in the last 12 months. His previous meningioma (which was excised 3 years ago) has shown no sign of recurrence but he has been left with a chronically low sodium level (usually 124–126 mmol/L) from SIADH which he controls by fluid restriction without sequelae.

His current medications are:

PARACETAMOL 1 G UP TO 6-HOURLY AS REQUIRED

PHENYTOIN 150 MG ORAL DAILY

You send for some routine blood tests:

	Value	Normal range		Value	Normal range
WCC	8×10^9/L	(4–11×10^9/L)	Ur	5 mmol/L	(3–7 mmol/L)
Neut.	7×10^9/L	(2–8×10^9/L)	Cr	87 µmol/L	(60–125 µmol/L)
Lymph.	1.0×10^9/L	(1–4.8×10^9/L)	Na	124 mmol/L	(135–145 mmol/L)
Hb	138 g/L	(135–175 g/L (male))	K	4.1 mmol/L	(3.5–5.0 mmol/L)
MCV	91 fL	(76–99 fL)	CRP	5 mg/L	(<5 mg/L)
Phenytoin	22 µmol/L	(40–80 µmol/L)			

Urinalysis: normal

Question: Select the *most appropriate* treatment option and mark it with a tick.

DECISION OPTIONS

A	INCREASE PHENYTOIN TO 175 MG ORAL DAILY	☐
B	INCREASE PHENYTOIN TO 200 MG ORAL DAILY	☐
C	STOP PHENYTOIN AND START CARBAMAZEPINE	☐
D	CONTINUE PHENYTOIN 150 MG DAILY AND START CARBAMAZEPINE	☐
E	DECREASE PHENYTOIN TO 125 MG ORAL DAILY	☐

Question 10.13 Data interpretation item worth 2 marks

CASE PRESENTATION

An obese 43-year-old is admitted for elective cholecystectomy, following a previous episode of cholecystitis. She is first on the theatre list tomorrow. It is midnight and the nurses call you to prescribe fluids because she is nil by mouth from midnight. She has not had routine biochemistry performed and previous results are not available to you.

Question: Select the *most appropriate* option and mark it with a tick.

DECISION OPTIONS

A	1 L 0.9% SALINE WITH 20 MMOL KCL OVER 12 HOURS	☐
B	1 L 0.9% SALINE WITH 20 MMOL KCL OVER 8 HOURS	☐
C	1 L 5% DEXTROSE WITH 20 MMOL KCL OVER 24 HOURS	☐
D	1 L 5% DEXTROSE WITH 40 MMOL KCL OVER 12 HOURS	☐
E	1 L 5% DEXTROSE WITH 40 MMOL KCL OVER 6 HOURS	☐

Question 10.14 Data interpretation item worth 2 marks

CASE PRESENTATION

A 32-year-old woman has been resident on the secure psychiatry ward following postnatal psychosis. She is clinically improving and required no drugs for over a week prior to discharge; the consultant wants routine bloods performed.

	Last week	Today	Normal range
Na	138 mmol/L	141 mmol/L	(135–145 mmol/L)
K	4.2 mmol/L	7.1 mmol/L	(3.5–5.0 mmol/L)
Ur	6 mmol/L	5.6 mmol/L	(3–7 mmol/L)
Cr	58 µmol/L	55 µmol/L	(60–125 µmol/L)

Her observations (including heart rate and lying–standing BP) are normal, as are the ECG and blood glucose. The consultant psychiatrist is very worried about the results—he asks you to sort this and keep him informed.

Question: Select the *most appropriate* option and mark it with a tick.

DECISION OPTIONS

A	1 L 0.9% SALINE WITH 20 MMOL KCL OVER 12 HOURS	☐
B	10 ML 10% IV CALCIUM GLUCONATE	☐
C	10 ML 10% IV CALCIUM GLUCONATE AND 10 UNITS ACTRAPID® INSULIN WITH 100 ML 20% IV DEXTROSE	☐
D	10 ML 10% IV CALCIUM GLUCONATE AND 10 UNITS ACTRAPID® INSULIN WITH 100 ML 20% IV DEXTROSE AND NEBULIZED SALBUTAMOL	☐
E	REPEAT BIOCHEMISTRY	☐

Question 10.15 Planning management item worth 2 marks

CASE PRESENTATION

You are called urgently to see a 30-year-old female who has become acutely breathless during her first infusion of IV co-amoxiclav for pyelonephritis. She has no other past medical history.

She is breathless at rest with a respiratory rate of 30/min. Blood pressure is 160/70 mmHg, heart rate 120/min. She is alert and able to converse in partial sentences. You note a diffuse urticarial rash over her entire body and widespread expiratory polyphonic wheeze on auscultating her lungs.

Question: Select the one *most appropriate* management option at this stage and mark it with a tick.

DECISION OPTIONS

A	CHANGE CO-AMOXICLAV TO MEROPENEM	☐
B	15 L/MINUTE OXYGEN VIA NON-REBREATHER MASK	☐
C	CHLORPHENAMINE 4 MG ORAL	☐
D	500 ML 0.9% SALINE IV OVER 30 MINUTES	☐
E	1 MG OF 1:10 000 ADRENALINE IM	☐

Question 10.16 Planning management item worth 2 marks

CASE PRESENTATION

An 80-year-old gentleman with chronic kidney disease (eGFR 26) presents to his GP for a well-person check. He has been found to have an elevated random blood sugar of 12 mmol/L.

He is seen by the dietician and commenced on a weight loss regimen and the GP organizes further blood tests two months later. They are as follows:

	Value	Normal range
Hb	145 g/L	(135–175 g/L (male))
Na	135 mmol/L	(135–145 mmol/L)
K	4.5 mmol/L	(3.5–5.0 mmol/L)
Ur	15 mmol/L	(3–7 mmol/L)
Cr	200 μmol/L	(60–125 μmol/L)
Fasting glucose	8 mmol/L	
HbA1c	52 mmol/mol	(<48 mmol/mol)

Question: Select the *most appropriate* management option at this stage and mark it with a tick.

DECISION OPTIONS

A	REVIEW BY DIETICIAN AND WEIGHT LOSS REGIMEN	☐
B	METFORMIN 500 MG ORAL TWICE DAILY	☐
C	GLICLAZIDE 40 MG ORAL ONCE DAILY	☐
D	MIXTARD 30® INSULIN (30% SOLUBLE AND 70% ISOPHANE) S/C TWICE DAILY	☐
E	LONG ACTING INSULIN (GLARGINE) S/C ONCE DAILY	☐

Question 10.17 Planning management item worth 2 marks

CASE PRESENTATION

A 65-year-old man presents to his GP with ongoing lower back pain that he has endured for many years, but he has now 'had enough' and wants it gone. He has no other medical history but reports indigestion, constipation and low mood on systems review. His neurological examination is unremarkable and MRI scans of his whole spine show degenerative change only with no evidence of cord or nerve root compression.

He is currently prescribed regular paracetamol 1 g 4 times daily and atorvastatin 10 mg daily. He describes ongoing back pain.

Question: Select the one *most appropriate* management option at this stage and mark it with a tick.

DECISION OPTIONS

A	ADD AMITRIPTYLINE 100 MG ORAL NIGHTLY	☐
B	STOP PARACETAMOL AND START CO-CODAMOL (8/500) TWO TABLETS 4-HOURLY	☐
C	ADD CODEINE 30 MG 4 TIMES DAILY WITH AS-REQUIRED MORPHINE SULPHATE (ORAMORPH® 10 MG/5 ML)	☐
D	ADD NAPROXEN 500 MG ORAL 8-HOURLY	☐
E	TENS	☐

Question 10.18 Planning management item worth 2 marks

CASE PRESENTATION

A 63-year-old female is admitted to the surgical ward with a distended abdomen, bilious vomiting and absolute constipation for 24 h. Her only significant past medical history is a left hemicolectomy for a Dukes' B colonic cancer some 12 months ago.

On clinical examination her abdomen is distended and tender in the left iliac fossa with no obvious guarding or rebound. Bowel sounds are tinkling. Rectal examination reveals an empty rectum. Abdominal X-ray reveals multiple loops of dilated small bowel with no free air. She is vomiting large volumes of bilious vomitus and feels constantly nauseated. She is otherwise clinically stable.

Question: Select the *most appropriate* management option whilst awaiting CT scan and mark it with a tick.

	DECISION OPTIONS	
A	METOCLOPRAMIDE 10 MG IV	☐
B	HALOPERIDOL 500 MICROGRAMS S/C	☐
C	CYCLIZINE 50 MG ORALLY	☐
D	LARGE BORE NASOGASTRIC TUBE	☑
E	ONDANSETRON 4 MG ORALLY	☐

Question 10.19 Planning management item worth 2 marks

CASE PRESENTATION

A 75-year-old gentleman is admitted to A&E with worsening breathlessness and wheeze. He was recently an inpatient requiring non-invasive ventilation (NIV) for an exacerbation of COPD.

On examination he is short of breath at rest but able to talk in partial sentences. He has a diffuse expiratory polyphonic wheeze on auscultation but no other abnormal clinical findings. SaO$_2$ 82% on air, respiratory rate 20/min. Chest X-ray shows hyperinflated lungs but no focal consolidation. A nurse has set up a salbutamol nebulizer and hands you the following ABG results:

	Value	Normal range
pH	7.30	(7.35–7.45)
PaO$_2$	8.9 kPa	(10.5–13.5 kPa)
PaCO$_2$	6.9 kPa	(4.5–6.0 kPa)
HCO$_3$	25 mEq/L	(22–26 mEq/L)

Question: Select the *most appropriate* management option at this stage and mark it with a tick.

	DECISION OPTIONS	
A	IPRATROPIUM BROMIDE 500 MICROGRAMS NEB	☐
B	PREDNISOLONE 30 MG ORALLY	☐
C	INTENSIVE CARE REVIEW FOR CONSIDERATION OF CONTINUOUS POSITIVE AIRWAYS PRESSURE (CPAP) NIV	☐
D	OXYGEN (60%) VIA VENTURI MASK	☐
E	IV AMINOPHYLLINE INFUSION	☐

Question 10.20 Planning management item worth 2 marks

CASE PRESENTATION

A 52-year-old obese female is admitted with severe epigastric tenderness. She has a history of gallstones.

On examination her abdomen is soft with severe epigastric tenderness and localised rebound tenderness. Bowel sounds are present but scanty. Clinically she is dehydrated with dry mucous membranes. Having been catheterized her urine output has been on average 20 mL per hour. Normal saline (500 mL) was given in A&E when she was found to be hypotensive (83/62 mmHg) with good response in blood pressure.

Her blood pressure is now 78/70 mmHg with heart rate of 120/min.

Initial blood tests show:

	Value	Normal range
Na	135 mmol/L	(135–145 mmol/L)
K	4.5 mmol/L	(3.5–5.0 mmol/L)
Ur	15 mmol/L	(3–7 mmol/L)
Cr	100 µmol/L	(60–125 µmol/L)
Amylase	2000 U/L	(<120 U/L)

Question: Select the *most appropriate* management option at this stage and mark it with a tick.

DECISION OPTIONS

A	1 L 5% DEXTROSE IV OVER 4 HOURS	☐
B	1 L 0.9% SALINE IV OVER 4 HOURS	☐
C	500 ML 5% HUMAN ALBUMIN SOLUTION IV OVER 30 MINUTES	☐
D	FLUID CHALLENGE OF 500 ML GELOFUSINE IV OVER 30 MINUTES	☐
E	1 L 0.9% SALINE IV OVER 12 HOURS	☐

Question 10.21 Planning management item worth 2 marks

CASE PRESENTATION

You are asked to see a 50-year-old gentleman in A&E with a known nut allergy. He has been out for dinner, following which he has developed widespread urticaria and swollen lips and hands. The paramedic has already administered 500 micrograms (1:1000) adrenaline IM and put him on high-flow oxygen.

He is comfortable at rest and is starting to feel better. His chest is clear with saturations of 100% on high-flow oxygen and a respiratory rate of 15/min. Blood pressure is 140/70 mmHg and heart rate is 120/min. His face remains swollen as do his hands and he has widespread uriticaria.

Question: Select the one *most appropriate* management option at this stage and mark it with a tick.

DECISION OPTIONS

A	HYDROCORTISONE 200 G IM STAT.	☐
B	SALBUTAMOL 5 MG NEB STAT.	☐
C	1 L 0.9% SALINE IV OVER 12 HOURS	☐
D	CHLORPHENAMINE 10 MG IV STAT.	☐
E	ADRENALINE 500 MICROGRAMS OF 1:1000 IM	☐

Question 10.22 Planning management item worth 2 marks

CASE PRESENTATION

A 90-year-old man is admitted to A&E with acute shortness of breath on waking up this morning.
His JVP is raised to 5 cm with coarse bilateral inspiratory crepitations to both mid-zones and peripheral oedema to both knees. Oxygen saturations are 80% on room air with a respiratory rate of 20/min. Blood pressure is 170/90 mmHg. Chest X-ray reveals bilateral interstitial shadowing, upper lobe diversion and cardiomegaly.

Question: Select the *most appropriate* management option at this stage and mark it with a tick.

DECISION OPTIONS

A	FUROSEMIDE 80 MG IV STAT.	☐
B	REFERRAL FOR NONINVASIVE VENTILATION (NIV)	☐
C	SPIRONOLACTONE 25 MG ORAL STAT.	☐
D	CO-AMOXICLAV 1.2 G IV 8-HOURLY	☐
E	BENDROFLUMETHIAZIDE 2.5 MG ORAL STAT.	☐

Question 10.23 Communicating information item worth 2 marks

CASE PRESENTATION

A 60-year-old female with type 2 diabetes mellitus, hypertension and heavy proteinuria is seen in her GP surgery. She is commenced on ramipril 2.5 mg once daily. You are asked to discuss this new medication with the patient.

Question: Select the *one* most appropriate piece of information to communicate to the patient and mark it with a tick.

DECISION OPTIONS

A	RISK OF HYPERKALAEMIA IS LOW WITH RAMIPRIL COMPARED TO OTHER ANTIHYPERTENSIVES	☐
B	COUGH IS A COMMON SIDE EFFECT WITH ACE-INHIBITORS AND TRIAL OF AN ANGIOTENSIN RECEPTOR BLOCKER INSTEAD IS INDICATED IF COUGH DEVELOPS	☐
C	NO PRECAUTIONS NEED TO BE TAKEN IF THE PATIENT DEVELOPS DIARRHOEA OR VOMITING	☐
D	ANGIO-OEDEMA ASSOCIATED WITH ACE-INHIBITORS ALWAYS OCCURS IN THE FIRST 24 HOURS	☐
E	REPEAT BLOOD TESTS LOOKING AT RENAL FUNCTION AND ELECTROLYTES 6 MONTHS AFTER INITIATION ARE ESSENTIAL	☐

Question 10.24 Communicating information item worth 2 marks

CASE PRESENTATION

A 19-year-old girl is admitted to hospital with a first presentation of diabetic ketoacidosis and is diagnosed with type 1 diabetes mellitus. She is converted from an insulin sliding scale to a basal–bolus regimen. You are asked to discuss insulin therapy with the patient.

Question: Select the *one* most appropriate piece of information to communicate to the patient and mark it with a tick.

DECISION OPTIONS

A	WHEN UNWELL THE PATIENT'S TOTAL DAILY INSULIN DOSAGE SHOULD BE DECREASED	☐
B	HYPOGLYCAEMIA SHOULD BE TREATED WITH A BOTTLE OF WATER	☐
C	LIPODYSTROPHY IS CAUSED BY REPEATED USE OF THE SAME INJECTION SITES	☐
D	HBA1C IS A SUITABLE WAY TO MONITOR BLOOD SUGARS FROM DAY TO DAY	☐
E	EXCESSIVE ALCOHOL INTAKE CAN CAUSE HYPERGLYCAEMIA	☐

Question 10.25 Communicating information item worth 2 marks

CASE PRESENTATION

A 25-year-old male is seen in the gastroenterology clinic for ongoing follow-up of his ulcerative colitis for which he takes mesalazine. Over the last week he has complained of increasing stool frequency (3–4 times per day with occasional blood and mucus). It is felt he is having a mild flare of his colitis and is commenced on oral prednisolone 30 mg once daily and prednisolone enemas. You are asked to discuss steroid treatment with him.

Question: Select the *one* most appropriate piece of information to communicate to the patient and mark it with a tick.

DECISION OPTIONS

A	PROLONGED COURSES OF STEROIDS SHOULD NEVER BE STOPPED SUDDENLY	☐
B	STEROIDS REDUCE THE RISK OF OSTEOPOROSIS	☐
C	RISK OF GASTRIC/DUODENAL ULCERS IS LOWER WHEN ON STEROID THERAPY	☐
D	STEROIDS DO NOT INCREASE THE RISK OF DIABETES MELLITUS	☐
E	PATIENTS ARE AT RISK OF HYPOTENSION WITH STEROID THERAPY	☐

Question 10.26 Communicating information item worth 2 marks

CASE PRESENTATION

A 50-year-old woman is seen at the rheumatology clinic with known giant cell arteritis. She is currently on a reducing regimen of prednisolone and is commenced on methotrexate. You are asked to discuss this medication with her.

Question: Select the *one* most appropriate piece of information to communicate to the patient and mark it with a tick.

DECISION OPTIONS

A	ONCE ON A STABLE DOSE, BLOOD TESTS ARE NOT REQUIRED	☐
B	METHOTREXATE SHOULD BE TAKEN DAILY	☐
C	METHOTREXATE IS SAFE TO USE IN PREGNANCY	☐
D	THERE IS NO ASSOCIATION BETWEEN METHOTREXATE AND PULMONARY FIBROSIS	☐
E	TRIMETHOPRIM SHOULD NOT BE USED FOR TREATMENT OF INFECTION	☐

Question 10.27 Communicating information item worth 2 marks

CASE PRESENTATION

A 75-year-old gentleman is admitted with left-sided upper limb weakness for 2 hours that then completely resolves. He is seen by the stroke team who diagnose a transient ischaemic attack and suggest simvastatin 40 mg, amongst other medication, for secondary prevention. You are asked to discuss this with him.

Question: Select the *one* most appropriate piece of information to communicate to the patient and mark it with a tick.

DECISION OPTIONS

A	WHEN TAKING CLARITHROMYCIN THE STATINS SHOULD BE STOPPED	☐
B	STATINS ARE MOST EFFECTIVE WHEN TAKEN IN THE MORNING	☐
C	IF MUSCLE CRAMPS DEVELOP THE DOSE SHOULD BE INCREASED	☐
D	STATINS ARE SAFE TO USE IN ACTIVE LIVER DISEASE	☐
E	THERE ARE NO DIETARY RESTRICTIONS WITH STATIN THERAPY	☐

Question 10.28 Communicating information item worth 2 marks

CASE PRESENTATION

A 60-year-old female with type 2 diabetes mellitus, hypertension and heavy proteinuria is seen in her GP surgery. She is commenced on ramipril 2.5 mg once daily. You are asked to discuss this new medication with the patient.

Question: Select the *one* most appropriate piece of information to communicate to the patient and mark it with a tick.

DECISION OPTIONS

A	RISK OF HYPERKALAEMIA IS LOW WITH RAMIPRIL COMPARED TO OTHER ANTIHYPERTENSIVES	☐
B	DRY COUGH IS A COMMON SIDE EFFECT WITH ACE-INHIBITORS AND WARRANTS TRIAL OF AN ANGIOTENSIN RECEPTOR BLOCKER INSTEAD	☐
C	NO PRECAUTIONS NEED TO BE TAKEN IF THE PATIENT DEVELOPS DIARRHOEA OR VOMITING	☐
D	ANGIO-OEDEMA ASSOCIATED WITH ACE-INHIBITORS ALWAYS OCCURS IN THE FIRST 24 HOURS	☐
E	REPEAT BLOOD TESTS LOOKING AT RENAL FUNCTION AND ELECTROLYTES 6 MONTHS AFTER INITIATION ARE ESSENTIAL	☐

> You may use a calculator at any time

Question 10.29 Calculation skills item worth 2 marks

CASE PRESENTATION

A patient is prescribed 187.5 micrograms of digoxin daily for the treatment of atrial fibrillation (AF).

Calculation: Using your knowledge of the available tablet strengths (you may refer to the BNF), how will you administer this dose? Write your answer in the box.

Answer

> You may use a calculator at any time

Question 10.30 Calculation skills item worth 2 marks

CASE PRESENTATION

You are asked by your registrar to prescribe an IV infusion of magnesium sulphate for the treatment of an arrhythmia in a 67-year-old patient. The recommended dose is 8 mmol. Magnesium sulphate is available in 10 mL ampoules, which contain 5 g (20 mmol) of magnesium sulphate.

Calculation: What volume of solution do you need to give? Write your answer in the box.

Answer

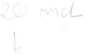

You may use a
calculator at any time

Question 10.31 Calculation skills item worth 2 marks

CASE PRESENTATION

Regarding the previous scenario, the hospital protocol states that magnesium sulphate should not be administered at a concentration exceeding 200 mg/mL.

Calculation: What is the minimum volume of diluent that would give a 200 mg/mL solution for administration to your patient? Write your answer in the box.

Answer

You may use a
calculator at any time

Question 10.32 Calculation skills item worth 2 marks

CASE PRESENTATION

Regarding the same scenario, the hospital protocol states that magnesium sulphate should not be administered at a rate exceeding 150 mg/min.

Calculation: To the nearest minute, what is the minimum infusion time for a dose of 8 mmol? Write your answer in the box.

Answer

You may use a
calculator at any time

Question 10.33 Calculation skills item worth 2 marks

CASE PRESENTATION

A 68-year-old patient presents to A&E complaining of urinary frequency, loin pain and a fever. Her urine dipstick is positive for leukocytes, blood and nitrites. She tells you that she takes regular immunosuppression for rheumatoid arthritis including 5 mg prednisolone daily as one tablet and a weekly dose of methotrexate. You admit her for management of severe sepsis.

Calculation: How many of her current prednisolone tablets should she take daily during her inpatient stay. Write your answer in the box.

Answer

Question 10.34 Calculation skills item worth 2 marks

CASE PRESENTATION

A 60-year-old woman in ITU has new-onset atrial fibrillation with mild signs of heart failure following major abdominal surgery. You decide to give a dose of 300 mg amiodarone. You ask the nurse to give this over 1 hour diluted in 250 mL of glucose 5%.

Calculation: What rate does this infusion (mL/min) run at? Write your answer in the box.

Answer

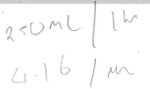

250 mL / 1 hr

4.16 / m

Question 10.35 Calculation skills item worth 2 marks

CASE PRESENTATION

You are asked by the medical registrar to switch a patient's antibiotic regimen to meropenem, following microbiology advice. The BNF indicates a daily dose of 2 g in four divided doses.

Calculation: What dose of IV meropenem should you prescribe, and at what rate? Write your answer in the box.

Answer 500 mg every ___6___ hours

Question 10.36 Calculation skills item worth 2 marks

CASE PRESENTATION

A 19-year-old woman presents to A&E during a holiday on the coast. She has an allergy to wasp stings and has been stung on the beach. She is now clinically stable in A&E and you are asked by the consultant to give her 10 mg chlorphenamine intravenously. It is only available as a 1% solution in 1 mL vials.

Calculation: What volume should be administered intravenously? Write your answer in the box.

Answer

Question 10.37 Prescribing item worth 10 marks

CASE PRESENTATION

A 52-year-old patient is recovering from a knee replacement in hospital and complains of indigestion since the operation. He is currently taking paracetamol, ibuprofen and codeine. He denies weight loss, anorexia or melaena.
After surgery an alginate-containing dressing was applied to his knee, but quickly removed because it produced an allergic rash.
Examination is unremarkable including a digital rectal examination.
His haemoglobin is 146 g/L.
You stop his ibuprofen but he says he wants something to give immediate relief.

Prescribing request: Write a prescription to provide immediate relief of dyspepsia. *(Use the 'once only' prescription chart provided.)*

ONCE ONLY MEDICINES

Date	Time	Medicine (approved name)	Dose	Route	Prescriber – sign + print	Time given	Given by
23.01.14	20.30	OMEPRAZOLE	20 mg	PO			

Question 10.38 Prescribing item worth 10 marks

CASE PRESENTATION

A 73-year-old male is admitted with pneumonia.

PAST MEDICAL HISTORY

Deep vein thrombosis 2 years ago (and finished warfarin 18 months ago) and diabetes. He is treated with IV antibiotics and requires 60% oxygen.
On examination he has right basal coarse crepitations. You are unable to palpate dorsalis pedis nor posterior tibialis pulses bilaterally, but the foot is warm and he denies pain. There is no evidence of acute limb ischaemia.
Your registrar spots that he has not been prescribed thromboprophylaxis.

Prescribing request: Write a prescription for ONE method of thromboprophylaxis. *(Use the hospital 'regular medicines' prescription chart provided.)*

REGULAR MEDICATION		Date					
		Time					
Drug (Approved name)		6					
		8					
Dose	Route	12					
Prescriber – sign + print	Start date	14					
		18					
Notes	Frequency	22					

Question 10.39 Prescribing item worth 10 marks

CASE PRESENTATION

A 43-year-old woman with a history of rheumatoid arthritis and hypertension is seen in A&E minors complaining of dysuria and urinary frequency. She has a mild fever but otherwise normal observations and no renal angle tenderness. She is allergic to penicillin.

Her current medications are as follows:

LISINOPRIL 10 MG ORAL DAILY
METHOTREXATE 15 MG ORAL WEEKLY
FOLIC ACID 5 MG ORAL WEEKLY

Her urinalysis is as follows:

Protein	++
Leucocytes	+++
Blood	++
Nitrite	+

Her blood tests show neutrophilia and raised CRP. You inform her that she has a urinary tract infection and can go home with antibiotics.

Prescribing request: Write a prescription for ONE drug to treat the cause of her symptoms. *(Use the hospital antibiotic prescription chart provided.)*

ANTIBIOTIC			Date						
			Time						
Drug (Approved name)			**6**						
			8						
Dose	Frequency	Route	**12**						
Prescriber – sign + print		Start date	**14**						
			18						
Indication		Review/stop date	**22**						

Question 10.40 Prescribing item worth 10 marks

CASE PRESENTATION

A 27-year-old is admitted for investigation of episodes of dizziness. Her PMH includes asthma only. She is pain free but reports occasional headaches. Your consultant asks you to prescribe appropriate analgesia to prevent the on-call doctor being called to do it should a headache begin.
She weighs 63 kg.

Prescribing request: Write a prescription for ONE drug for analgesia. *(Choose between the hospital 'regular medicines' or 'as required' prescription charts provided.)*

REGULAR MEDICATION

Drug (Approved name)		Date							
		Time							
Drug (Approved name)		6							
		8							
Dose	Route	12							
Prescriber – sign + print	Start date	14							
		18							
Notes	Frequency	22							

AS REQUIRED MEDICATION

Drug (Approved name)							
Drug (Approved name) *(paracetamol)*		Date					
		Time					
Dose *1 g*	Route *PO*	Route					
Prescriber – sign + print	Start date	Given by					
Indication *Headache*	Frequency	Sign					

Question 10.41 Prescribing item worth 10 marks

CASE PRESENTATION

You are called to urgently review a 70-year-old male who has been an inpatient for 3 weeks after a large ischaemic stroke. He is nil by mouth and fed by a nasogastric tube due to an unsafe swallow. The nurses report that he has become increasingly dyspnoeic and febrile. He has no allergies but reports profuse diarrhoea following treatment with both cefotaxime and ciprofloxacin on a previous admission.

Temperature	38.4°C ↑
Heart rate	126 b.p.m. ↑
BP	83/52 mmHg ↓
Respiratory rate	36/min ↑
SaO$_2$	82% (on air) ↓

IV fluids are started by the critical care outreach nurse who has ordered a CXR.

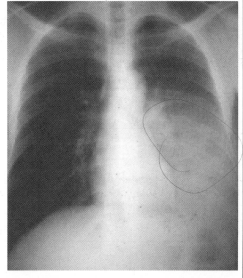

Prescribing request: Write a prescription for ONE drug to treat the cause of his symptoms. *(Use the hospital antibiotic prescription chart provided.)*

ANTIBIOTICS

			Date					
			Time					
Drug (Approved name)			**6**					
			8					
Dose	**Frequency**	**Route**	**12**					
Prescriber – sign + print		**Start date**	**14**					
			18					
Indication		**Review/stop date**	**22**					

Question 10.42 Prescribing item worth 10 marks

CASE PRESENTATION

One of your patients, a 68-year-old lady making a good recovery from hip surgery, requests a laxative as she has not opened her bowels for 4 days. She is now mobilizing, but you attribute her constipation to recent immobility. She reports feeling slightly bloated but denies cramps. An abdominal X-ray reveals no evidence of obstruction and a digital rectal examination reveals fairly soft stool. She says she would prefer something by the oral route in the first instance.

Prescribing request: Write a prescription for ONE drug to treat the constipation. *(Use the hospital regular medication prescription chart provided.)*

REGULAR MEDICATION		Date							
		Time							
Drug (Approved name) SENNA		**6**							
		8							
Dose 7.5 Mg	Route PO	**12**							
Prescriber – sign + print	Start date	**14**							
		18							
Notes	Frequency	**22**							

Question 10.43 Prescribing item worth 10 marks

CASE PRESENTATION

A 42-year-old complains of constant pain following a knee replacement. He has no other medical history. His current medication is listed below:

PARACETAMOL   1 G ORAL 6-HOURLY REGULARLY
IBUPROFEN   400 MG ORAL 6-HOURLY REGULARLY

Prescribing request: Write a prescription for ONE additional drug for analgesia. *(Choose between the hospital 'regular medicines' or 'as required' prescription charts provided.)*

REGULAR MEDICATION		Date							
		Time							
Drug (Approved name) CODEINE PHOSPHATE		**6**							
		8							
Dose 30 mg	Route PO	**12**							
Prescriber – sign + print	Start date	**14**							
		18							
Notes	Frequency 4 hrs	**22**							

AS REQUIRED MEDICATION								
Drug (Approved name)		Date						
		Time						
Dose	Route	Route						
Prescriber – sign + print	Start date	Given by						
Indication	Frequency	Sign						

Question 10.44 Prescribing item worth 10 marks

CASE PRESENTATION

A 36-year-old woman complains of occasional abdominal pain. She is on antibiotics and IV fluid for cholecystitis. Except for a peptic ulcer, she has no other medical history; beyond the pain, she is making a good recovery. Her current medication is listed below:

PARACETAMOL   1G ORAL 6-HOURLY REGULARLY
CO-AMOXICLAV 1.2 G IV 8-HOURLY

no NSAIDS

She reports no allergies.

Prescribing request: Write a prescription for ONE additional drug for analgesia. *(Choose between the hospital 'regular medicines' or 'as required' prescription charts provided.)*

REGULAR MEDICATION

		Date					
		Time					
Drug (Approved name)		6					
		8					
Dose	Route	12					
Prescriber – sign + print	Start date	14					
		18					
Notes	Frequency	22					

AS REQUIRED MEDICATION

Drug (Approved name) *CODEINE PHOSPHATE*		Date					
		Time					
Dose *30 mg*	Route *PO*	Route					
Prescriber – sign + print	Start date *23·01·16*	Given by					
Indication *Pain PO*	Frequency *6hrly*	Sign					

Question 10.45 Drug monitoring item worth 2 points

CASE PRESENTATION

An aminophylline infusion is commenced for a patient with severe asthma when nebulized medication and steroids prove inadequate.

Question: Which *one* option would be most beneficial in monitoring aminophylline's therapeutic effect? Mark it with a tick in the column provided.

	DECISION OPTIONS	
A	HEART RATE	☐
B	BLOOD PRESSURE	☐
C	OXYGEN SATURATION	☐
D	SERUM THEOPHYLLINE LEVEL	☐
E	GLASGOW COMA SCALE (GCS)	☐

Question 10.46 Drug monitoring item worth 2 points

CASE PRESENTATION

A 59-year-old female patient is admitted to the Emergency Admissions Unit with productive cough and fever. Clinically she has coarse left basal crepitations and associated dullness to percussion. Chest X-ray shows left lower lobe consolidation. She is commenced on IV piperacillin/tazobactam as per local protocol.

Question: Which *one* option would most adequately assess response to antibiotics whilst an inpatient?

	DECISION OPTIONS	
A	CHEST X-RAY	☐
B	RESPIRATORY RATE	☐
C	BLOOD PRESSURE	☐
D	RESOLUTION OF CREPITATIONS ON AUSCULTATION	☐
E	FLUID BALANCE	☐

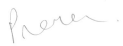

Question 10.47 Drug monitoring item worth 2 points

CASE PRESENTATION

A 41-year-old male patient is prescribed prednisolone and tacrolimus (Prograf®) after renal transplantation to prevent graft rejection.

Question: Which *one* of the following could you measure/monitor to ascertain whether the tacrolimus level is within the normal reference range?

	DECISION OPTIONS	
A	TACROLIMUS LEVEL ('PEAK' LEVEL 1 HOUR AFTER MORNING DOSE)	☐
B	SERUM ALT	☐
C	PRESENCE OF TREMOR	☐
D	TACROLIMUS LEVEL ('TROUGH' LEVEL PRIOR TO MORNING DOSE)	☐
E	PRESENCE OF GUM HYPERPLASIA	☐

Question 10.48 Drug monitoring item worth 2 points

CASE PRESENTATION

A 27-year-old male patient is commenced on fluoxetine for the treatment of depression. His GP asks him to make another appointment in 2 weeks' time to assess how he is getting on with the new prescription.

Question: Which *one* of the following would be the most appropriate for the GP to assess/monitor at his next appointment?

	DECISION OPTIONS	
A	BLOOD PRESSURE	☐
B	ASSESSMENT FOR SIGNS OF SUICIDAL IDEATION	☐
C	FULL BLOOD COUNT	☐
D	ASSESS FOR EFFICACY	☐
E	SERUM CREATININE	☐

Question 10.49 Drug monitoring item worth 2 points

CASE PRESENTATION

A 47-year-old female patient with type 1 diabetes mellitus is admitted to the A&E department with a 3-day history of productive cough and fever. A chest X-ray shows left lower lobe pneumonia. Blood results are as follows:

	Value	Normal range
Glucose	45 mmol/L	
pH	7.1	(7.35–7.45)
HCO_3-	12 mmol/L	(22–26 mmol/L)
Serum ketones	4.5 mmol/L	(0.05–0.29 mmol/L)

She is diagnosed with pneumonia and diabetic ketoacidosis, commenced on IV antibiotics and an insulin sliding scale and aggressively rehydrated. She is transferred to the high dependency unit. You are asked to review her overnight.

Question: Which *one* option would best suggest response to DKA treatment?

DECISION OPTIONS

A	SERUM GLUCOSE	☐
B	BLOOD PRESSURE	☐
C	URINARY GLUCOSE	☐
D	SERUM KETONES	☐
E	URINARY OUTPUT	☐

Question 10.50 Drug monitoring item worth 2 points

CASE PRESENTATION

An 85-year-old female patient is admitted to the emergency assessment unit with shortness of breath and a wheeze. She has smoked 20 cigarettes per day for 30 years but has never seen a doctor for her wheeze and dyspnoea. Chest X-ray shows hyperexpanded lung fields. Her saturations are 79% on air. Arterial blood gas (taken on air) is as follows:

	Value	Normal range
pH	7.4	(7.35–7.45)
PaO_2	7.2 kPa	(10.5–13.5 kPa)
$PaCO_2$	7.5 kPa	(4.5–6.0 kPa)
HCO_3-	35 mmol/L	(22–26 mmol/L)

She is commenced on oxygen via a venturi mask (35%).

Question: Which *one* option would be most helpful in monitoring her response to oxygen therapy?

DECISION OPTIONS

A	GLASGOW COMA SCALE (GCS)	☐
B	RESPIRATORY RATE	☐
C	BLOOD PRESSURE	☐
D	PULSE OXIMETRY	☐
E	VENOUS BLOOD GAS (VBG)	☐

Question 10.51 Drug monitoring item worth 2 points

CASE PRESENTATION

A 46-year-old Caucasian male with diabetes is diagnosed with stage 1 hypertension. A decision is made to start him on ramipril and to up-titrate the dose gradually to achieve a target blood pressure below 140/90 mmHg.

Question: Before prescribing ramipril, which *one* of the following parameters would be the most important for you to check in primary care?

	DECISION OPTIONS	
A	SERUM ALT	☐
B	SERUM CREATININE	☐
C	URINE OUTPUT	☐
D	SERUM CALCIUM	☐
E	WHITE BLOOD CELL COUNT	☐

Question 10.52 Drug monitoring item worth 2 points

CASE PRESENTATION

A 65-year-old female patient is prescribed vancomycin 1 g twice daily by IV infusion for the treatment of a staphylococcal skin infection. A 'trough' level taken prior to the third dose is reported by the biochemistry laboratory to be 10 mg/L.

Question: Which *one* of the following statements is true about this patient's antibiotic therapy?

	DECISION OPTIONS	
A	1 G TWICE DAILY IS A SUITABLE DOSE FOR THIS PATIENT	☐
B	1 G TWICE DAILY IS TOO HIGH A DOSE AND SHOULD BE REDUCED	☐
C	1 G TWICE DAILY IS TOO LOW A DOSE AND SHOULD BE INCREASED	☐
D	A 'POST' DOSE LEVEL IS REQUIRED IN ORDER TO ASCERTAIN THE SUITABILITY OF THIS DOSE FOR THIS PATIENT	☐
E	LIVER FUNCTION OUGHT TO BE CHECKED REGULARLY DURING THERAPY WITH VANCOMYCIN	☐

Question 10.53 Adverse drug reactions item worth 2 marks

CASE PRESENTATION

A 58-year-old woman attends a routine follow-up appointment after starting an ACE-inhibitor for the treatment of hypertension 4 weeks earlier.

On questioning, you establish that she feels more tired than usual since beginning the prescription.

Question: Based on the known adverse effect profile of lisinopril, select the *one* most appropriate blood test. Mark it with a tick in the column provided.

DECISION OPTIONS

A	SERUM CREATININE	☐
B	NEUTROPHIL COUNT	☐
C	SERUM SODIUM	☐
D	SERUM ALBUMIN	☐
E	SERUM MAGNESIUM	☐

Question 10.54 Adverse drug reactions item worth 2 marks

CASE PRESENTATION

A 48-year-old man with a history of hypertension attends the GP complaining of 'overheating', having noticed facial flushing recently. He wonders if it is related to a new prescription he started last month.

His current medication is listed.

Question: Select the *one* drug from the list most likely to cause this new problem. Mark it with a tick in the column provided.

CURRENT PRESCRIPTIONS

Drug name	Dose	Route	Freq.	
LISINOPRIL	5 MG	ORAL	DAILY	☐
AMLODIPINE	5 MG	ORAL	DAILY	☐
BENDROFLUMETHIAZIDE	2.5 MG	ORAL	DAILY	☐
PARACETAMOL	1 G	ORAL	6-HOURLY	☐
CODEINE	30 MG	ORAL	6-HOURLY	☐

Question 10.55 Adverse drug reactions item worth 2 marks

CASE PRESENTATION

A 68-year-old woman is being treated as an inpatient for renal colic. Her baseline creatinine, on admission, was recorded as 112 µmol/L; however, on day 3 of her admission it is reported to be 220 µmol/L.

She has no history of renal impairment. You are asked to review the medication chart.

Question: Select the one drug that is most likely to have caused the deterioration in this patient's renal function. Mark it with a tick in the column provided.

CURRENT PRESCRIPTIONS

Drug name	Dose	Route	Freq.	
CO-AMOXICLAV	625 MG	IV	8-HOURLY	☐
PARACETAMOL	1 G	ORAL	6-HOURLY	☐
OMEPRAZOLE	20 MG	ORAL	DAILY	☐
VITAMIN B	1 TABLET	ORAL	DAILY	☐
DICLOFENAC	100 MG	PR	DAILY	☐

Question 10.56 Adverse drug reactions item worth 2 marks

CASE PRESENTATION

A 55-year-old woman with a history of rheumatoid arthritis, for which she currently takes methotrexate, visits her GP complaining of ongoing constipation following a recent knee replacement. A list of her newly prescribed medication is provided.

Question: Select the one drug most likely to have caused her constipation. Mark it with a tick in the column provided.

CURRENT PRESCRIPTIONS

Drug name	Dose	Route	Freq.	
CO-DYDRAMOL 10/500	2 TABLETS	ORAL	6-HOURLY	☐
IBUPROFEN	400 MG	ORAL	8-HOURLY	☐
AMLODIPINE	5 MG	ORAL	DAILY	☐
TRIMETHOPRIM	200 MG	ORAL	12-HOURLY	☐
CYCLIZINE	50 MG	ORAL	AS REQUIRED	☐

Question 10.57 Adverse drug reactions item worth 2 marks

CASE PRESENTATION

A 68-year-old woman is admitted to the coronary care unit with a diagnosis of worsening congestive cardiac failure. On day 3 of her admission she is stable enough to be transferred to a general ward.

She calls for the doctor before transfer complaining of an ongoing dry mouth and some blurred vision.

Question: Select the *one* drug that is most likely to have caused this patient's side effects. Mark it with a tick in the column provided.

CURRENT PRESCRIPTIONS

Drug name	Dose	Route	Freq.	
LISINOPRIL	5 MG	ORAL	DAILY	☐
CYCLIZINE	50 MG	ORAL	8-HOURLY	☐
MORPHINE SULPHATE 10 MG/5 ML	5 MG	ORAL	8-HOURLY AS REQUIRED	☐
ASPIRIN	75 MG	ORAL	DAILY	☐
CARVEDILOL	6.25 MG	ORAL	DAILY	☐

Question 10.58 Adverse drug reactions item worth 2 marks

CASE PRESENTATION

An 80-year-old man is brought to A&E. He has frank haematuria after catheterization by the GP.

He is currently taking warfarin for thromboprophylaxis as he has a diagnosis of AF. You request an emergency INR, which is reported as 5.2.

Question: Which *one* of the following would be the most appropriate course of action? Mark it with a tick in the column provided.

DECISION OPTIONS

A	CONTINUE WARFARIN	☐
B	GIVE VITAMIN K BY MOUTH	☐
C	GIVE VITAMIN K BY SLOW IV INJECTION	☐
D	WITHHOLD 1–2 DOSES OF WARFARIN AND RESTART AT LOWER DOSE	☐
E	GIVE PROTAMINE BY SLOW IV INJECTION	☐

Question 10.59 Adverse drug reactions item worth 2 marks

CASE PRESENTATION

You are called to a ward to review a 32-year-old woman who appears to be suffering from an allergic reaction after receiving piperacillin with tazobactam (Tazocin®) for the treatment of pneumonia.

Her symptoms are limited to pruritis and a macular rash on her trunk.

Question: Which *one* of the following would be the most appropriate immediate course of action? Mark it with a tick in the column provided.

	DECISION OPTIONS	
A	SWITCH TO CO-AMOXICLAV	☐
B	ATTEMPT TO INDUCE EMESIS	☐
C	ADMINISTER ORAL CHLORPHENAMINE	☐
D	ADMINISTER IV HYDROCORTISONE	☐
E	ADMINISTER IM ADRENALINE	☐

Question 10.60 Adverse drug reactions item worth 2 marks

CASE PRESENTATION

A 78-year-old male patient on your ward is prescribed oral gliclazide 80 mg 12-hourly for the treatment of type 2 diabetes. He is currently nil by mouth following minor surgery.

His blood glucose is 2.9, he is responding appropriately to questions, but appears drowsy. He has just had a further gliclazide dose for the morning.

Question: Which one statement regarding management of hypoglycaemic patients should guide your treatment? Mark it with a tick in the column provided.

	DECISION OPTIONS	
A	A CONSCIOUS PATIENT COULD BE GIVEN ORANGE JUICE	☐
B	AN UNCONSCIOUS PATIENT SHOULD BE GIVEN AN IV INFUSION OF 50% GLUCOSE	☐
C	DRUG-INDUCED HYPOGLYCAEMIA CAN BE MANAGED WITHOUT HOSPITAL ADMISSION	☐
D	UNCONSCIOUS PATIENTS SHOULD BE GIVEN 50 MG OF IV GLUCAGON	☐
E	DRUG-INDUCED HYPOGLYCAEMIA IS LESS LIKELY TO OCCUR IN PATIENTS ON SULPHONYLUREAS THAN IN PATIENTS ON METFORMIN	☐

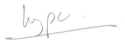

Question 10.1 Answer, see ticks beside current prescriptions chart

Antiplatelets (aspirin), anticoagulants (heparin) and the contraceptive pill should be stopped without alternatives sought. Metformin (an oral hypoglycaemic) is stopped the day before surgery, due to the risk of lactic acidosis in the event of renal compromise during surgery. Diabetic patients are all considered for initiation of insulin infusion by 'sliding scale' in the perioperative period.

Insulin (including Novomix 30) should also be stopped and converted to a sliding scale.

Remember, most drugs are not stopped during surgery, and stopping beta-blockers and calcium-channel blockers before surgery can actually be harmful.

CURRENT PRESCRIPTIONS

Drug name	Dose	Route	Freq.	A	B
METFORMIN	1 G	ORAL	12-HOURLY	☐	✓
MICROGYNON 30 ED®	ONE	ORAL	DAILY	✓	☐
ENOXAPARIN	40 MG	S/C	DAILY	✓	☐
ASPIRIN	75 MG	ORAL	DAILY	✓	☐
BISOPROLOL	5 MG	ORAL	DAILY	☐	☐
NOVOMIX 30®	15 UNITS	S/C	12-HOURLY	☐	✓
PARACETAMOL	1 G	ORAL	6-HOURLY	☐	☐
LANSOPRAZOLE	30 MG	ORAL	DAILY	☐	☐

Question 10.2 Answer, see ticks beside current prescriptions chart

This patient is taking too much paracetamol (max. 4 g/day). You are probably spotting a trend here – this is a very common exam question! As the patient is in pain it would be sensible to stop the paracetamol rather than the co-codamol (which obviously also contains paracetamol).

The simvastatin dose is one thousand times what it should be (20 g instead of 20 mg) and hence should be amended. Tamoxifen is most commonly used in breast cancer; while it is occasionally used in men with breast or prostate cancer, neither are in this patient's medical history, and hence this drug is not indicated and should be stopped (the most common cause for such an error is not checking the patient name on a drug label.)

The daily dose of alendronic acid is 10 mg, not 70 mg. The 70 mg preparation is licensed for the treatment of post-menopausal osteoporosis (i.e. in women) and is given once weekly.

CURRENT PRESCRIPTIONS

Drug name	Dose	Route	Freq.	A
BENDROFLUMETHIAZIDE	2.5 MG	ORAL	DAILY	☐
PARACETAMOL	500 MG	ORAL	AS REQUIRED UP TO 6-HOURLY	✓
SIMVASTATIN	20 G	ORAL	NIGHTLY	✓
TAMOXIFEN	20 MG	ORAL	DAILY	✓
AMOXICILLIN (FOR 7 DAYS)	500 MG	ORAL	8-HOURLY	☐
LISINOPRIL	10 MG	ORAL	NIGHTLY	☐
CO-CODAMOL 30/500	2 TABLETS	ORAL	6-HOURLY	☐
ALENDRONIC ACID	70 MG	ORAL	DAILY	✓

Question 10.3 Answer, see ticks beside current prescriptions chart

This patient's history (dizziness due to hypotension with dry cough) would point towards ACE-inhibitor side effects, and sure enough he is taking lisinopril which should be stopped.

The aspirin is not contraindicated in this scenario, but the dose certainly is: 300 mg is the treatment dose (for stroke and acute coronary syndromes) which is rarely given beyond 2 weeks. The standard prophylactic dose is 75 mg. Therefore, this is a drug error and should be stopped.

The GTN spray is as required and has not been required for years, so unlikely to be contributing to his hypotension. One could argue that its use may worsen his hypotension (and therefore dizziness), but the aspirin is a bigger priority.

St John's Wort is an antidepressant. Its main problems reflect its widespread interactions with other drugs. Unusually, however, it does not interact with any drugs in this list so should not be stopped (Note: look it up in the BNF—the authors certainly had to! It will be available in your exam so get used to doing it now.)

CURRENT PRESCRIPTIONS

Drug name	Dose	Route	Freq.	A
ASPIRIN	375 MG	ORAL	DAILY	✓
LISINOPRIL	20 MG	ORAL	NIGHTLY	✓
GTN SPRAY	1 SPRAY	SUBLINGUAL	AS REQUIRED UP TO 1-HOURLY	☐
CLOPIDOGREL	75 MG	ORAL	DAILY	☐
ST JOHN'S WORT	5 MG	ORAL	DAILY	☐
PRAVASTATIN	10 MG	ORAL	NIGHTLY	☐
PARACETAMOL	1 G	ORAL	6-HOURLY	☐

Question 10.4 Answer, see ticks beside current prescriptions chart

Each tablet of co-codamol contains 500 mg of paracetamol, i.e. he can only take 2 tablets (1 g) 4 times per day (6-hourly) not 6 times per day (4-hourly). This case was included to emphasize the difference between 'hourly' and 'every' in a prescription.

Qlaira® is a combined oral contraceptive pill and a male patient should not be taking this. (Patients commonly turn up with their partner's medication so be careful). If you do not recognize a drug, look it up in the BNF which you will have access to in the exam.

While enalapril (an ACE-inhibitor) may be best given in the evening to minimize the effects of postural hypotension (which is not widespread practice), it is clearly not the priority in this case: the question asks for the two major drug errors.

CURRENT PRESCRIPTIONS

Drug name	Dose	Route	Freq.	A
CO-CODAMOL 8/500	2 TABLETS	ORAL	4-HOURLY	✓
AMLODIPINE	5 MG	ORAL	DAILY	☐
ASPIRIN	75 MG	ORAL	DAILY	☐
ENALAPRIL	10 MG	ORAL	DAILY	☐
PROPRANOLOL	40 MG	ORAL	8-HOURLY	☐
QLAIRA®	1 TABLET	ORAL	DAILY	✓
IBUPROFEN	200 MG	ORAL	AS REQUIRED UP TO 8-HOURLY	☐

Question 10.5 Answer, see ticks beside current prescriptions chart

This patient has developed acute renal failure; drugs are a common cause. Of the new drugs, ibuprofen is the most likely culprit and should therefore be stopped. While she has acute renal failure (and particularly a raised potassium) the ACE-inhibitor lisinopril (which can cause hyperkalaemia and renal failure anyway) should also be withheld. Remember that while aspirin is an NSAID, it does not cause renal failure and so should be continued.

Her drowsiness probably reflects the accumulation of diazepam and co-codamol in her blood owing to reduced excretion in the urine due to the new renal failure. While the original dose of diazepam may have been appropriate, it is now having a significantly excessive effect (i.e. reduced consciousness level and respiratory rate) and should therefore be stopped. Codeine (a weak opioid) should also be stopped as this can also cause drowsiness and respiratory depression.

CURRENT PRESCRIPTIONS

Drug name	Dose	Route	Freq.	A
COCODAMOL 8/500	2 TABLETS	ORAL	6-HOURLY	✓
DIAZEPAM	2 MG	ORAL	12-HOURLY	✓
LISINOPRIL	10 MG	ORAL	NIGHTLY	✓
ASPIRIN	75 MG	ORAL	DAILY	☐
IBUPROFEN	400 MG	ORAL	8-HOURLY	✓
TRIMETHOPRIM	200 MG	ORAL	12-HOURLY	☐

Question 10.6 Answers, see ticks beside current prescriptions chart

Naproxen (a NSAID) inhibits the prostaglandin synthesis needed for gastric mucosal protection from acid. The gastric mucosa is therefore at risk of inflammation and ulceration. Oral steroids inhibit gastric epithelial renewal thus predisposing to ulceration.

Prednisolone (a corticosteroid) is often used to reduce inflammation in acute flares of asthma, COPD and inflammatory bowel disease (to name a few). Through multiple mechanisms it may cause hyperglycaemia, particularly by promoting hepatic gluconeogenesis and impairing cellular uptake of glucose in response to insulin. Patients with diabetes should be warned about this and alter their oral hypoglycaemic or insulin regimens accordingly.

Erythromycin (a macrolide) is a P-450 enzyme inhibitor and is likely to be responsible for the excessively high INR (through reducing warfarin breakdown and thus increasing its accumulation).

CURRENT PRESCRIPTIONS

Drug name	Dose	Route	Freq.	A	B	C
PARACETAMOL	1 G	ORAL	6-HOURLY	☐	☐	☐
NAPROXEN	500 MG	ORAL	12-HOURLY	✓	☐	☐
WARFARIN	2 MG	ORAL	DAILY	☐	☐	☐
PREDNISOLONE	30 MG	ORAL	DAILY	✓	✓	☐
RAMIPRIL	2.5 MG	ORAL	NIGHTLY	☐	☐	☐
ALLOPURINOL	100 MG	ORAL	DAILY	☐	☐	☐
ERYTHROMYCIN	500 MG	ORAL	6-HOURLY	☐	☐	✓

Question 10.7 Answer, see ticks beside current prescriptions chart

Antiplatelets (in this case aspirin) are usually stopped before surgery (as are anticoagulants) to prevent excessive intraoperative bleeding. Bendroflumethiazide is a thiazide diuretic. This can cause gout, so should be stopped anyway. Furthermore, the patient's blood pressure is low with a heart rate at the upper limit of normal; therefore, one of his antihypertensives should be stopped – when given the choice of stopping the diuretic (with no impact on heart rate) or the beta-blocker (which slows the heart rate) it would be sensible to pick the diuretic as the patient may become tachycardic without the beta-blocker. We try to avoid altering beta-blocker and calcium-channel blocker drugs preoperatively as it can cause intraoperative complications (obviously if a patient is profoundly bradycardic or hypotensive then they should be omitted, but stopping the diuretic should resolve the hypotension here anyway). Lithium should be omitted the day before surgery.

This patient is on long-term steroids for polymyalgia rheumatica so may have adrenal atrophy; he may therefore be unable to mount an adequate physiological ('stress') response to surgery, resulting in profound hypotension. The anaesthetist will need to be made aware so that supplementary IV steroids can be given at induction.

CURRENT PRESCRIPTIONS

Drug name	Dose	Route	Freq.	A
ALLOPURINOL	100 MG	ORAL	DAILY	☐
BENDROFLUMETHIAZIDE	5 MG	ORAL	DAILY	✓
LITHIUM CARBONATE MR	600 MG	ORAL	12-HOURLY	✓
ASPIRIN	75 MG	ORAL	DAILY	✓
BISOPROLOL	5 MG	ORAL	DAILY	☐
PREDNISOLONE	5 MG	ORAL	DAILY	✓
PARACETAMOL	1 G	ORAL	6-HOURLY	☐
LANSOPRAZOLE	30 MG	ORAL	DAILY	☐

Question 10.8 Answer, see ticks beside current prescriptions chart

LMW heparin is used subcutaneously for treating PE/DVT and acute coronary syndromes (i.e. unstable angina and myocardial infarctions); it is also used (at a much lower dose) for DVT prophylaxis in a significant proportion of inpatients. There are three LMW heparins available (enoxaparin, dalteparin and tinzaparin). The dose of enoxaparin prescribed is the prophylactic dose, and is inadequate for treating a DVT (i.e. as the patient is 60 kg we would expect her to be prescribed 90 mg daily, i.e. 1.5 mg/kg pending adequate renal function). You can prescribe any LMW heparin in units or mg. Unfractionated heparin is used intravenously when tighter control is needed (i.e. much less commonly). You are not expected to remember these doses, but you are expected to use the BNF to check!

The units for paracetamol are incorrect (i.e. should be 1 g (not 1 mg) 6-hourly and in reality the nurses would highlight this as they cannot administer 1 mg).

Yasmin® is a combined oral contraceptive: these are contraindicated in patients with migraine with aura because there is a significantly increased risk of stroke. The combined oral contraceptive is also prothrombotic and contraindicated in patients with a history of venous thromboembolism: given her DVT this is a further reason to stop this.

The absence of urine (anuria) suggests renal failure; the absence of a palpable bladder or hydronephrosis suggests a pre- or intrarenal cause (see Chapter 3). She has just started ibuprofen which is a common cause of acute renal failure, and this should therefore be withheld.

She is on propranolol as migraine prophylaxis.

CURRENT PRESCRIPTIONS

Drug name	Dose	Route	Freq.	A
ENOXAPARIN	40 MG	S/C	DAILY	✓
PARACETAMOL	1 MG	ORAL	6-HOURLY	✓
YASMIN®	1 TABLET	ORAL	DAILY	✓
IBUPROFEN	200 MG	ORAL	8-HOURLY	✓
PROPRANOLOL	40 MG	ORAL	12-HOURLY	☐
CYCLIZINE	50 MG	ORAL	AS REQUIRED UP TO 8-HOURLY	☐

Question 10.9 Answer

This patient has symptoms and plasma levels suggesting severe (late) lithium toxicity:
- Mild lithium toxicity – tremor
- Moderate lithium toxicity – lethargy
- Severe lithium toxicity – arrhythmias, seizures, coma and renal failure.

As the dose has not changed, you must look for drugs that may have increased the plasma levels. As there are no enzyme inhibitors which have recently been started, one should consider whether there is reduced excretion: certainly there is evidence of mild renal failure, but this probably would not account for it, which in fact is a consequence of the lithium toxicity.

Lithium excretion is significantly reduced by ACE-inhibitors in this case lisinopril, diuretics (and particularly thiazides, in this case bendroflumethiazide) and NSAIDs (not given here). If a diuretic must be given, loop diuretics (e.g. furosemide) are the safest.

The presence of arrhythmias suggested by the episode of palpitations, renal failure or seizures suggests dialysis is required. In the meantime, the lithium and the two drugs which caused the toxicity should be stopped, particularly as she is not currently hypertensive and has mild acute kidney injury.

DECISION OPTIONS

A	REDUCE LITHIUM	☐
B	STOP LITHIUM	☐
C	REDUCE LITHIUM, STOP BENDROFLUMETHIAZIDE	☐
D	STOP LITHIUM, STOP BENDROFLUMETHIAZIDE	☐
E	STOP LITHIUM, STOP BENDROFLUMETHIAZIDE, STOP LISINOPRIL	✓

Question 10.10 Answer

This patient has clinical evidence of hyperthyroidism and is on thyroid replacement. Her clinical features and TSH result suggest she is receiving too much levothyroxine. Remember, that in hyperthyroidism most things speed up (including gut motility, heart rate, alertness, etc.) although menstrual blood loss decreases.

Hypothyroidism should be monitored by clinical response and TFT. The most important TFT for monitoring is the TSH and a range of 0.5–5.0 µIU/L is targeted (remember that in primary hyper- and hypothyroidism (which are the most common scenarios) the TSH is inversely proportional to the T4 or T3 because the pituitary gland (which produces the TSH) is trying to alter the production of thyroxine from a 'faulty' thyroid gland by increasing TSH production (with hypothyroidism) or decreasing TSH production (with hyperthyroidism)). Thus, the symptoms and TFT evidence of hyperthyroidism warrant a reduction in levothyroxine dose. A quick look in the BNF reveals that dose changes when up-titrating levothyroxine are in 25–50 microgram increments, and this is the same when decreasing the dose. We also know that as a general rule in this type of question, in the absence of signs of toxicity, one should amend the dose by the smallest increment possible making option D the most appropriate.

Increasing the loperamide would not address the underlying problem, and would also result in a dose above the maximum recommended in the BNF.

DECISION OPTIONS

A	INCREASE LOPERAMIDE	☐
B	INCREASE LEVOTHYROXINE TO 250 MICROGRAMS DAILY	☐
C	INCREASE LEVOTHYROXINE TO 300 MICROGRAMS DAILY	☐
D	DECREASE LEVOTHYROXINE TO 150 MICROGRAMS DAILY	✓
E	DECREASE LEVOTHYROXINE TO 100 MICROGRAMS DAILY	☐

Question 10.11 Answer

This patient's biochemistry (and ability to drink) suggest an improvement from his renal failure. However, as part of the recovery, patients may enter a 'polyuric phase' in which their urine output increases and fluid input may not keep pace, resulting in dehydration and electrolyte abnormalities. Urine output exceeding 200 mL/h should always prompt consideration of this phenomenon.

Fluid balance is not nearly as complicated as fluid charts insinuate; there is one simple rule: the input should be similar to the output (allowing say 10–15% difference for insensible losses such as sweating) unless there is a good reason for discrepancy. The most common reason is whilst being rehydrated following dehydration or renal failure (when input will exceed output). In this example it is wise to calculate the balance as shown (see the balance column in case presentation). In this example the input originally exceeds the output as we would expect while he is being rehydrated, and then normalizes by day 3 (when the bloods are taken). However, the next day's urine output is 250 mL/hour (6 L in 24 hours) and causes a significant negative balance – this patient's oral intake of 500 mL is grossly inadequate, so option A is definitely not correct.

The hypokalaemia warrants replacement and the sodium is at the upper end of normal making 5% dextrose with KCl the most appropriate choice. Given that the patient is losing 1 L every 4 hours (24/6) the input should match, so a 1 L bag over 4 hours would be most appropriate.

One could argue that his negative balance yesterday requires an input rate that exceeds his output because he is dehydrated, but option E includes 40 mmol KCl over 1 hour: this should never be given at more than 20 mmol/hour, making option D the most appropriate.

DECISION OPTIONS

A	ENCOURAGE ORAL FLUIDS	☐
B	GIVE 1 L 0.9% SALINE WITH 20 MMOL KCL OVER 12 HOURS	☐
C	GIVE 1 L 5% DEXTROSE WITH 20 MMOL KCL OVER 12 HOURS	☐
D	GIVE 1 L 5% DEXTROSE WITH 20 MMOL KCL OVER 4 HOURS	✓
E	GIVE 1 L 5% DEXTROSE WITH 40 MMOL KCL OVER 1 HOURS	☐

Question 10.12 Answer

Antiepileptic drugs should never be abruptly stopped (even if an alternative is given) unless the patient is toxic and in a hospital environment where emergency seizure treatment may be instigated.

Carbamazepine is a key cause of SIADH and hence is not appropriate here as it would likely lower the sodium further which in itself would increase the risk of seizures. Thus we are left with changing the phenytoin dose: given the subtherapeutic clinical effect (i.e. still having seizures) and plasma level, the dose should be increased particularly as there is no mention of toxicity.

Phenytoin has zero-order kinetics and hence a very narrow therapeutic index (i.e. a small range of plasma concentration over which the drug will be therapeutic and therefore a greater chance of toxicity with any dose increases). Thus (as with most PSA questions) we should increase the dose by the minimum increment possible.

DECISION OPTIONS

A	INCREASE PHENYTOIN TO 175 MG ORAL DAILY	✓
B	INCREASE PHENYTOIN TO 200 MG ORAL DAILY	☐
C	STOP PHENYTOIN AND START CARBAMAZEPINE	☐
D	CONTINUE PHENYTOIN 150 MG DAILY AND START CARBAMAZEPINE	☐
E	DECREASE PHENYTOIN TO 125 MG ORAL DAILY	☐

Question 10.13 Answer

This patient requires maintenance fluids. Adults (obese or not) generally require 3 L IV maintenance fluids per day (equating to 8-hourly bags); the elderly or very underweight require 2 L (i.e. 12-hourly bags).
Adults require 40–60 mmol KCl per day when nil by mouth.
The absence of biochemistry results is not ideal, but sometimes realistic! Assuming they are normal (and there is no particular reason to suspect otherwise) maintenance fluids should comprise 'two salt (2 L 0.9% saline) and one sweet (1 L 5% dextrose)' every 24 h with 40–60 mmol KCl per day.
That B is the only option that is 8-hourly makes this answer the *most appropriate* and quite straightforward. Options D and E are not appropriate because 40 mmol KCl is generally reserved for patients who are hypokalaemic while options A and C are too slow.

DECISION OPTIONS

A	1 L 0.9% SALINE WITH 20 MMOL KCL OVER 12 HOURS	☐
B	1 L 0.9% SALINE WITH 20 MMOL KCL OVER 8 HOURS	✓
C	1 L 5% DEXTROSE WITH 20 MMOL KCL OVER 24 HOURS	☐
D	1 L 5% DEXTROSE WITH 40 MMOL KCL OVER 12 HOURS	☐
E	1 L 5% DEXTROSE WITH 40 MMOL KCL OVER 6 HOURS	☐

Question 10.14 Answer

The only abnormality in this patient's blood tests is the hyperkalaemia. This scenario reiterates three things:

1. Any results should be interpreted in the context of the patient's condition (in this case very well and on no medication);
2. Biochemistry results should be interpreted by comparison to previous results: in the absence of a physiological reason the potassium has increased by 2.9 mmol/L – this seems unlikely;
3. Of any result, the potassium is the most likely to be artefactually abnormal. Remember the causes of hyperkalaemia (DREAD: **d**rugs (she is not taking any), **r**enal failure (normal creatinine here), **e**ndocrine (lack of postural hypotension makes Addison's disease unlikely), **a**rtefact, and **d**iabetic ketoacidosis (blood sugar normal)).

Therefore, the correct answer is E, to repeat the test. If one were presented with the option to give calcium gluconate (which stabilizes the myocardium to prevent arrhythmias) *and* re-check the results then this might also be an appropriate option, but this is not the case. Option D outlines the correct treatment for (true) hyperkalaemia.

DECISION OPTIONS

A	1 L 0.9% SALINE WITH 20 MMOL KCL OVER 12 HOURS	☐
B	10 ML 10% IV CALCIUM GLUCONATE	☐
C	10 ML 10% IV CALCIUM GLUCONATE AND 10 UNITS ACTRAPID® INSULIN WITH 100 ML 20% IV DEXTROSE	☐
D	10 ML 10% IV CALCIUM GLUCONATE AND 10 UNITS ACTRAPID® INSULIN WITH 100 ML 20% IV DEXTROSE AND NEBULIZED SALBUTAMOL	☐
E	REPEAT BIOCHEMISTRY	✓

Question 10.15 Answer

A	The patient has had an anaphylactic reaction to a penicillin; thus a non-penicillin based antibiotic would be appropriate as replacement. Stopping the co-amoxiclav infusion would be the first management, but this is not offered as an option, changing antibiotics at present would not be the priority. Furthermore, the cross reactivity with carbapenems such as meropenem (10%) would make this a less favourable (though not strictly contraindicated) option.
B	**Correct:** high flow oxygen is an important first line intervention to optimize oxygenation in this patient with anaphylaxis.
C	Chlorphenamine is part of the anaphylaxis management pathway; however, 10 mg intravenously is used in anaphylaxis, while 4 mg orally is used for symptomatic relief of allergy.
D	IV fluids in anaphylaxis management are important but oxygen is a part of 'airway' or 'breathing' assessment and thus comes before 'circulation' in your **ABC** approach to the sick patient.
E	The patient is having an anaphylactic reaction and adrenaline is a vital part of anaphylactic drug management (comprising adrenaline, hydrocortisone and chlorphenamine). However, the dosing is incorrect: anaphylaxis dosing is 500 micrograms (0.5 mg) of 1:1000 adrenaline intramuscularly. The dose offered is that used intravenously in cardiac arrest.

DECISION OPTIONS

A	CHANGE CO-AMOXICLAV TO MEROPENEM	☐
B	15 L/MINUTE OXYGEN VIA NON-REBREATHER MASK	✓
C	CHLORPHENAMINE 4 MG ORAL	☐
D	500 ML 0.9% SALINE IV OVER 30 MINUTES	☐
E	1 MG OF 1:10 000 ADRENALINE IM	☐

Question 10.16 Answer

A	An essential part of a new diagnosis of type two diabetes mellitus. Many type two diabetics can be managed with diet and weight loss alone. If patients fail to improve their blood sugar control they should be commenced on an appropriate oral hypoglycaemic drug, but should also continue with their diet. In this instance, dietary measures appear to have proved inadequate necessitating drug therapy.
B	A biguanide, metformin is usually the first-line drug treatment in type II diabetes mellitus when diet and exercise are inadequate; however it is contraindicated in patients with an eGFR <30 mL/minute/1.73 m^2 and should be used with caution if <45 mL/minute/1.73 m^2) given the increased risk of lactic acidosis.
C	**Correct:** gliclazide is a sulphonylurea, and would be the first-line choice for drug therapy given his chronic kidney disease. There is an increased risk of hypoglycaemia with gliclazide compared to metformin.
D	A standard insulin regimen in type 2 diabetes; however, insulin would not be first-line management.
E	Once-daily regimens can also be used in type 2 diabetes mellitus, but again would not be first-line treatment.

DECISION OPTIONS

A	REVIEW BY DIETICIAN AND WEIGHT LOSS REGIMEN	☐
B	METFORMIN 500 MG ORAL TWICE DAILY	☐
C	GLICLAZIDE 40 MG ORAL ONCE DAILY	✓
D	MIXTARD 30® INSULIN (30% SOLUBLE AND 70% ISOPHANE) S/C TWICE DAILY	☐
E	LONG ACTING INSULIN (GLARGINE) S/C ONCE DAILY	☐

Question 10.17 Answer

A	Tricyclic antidepressants are sometimes used to treat pain, particularly when an element of depression is present (as here); however, 100 mg is 10 times the normal starting dose and is thus inappropriate.
B	Co-codamol contains paracetamol and codeine. While adding a weak opioid would be sensible as a next step, two tablets (each containing 500 mg paracetamol) 4-hourly (i.e. 6 times per day) would result in 6 g paracetamol daily, 50% more than the maximum 4 g. Watch out for this trick – 4-hourly is not the same as 4 times per day (which would be 6-hourly).
C	Adding a weak opioid would be sensible plus giving an 'as required' dose of a stronger opioid (morphine sulphate) would also be wise. However, opioids are constipating; as we are told he is constipated, in the absence of a laxative, they should be avoided.
D	Using an NSAID might be helpful, but is contraindicated by his indigestion.
E	**Correct:** non-pharmacological treatments should be considered for pain relief if they have adequate evidence; while junior doctors rarely utilize TENS, the absence of a safe other option make this the default option and emphasizes the need to use non drug treatments.

DECISION OPTIONS

A	ADD AMITRIPTYLINE 100 MG ORAL NIGHTLY	☐
B	STOP PARACETAMOL AND START CO-CODAMOL (8/500) TWO TABLETS 4-HOURLY	☐
C	ADD CODEINE 30 MG 4 TIMES DAILY WITH AS-REQUIRED MORPHINE SULPHATE (ORAMORPH® 10 MG/5 ML)	☐
D	ADD NAPROXEN 500 MG ORAL 8-HOURLY	☐
E	TENS	✓

Question 10.18 Answer

A	This patient's history and investigations suggest small bowel obstruction, which has probably been caused by adhesions from her previous abdominal surgery. Metoclopramide 10 mg IV is a prokinetic type antiemetic and thus would not be appropriate in a patient with bowel obstruction or in the first few days following abdominal surgery.
B	Haloperidol is a dopamine antagonist and is primarily used as a sedating agent but can also be used as an antiemetic particularly in palliative care. This would not be the most appropriate first-line antiemetic in this case.
C	Cyclizine is an antihistamine-based antiemetic and is beneficial in most causes of nausea. However, in bowel obstruction oral administration would be ineffective.
D	**Correct:** in bowel obstruction the most effective way of relieving nausea is to remove the obstruction or decompress the system with a nasogastric tube; concomitant IV fluids should be given to prevent dehydration while nil by mouth, hence the term 'drip and suck'. If the patient is still nauseated or a nasogastric tube/surgical intervention is not possible then antiemetic medications should be used.
E	Ondansetron is a $5HT_3$ antagonist and an effective antiemetic for most causes of nausea. It is particularly effective for chemically induced nausea including chemotherapy. Although ondansetron would be an appropriate choice, giving it orally would be ineffective as it would be either vomited (if administered before the nasogastric tube is placed) or aspirated through the nasogastric tube once sited.

DECISION OPTIONS

A	METOCLOPRAMIDE 10 MG IV	☐
B	HALOPERIDOL 500 MICROGRAMS S/C	☐
C	CYCLIZINE 50 MG ORALLY	☐
D	LARGE BORE NASOGASTRIC TUBE	✓
E	ONDANSETRON 4 MG ORALLY	☐

Question 10.19 Answer

A	**Correct:** ipratropium is an anticholinergic and effective in the management of exacerbations of COPD in conjunction with salbutamol.
B	Oral or intravenous steroids are effective in the management of exacerbations of COPD; however, out of the options ipratropium would be first choice because steroids take time to work.
C	Early intensive care review in patients not responding to treatment is important; however, initial management is still to be started with this patient. Furthermore, should NIV be required here, BPAP would be indicated as he has type-2 respiratory failure (i.e. low PaO_2 with high $PaCO_2$) while CPAP is generally reserved for type 1 respiratory failure (i.e. low PaO_2 with low/normal $PaCO_2$).
D	With the history of COPD, in particular CO_2 retention, and the non life-threatening observations and ABG results, 24% oxygen should be first choice and any increases thereafter carefully titrated with an arterial blood gas (ABG).
E	Aminophylline is used if patients fail to respond to initial management – this would not be appropriate at this stage. This therapy should be initiated under the direction of a senior colleague.

DECISION OPTIONS

A	IPRATROPIUM BROMIDE 500 MICROGRAMS NEB	✓
B	PREDNISOLONE 30 MG ORALLY	☐
C	INTENSIVE CARE REVIEW FOR CONSIDERATION OF CONTINUOUS POSITIVE AIRWAYS PRESSURE (CPAP) NIV	☐
D	OXYGEN (60%) VIA VENTURI MASK	☐
E	IV AMINOPHYLLINE INFUSION	☐

Question 10.20 Answer

A	This patient is in hypotensive shock; thus the fluid choice should be a colloid (as systolic BP <90 mmHg) and in the form of a fluid challenge (stat. or up to 1 h). Furthermore, the sodium is at the lower end of normal, so 5% dextrose would not seem sensible.
B	0.9% saline is one of the main fluids used in resuscitation along with Hartmann's and colloids. It is important to reassess fluid status in acutely unwell patients. Patients with pancreatitis require large volumes of fluid. This shocked patient requires fluids at a rate faster than 250 mL/h.
C	HAS would not be the first-choice fluid here. It is typically used in liver failure where low-sodium content is required (for replacement and maintenance).
D	**Correct:** the patient is clinically dehydrated and has responded to an initial bolus of crystalloid. A further bolus of fluid in the setting of dehydration, hypotension and low-urine output would certainly be the most appropriate action, and a colloid would stay intravascularly (and thus maintain blood pressure) for longer.
E	The speed of delivery would be inadequate given the clinical scenario.

DECISION OPTIONS

A	1 L 5% DEXTROSE IV OVER 4 HOURS	☐
B	1 L 0.9% SALINE IV OVER 4 HOURS	☐
C	500 ML 5% HUMAN ALBUMIN SOLUTION IV OVER 30 MINUTES	☐
D	FLUID CHALLENGE OF 500 ML GELOFUSINE IV OVER 30 MINUTES	✓
E	1 L 0.9% SALINE IV OVER 12 HOURS	☐

Question 10.21 Answer

A	After his initial management he is clinically improving and thus IV steroid and antihistamine would be appropriate next steps. However, option A gives the incorrect dose (should be 200 mg not 200 g) and route (should be IV not IM).
B	In the absence of any obvious wheeze (and thus clinically detectable bronchospasm), the bronchodilator salbutamol would not be helpful.
C	Fluid resuscitation is an important part of anaphylaxis management; however, this would not be the next most appropriate step particularly when prescribed over 12 hours (would require a faster rate given the tachycardia).
D	**Correct:** clinically he is improving after his initial management and a long-acting antihistamine would be the next appropriate step along with hydrocortisone.
E	As the patient is clinically improving, a further dose of adrenaline at this time would not be appropriate.

DECISION OPTIONS

A	HYDROCORTISONE 200 G IM STAT.	☐
B	SALBUTAMOL 5 MG NEB STAT.	☐
C	1 L 0.9% SALINE IV OVER 12 HOURS	☐
D	CHLORPHENAMINE 10 MG IV STAT.	✓
E	ADRENALINE 500 MICROGRAMS OF 1:1000 IM	☐

Question 10.22 Answer

A	**Correct:** IV loop diuretics will be the most effective way of improving respiratory function in this patient with pulmonary oedema.
B	NIV is an option for pulmonary oedema; however, patients should be optimized on oxygen first and only considered for NIV if they remain hypoxic on 100% oxygen via non-rebreather mask.
C	Spironolactone is an aldosterone antagonist and is used in chronic heart failure. It would not be first line in acute pulmonary oedema.
D	From the clinical history there is no evidence of a chest infection.
E	Bendroflumethiazide is a thiazide diuretic used in chronic hypertension and congestive cardiac failure, not acute pulmonary oedema.

DECISION OPTIONS

A	FUROSEMIDE 80 MG IV STAT.	✓
B	REFERRAL FOR NONINVASIVE VENTILATION (NIV)	☐
C	SPIRONOLACTONE 25 MG ORAL STAT.	☐
D	CO-AMOXICLAV 1.2 G IV 8-HOURLY	☐
E	BENDROFLUMETHIAZIDE 2.5 MG ORAL STAT.	☐

Question 10.23 Answer

A	ACE-inhibitors increase the risk of hyperkalaemia, particularly in the setting of acute kidney injury.
B	**Correct:** cough is very common with ACE-inhibitors and thought to be due to build up of bradykinin; it is often dose-dependent. If this occurs, a trial of an angiotensin receptor blocker is indicated.
C	Caution should be taken, particularly in the elderly who are unwell on ACE-inhibitors, as it increases risk of acute kidney injury.
D	Interestingly, angio-oedema related to ACE-inhibitors is often a delayed reaction needing time for accumulation of bradykinin. It is typically months later.
E	Monitoring renal function and potassium following initiation of ACE-inhibition is essential; if there is an acute deterioration in either then the medication may need to be stopped – tests should be performed 1–2 weeks after initiation of therapy.

DECISION OPTIONS

A	RISK OF HYPERKALAEMIA IS LOW WITH RAMIPRIL COMPARED TO OTHER ANTIHYPERTENSIVES	☐
B	COUGH IS A COMMON SIDE EFFECT WITH ACE-INHIBITORS AND TRIAL OF AN ANGIOTENSIN RECEPTOR BLOCKER INSTEAD IS INDICATED IF COUGH DEVELOPS	✓
C	NO PRECAUTIONS NEED TO BE TAKEN IF THE PATIENT DEVELOPS DIARRHOEA OR VOMITING	☐
D	ANGIO-OEDEMA ASSOCIATED WITH ACE-INHIBITORS ALWAYS OCCURS IN THE FIRST 24 HOURS	☐
E	REPEAT BLOOD TESTS LOOKING AT RENAL FUNCTION AND ELECTROLYTES 6 MONTHS AFTER INITIATION ARE ESSENTIAL	☐

Question 10.24 Answer

A	When unwell, basal blood glucose increases therefore higher doses of insulin are required. Failing to do so will increase the risk of diabetic ketoacidosis.
B	In the conscious patient, hypoglycaemia should be treated with glucose tablets, a sugary drink or glucose gel.
C	**Correct:** failing to rotate injection sites will result in lipodystrophy which can be uncomfortable but also varies the quantity of insulin absorbed.
D	HbA1c gives average glucose control over a 3-month period. In diabetic patients an HbA1c of under 48 mmol/mol is targeted.
E	Excessive alcohol intake can result in life-threatening hypoglycaemia, and is a common cause of hypoglycaemia in young diabetic adults.

DECISION OPTIONS

A	WHEN UNWELL THE PATIENT'S TOTAL DAILY INSULIN DOSAGE SHOULD BE DECREASED	☐
B	HYPOGLYCAEMIA SHOULD BE TREATED WITH A BOTTLE OF WATER	☐
C	LIPODYSTROPHY IS CAUSED BY REPEATED USE OF THE SAME INJECTION SITES	✓
D	HBA1C IS A SUITABLE WAY TO MONITOR BLOOD SUGARS FROM DAY TO DAY	☐
E	EXCESSIVE ALCOHOL INTAKE CAN CAUSE HYPERGLYCAEMIA	☐

Question 10.25 Answer

A	**Correct:** those on long courses of steroids should never have this medication stopped abruptly due to the risk of Addisonian crisis. All patients on steroids should hold a 'steroid therapy card' to warn health care professionals.
B	Steroids increase the risk of osteoporosis, particularly in the elderly. Patients should be prescribed a calcium tablet if not a bisphosphonate too.
C	Gastric protection should be considered whilst taking prednisolone due to the increased risk of gastric irritation and gastric/duodenal ulceration. Options include histamine (H2) antagonists or proton pump inhibitors.
D	Long-term steroid therapy increases the risk of diabetes mellitus and blood sugars should be monitored regularly.
E	Patients on steroids are at risk of hypertension and should be monitored regularly.

DECISION OPTIONS

A	PROLONGED COURSES OF STEROIDS SHOULD NEVER BE STOPPED SUDDENLY	✓
B	STEROIDS REDUCE THE RISK OF OSTEOPOROSIS	☐
C	RISK OF GASTRIC/DUODENAL ULCERS IS LOWER WHEN ON STEROID THERAPY	☐
D	STEROIDS DO NOT INCREASE THE RISK OF DIABETES MELLITUS	☐
E	PATIENTS ARE AT RISK OF HYPOTENSION WITH STEROID THERAPY	☐

Question 10.26 Answer

A	Regular blood tests every 3–4 weeks will be required to monitor full blood count, liver and renal function. Neutropenia is a common side effect.
B	It is essential that methotrexate is only taken once weekly. It should never be prescribed more than once a week for the treatment of non-oncological conditions.
C	Methotrexate is highly teratogenic and must never be used in pregnancy or when breast feeding.
D	Pulmonary fibrosis is a potential side effect of methotrexate therapy. The drug should be stopped if this is confirmed.
E	**Correct:** folate antagonists such as trimethoprim and co-trimoxazole should never be used with methotrexate as they will increase its effect as a folate antagonist and, therefore, put the patient at risk of severe side effects, particularly bone marrow suppression and thus neutropenic sepsis.

DECISION OPTIONS

A	ONCE ON A STABLE DOSE, BLOOD TESTS ARE NOT REQUIRED	☐
B	METHOTREXATE SHOULD BE TAKEN DAILY	☐
C	METHOTREXATE IS SAFE TO USE IN PREGNANCY	☐
D	THERE IS NO ASSOCIATION BETWEEN METHOTREXATE AND PULMONARY FIBROSIS	☐
E	TRIMETHOPRIM SHOULD NOT BE USED FOR TREATMENT OF INFECTION	✓

Question 10.27 Answer

A	**Correct:** statins should be stopped while taking clarithromycin (a CYP3A4 inhibitor) as they increase toxicity and associated side effects.
B	Most cholesterol metabolism occurs overnight, so conventionally most statins are taken at night.
C	Myositis is a potentially serious complication if left unaddressed; therefore, patients should be warned to seek medical assistance if they develop unusual aches or pains. The medication should be stopped.
D	Statins should not be used in those with active liver disease as this may potentially affect its metabolism.
E	Grapefruit should be avoided in those taking statins as it contains polyphenolic compounds that inhibit CYP3A4 and thus increase statin toxicity.

DECISION OPTIONS

A	WHEN TAKING CLARITHROMYCIN THE STATINS SHOULD BE STOPPED	✓
B	STATINS ARE MOST EFFECTIVE WHEN TAKEN IN THE MORNING	☐
C	IF MUSCLE CRAMPS DEVELOP THE DOSE SHOULD BE INCREASED	☐
D	STATINS ARE SAFE TO USE IN ACTIVE LIVER DISEASE	☐
E	THERE ARE NO DIETARY RESTRICTIONS WITH STATIN THERAPY	☐

Question 10.28 Answer

A	ACE-inhibitors increase the risk of hyperkalaemia, particularly in the setting of acute kidney injury (AKI).
B	**Correct**: cough is very common with ACE-inhibitors and is thought to be due to release of bradykinin and is often dose dependent. Trial of an ARB instead is an option if cough develops.
C	Caution should be taken, particularly in the elderly who are unwell when taking ACE-inhibitors as they increase the risk of AKI.
D	Interestingly angio-oedema related to ACE-inhibitors is often a delayed reaction due to time for accumulation of bradykinin. It typically occurs months after initiation.
E	Monitoring renal function and potassium following initiation of ACE-inhibition is essential. If there is an acute deterioration in either, then the medication may need to be stopped. Both parameters should be monitored 1–2 weeks after initiation of therapy.

DECISION OPTIONS

A	RISK OF HYPERKALAEMIA IS LOW WITH RAMIPRIL COMPARED TO OTHER ANTIHYPERTENSIVES	☐
B	DRY COUGH IS A COMMON SIDE EFFECT WITH ACE-INHIBITORS AND WARRANTS TRIAL OF AN ANGIOTENSIN RECEPTOR BLOCKER INSTEAD	✓
C	NO PRECAUTIONS NEED TO BE TAKEN IF THE PATIENT DEVELOPS DIARRHOEA OR VOMITING	☐
D	ANGIO-OEDEMA ASSOCIATED WITH ACE-INHIBITORS ALWAYS OCCURS IN THE FIRST 24 HOURS	☐
E	REPEAT BLOOD TESTS LOOKING AT RENAL FUNCTION AND ELECTROLYTES 6 MONTHS AFTER INITIATION ARE ESSENTIAL	☐

Question 10.29 Answer

Correct answer and working

This answer does not really need an explanation as it requires simple addition. This question has been included in order to reinforce the practicalities of dosage administration and to teach you to think about administration of a drug before you prescribe it.

Answer	One 125 microgram tablet and one 62.5 microgram tablet

Question 10.30 Answer

Use the equation: $(10 \div 20) \times 8$

Answer	4 mL

Question 10.31 Answer

Correct answer and working

20 mmol = 5 g, so using our equation, we can calculate that 8 mmol = 2 g
2000 mg in 10 mL = 200 mg/mL

Answer | 10 mL

Question 10.32 Answer

Correct answer and working

Use the equation: $(1 \div 150) \times 2000$. Note: this is to the nearest minute.

Answer | 13 min

Question 10.33 Answer

Correct answer and working

She takes one 5 mg daily of prednisolone for the management of rheumatoid arthritis. During episodes of sepsis, steroid prescriptions are doubled to meet physiological demand upon the hypothalamic pituitary adrenal axis (HPA axis), which is suppressed during long-term steroid treatment ('sick day rules').
Her prednisolone prescription should be doubled to 10 mg, or 2×5 mg tablets.

Clinical point

Note that methotrexate would be stopped in this scenario as it is contraindicated in the presence of active infection. The dihydrofolate reductase inhibitor trimethoprim should be avoided in the management of urinary tract infection in patients taking methotrexate, due to the risk of additive toxicity and bone marrow suppression.

Answer | 2 tablets

Question 10.34 Answer

Correct answer

250 mL total volume/60 min = 4.2 mL/min

Clinical point

Amiodarone is referred to as 'the Domestos of antiarrythmics' in undergraduate lectures because it can play a part in the management of many arrhythmias. This will not help you in an OSCE interrogation. The mechanistic answer is therefore that it is a class III antiarrhythmic – prolonging repolarization (phase III) of the cardiac action potential cycle. In short it slows conduction of each heartbeat. This is mediated by sodium and potassium channel activity. It is structurally similar to iodine, hence some of its side effects. Its name acknowledges iodine (amIODarone).

Answer   4.2 mL/min

Question 10.35 Answer

Correct answer

2 g = 2000 mg/4 = 500 mg
24 h/4 doses = every 6 h
You must prescribe 500 mg rather than 0.5 g

Answer   500 MG EVERY 6 HOURS

Question 10.36 Answer

Correct answer

A 1% solution contains 1 g in 100 mL.
Thus there are 10 mg in 1 mL.

Answer   1 mL

Question 10.37 Answer

A. Drug choice	Score	Feedback/justification	B. Dose, route, frequency	Score	Feedback/justification
1. MAGNESIUM CARBONATE	4	A suitable antacid which will give quick relief.	10 ML ORAL	4	
2. ALUMINIUM HYDROXIDE	4	As above	1 CAPSULE ORAL	4	
3. CO-MAGALDROX	4	As above	10 ML ORAL	4	
4. CO-MAGALDROX	4	As above	20 ML ORAL	4	
5. MAGNESIUM TRISILICATE	4	As above	1 TABLET ORAL (CHEWED)	4	
6. MAGNESIUM TRISILICATE	4	As above	2 TABLETS ORAL (CHEWED)	4	
7. MAGNESIUM TRISILICATE MIXTURE	4	As above	10 ML IN WATER ORAL	4	
8. MAGNESIUM TRISILICATE MIXTURE	4	As above	20 ML IN WATER ORAL	4	
9. ANY ALGINATE-CONTAINING DRUG, e.g. GAVISCON®, PEPTAC® OR ACIDEX®	0	Patient is allergic to alginate dressings so not sensible to give oral alginate!	N/A		
10. ANY PROTON PUMP INHIBITOR, e.g. LANSOPRAZOLE OR OMEPRAZOLE	1	May improve dyspepsia through antisecretory mechanism but this is not immediate.	CORRECT DOSE ACCORDING TO BNF	4	
11. ANY H2 RECEPTOR ANTAGONIST, E.G. RANITIDINE	1	As above	CORRECT DOSE ACCORDING TO BNF	4	

Marking guide for A and B.
4 marks: for an optimal answer that cannot be improved.
3 marks: for an answer that is good but is suboptimal on some grounds (e.g. cost-effectiveness, likely adherence)
2 marks: for an answer that is likely to provide benefit but is clearly suboptimal for more than one reason.
1 mark: for an answer that has some justification and deserves some credit.

C. Timing. Candidates will also be given **1 mark for correctly dating** (and timing) the prescription

D. Signature. Candidates will also be given **1 mark for signing** the prescription

For example, the prescription should appear as:

ONCE ONLY MEDICINES

Date	Time	Medicine (approved name)	Dose	Route	Prescriber – sign + print	Time given	Given by
01/02/13	13 30	MAGNESIUM CARBONATE	10 ML	ORAL	YOUR NAME AND SIGNATURE		

Question 10.38 Answer

A. Drug choice	Score	Feedback/justification	B. Dose, route, frequency	Score	Feedback/justification
1. DALTEPARIN (not Fragmin® (trade name))	4	Dalteparin, enoxaparin and tinzaparin are LMW heparins used for preventing DVT and PE (and at higher doses used for treating them, treating ACS and ischaemic limbs).	5000 UNITS S/C ONCE DAILY Most hospitals administer heparin at 6pm – this is solely for nursing staff convenience (i.e. take bulky syringes round only once daily).	4	This is the prophylactic dose (remember LMW heparin may be used for treatment or prophylaxis). Patients with low body weight or severe renal failure require a reduced dose.
2. ENOXAPARIN (not Clexane® (trade name))	4	As above	40 MG OR 4000 UNITS S/C ONCE DAILY (can be prescribed either way)	4	As above (it does not matter which of the three LMW heparins you selected; in real life it reflects hospital policy and dalteparin is cheapest at present!)
3. TINZAPARIN (not Innohep® (trade name))	4	As above	3500–4500 UNITS S/C ONCE DAILY	3	Strictly speaking, tinzaparin is only licensed for VTE prophylaxis in surgical patients. In this clearly medical admission, enoxaparin or dalteparin would be better choices. Note that a specific dose (not a range) must be prescribed e.g. 3500 units.
4. ALTEPLASE	0	Thrombolytics activate plasminogen to form plasmin, which degrades fibrin and so breaks up thrombi. Thrombolysis is definitely not warranted here: there is no thrombus to lyse!	N/A		
5. ASPIRIN	0	Aspirin is an antiplatelet and has no role in the prevention of PE or DVT.	N/A		
6. WARFARIN	0	Warfarin is the oral anticoagulant of choice. It antagonizes the effect of vitamin K, preventing formation of the vitamin K-dependent clotting factors (II, VII, IX and X). Hence prolonging the PT/INR. It is not used for thromboprophylaxis in the absence of AF.	N/A		
7. COMPRESSION STOCKINGS (or anti-embolism stockings)	0	While normally a sensible option for preventing DVT, these are contraindicated here because the pulses are not palpable suggesting peripheral arterial disease that might become critical if additional (external) pressure is applied.	N/A		

Marking guide for A and B.
4 marks: for an optimal answer that cannot be improved.
3 marks: for an answer that is good but is suboptimal on some grounds (e.g. cost-effectiveness, likely adherence).
2 marks: for an answer that is likely to provide benefit but is clearly suboptimal for more than one reason.
1 mark: for an answer that has some justification and deserves some credit.

C. Timing. Candidates will also be given **1 mark for correctly dating** (and timing) the prescription

D. Signature. Candidates will also be given **1 mark for signing** the prescription

For example, the prescription should appear as:

REGULAR MEDICATION		Date						
		Time						
Drug (Approved name) DALTEPARIN		**6**						
		8						
Dose 5000 UNITS	Route S/C	**12**						
Prescriber – sign + print *YOUR NAME AND SIGNATURE*	Start date 01/02/13	**14**						
		⑱						
Notes	Frequency DAILY	**22**						

Question 10.39 Answer

A. Drug choice	Score	Feedback/justification	B. Dose, route, frequency	Score	Feedback/justification
1. NITROFURANTOIN	4	The BNF (section 5.1.13) stipulates that nitrofurantoin is the only appropriate first line antibiotic here because amoxicillin is a penicillin (to which she is allergic) and trimethoprim is a folate antagonist, and is thus contraindicated in anyone taking methotrexate due to increased risk of bone marrow suppression.	50 MG 6-HOURLY ORAL FOR 3 DAYS. MUST have an indication (urinary tract infection) MUST have start date (today) MUST have a stop/review date (3 days time)	4	Antibiotics MUST have indications and stop/review dates. This prevents unnecessarily long courses which encourage complications (such as *Clostridium difficile* gastroenteritis) and antibiotic resistance.
2. NITROFURANTOIN	4	See above	50 MG ORAL DAILY	0	This is the UTI prophylaxis dose, i.e. incorrect.
3. DOXYCYCLINE	1	Many hospital trusts advocate using doxycycline, usually if due to MRSA; however, the BNF does not mention this as a first-line antibiotic, so unless your local antibiotic policy states otherwise, nitrofurantoin should be used instead. In the PSA exam you will not have access to your local antibiotic policy – therefore learn the first-line choices for common infections and then learn to use the BNF when complicated cases (such as this one) arise.	100 MG ORAL DAILY FOR 3 DAYS MUST have an indication (i.e. urinary tract infection) MUST have start date (today) MUST have a stop/review date (3 days time)	4	Doxycyline requires a stat dose of 200 mg oral on the first day then 100 mg oral daily for the remainder.
4. TRIMETHOPRIM	0	See above	N/A		
5. CO-AMOXICLAV	0	See above (co-AMOXIclav contains amoxicillin).	N/A		
6. AMOXICILLIN	0	See above	N/A		
7. ORAL CEPHALOSPORIN, PIVMECILLINAM *OR* A QUINOLONE	1	None are first-line according to the BNF, thus gaining less marks than with nitrofurantoin. Note that a proportion of people allergic to penicillin will also be allergic to cephalosporins; while not an absolute contraindication, it would be unwise to take this risk when a perfectly viable alternative is available.	CORRECT DOSE ACCORDING TO BNF MUST have an indication (urinary tract infection) MUST have start date (today) MUST have a stop/review date (3 days time)	4	

Question 10.39 Answer *(Cont'd)*

Marking guide for A and B.
4 marks: for an optimal answer that cannot be improved.
3 marks: for an answer that is good but is suboptimal on some grounds (e.g. cost-effectiveness, likely adherence).
2 marks: for an answer that is likely to provide benefit but is clearly suboptimal for more than one reason.
1 mark: for an answer that has some justification and deserves some credit.

C. Timing. Candidates will also be given **1 mark for correctly dating** (and timing) the prescription

D. Signature. Candidates will also be given **1 mark for signing** the prescription

For example, the prescription should appear as:

ANTIBIOTIC

	Date						
	Time						

Drug (Approved name) NITROFURANTOIN			⑥						
			8						
Dose 50 MG	Frequency 6-HOURLY	Route ORAL	⑫						
Prescriber – sign + print *YOUR SIGNATURE AND NAME*		Start date *TODAY'S DATE*	14						
			⑱						
Indication URINARY TRACT INFECTION		Review/stop date *TODAY'S DATE PLUS 3 DAYS*	㉒						

Question 10.40 Answer

A. Drug choice	Score	Feedback/justification	B. Dose, route, frequency	Score	Feedback/justification
1. PARACETAMOL	4	This is an appropriate first-line analgesic (see Chapter 2).	500 MG UP TO 4-HOURLY ORAL (maximum dose 4 g in 24 h) MUST have indication (pain or headache) MUST have frequency (4-hourly) – note this is a maximum frequency *up* to which the nurses will administer	4	This should be on the 'as required' chart because the patient is currently pain free so does not require regular (potentially harmful) drugs.
2. PARACETAMOL	4	As above	1 G UP TO 6-HOURLY ORAL (maximum 4 g in 24 h) MUST have indication (i.e. pain or headache) MUST have frequency (6-hourly)	4	As above
3. IBUPROFEN	0	She has asthma. Remember the cautions/contraindications for NSAIDs: renal failure, heart failure, asthma, indigestion, clotting dyscrasias.	N/A		
4. CODEINE	0	Using a mild opioid before paracetamol +/– NSAIDs is not appropriate (i.e. risks outweigh the benefits); furthermore, opioids should be avoided with primary headache (i.e. tension headache, migraine and cluster headache) as they can make them worse.	N/A		
5. TRAMADOL	0	As above	N/A		
6. ORAMORPH®	0	This is a stronger opioid and should definitely be avoided. Further, one should use the generic name (morphine sulphate), not the brand name.	N/A		

Marking guide for A and B.

4 marks: for an optimal answer that cannot be improved.

3 marks: for an answer that is good but is suboptimal on some grounds (e.g. cost-effectiveness, likely adherence).

2 marks: for an answer that is likely to provide benefit but is clearly suboptimal for more than one reason.

1 mark: for an answer that has some justification and deserves some credit.

C. Timing. Candidates will also be given **1 mark for correctly dating** (and timing) the prescription

D. Signature. Candidates will also be given **1 mark for signing** the prescription

Question 10.40 Answer *(Cont'd)*

For example, the prescription should appear as:

AS REQUIRED MEDICATION

Drug (Approved name) PARACETAMOL		Date						
		Time						
Dose 1G	Route ORAL	Route						
Prescriber – sign + print *YOUR SIGNATURE AND NAME*	Start date *TODAY'S DATE*	Given by						
Indication PAIN (or HEADACHE)	Frequency MAXIMUM 6-HOURLY*	Sign						

* Strictly speaking 1 g of paracetamol may be given every 4 hours providing no more than 4 g is given in 24 hours (i.e. one can take a dose 4 hours after the previous rather than waiting a further 2 hours but, to be clear, no more than 4 g can be taken per day).

A. Drug choice	Score	Feedback/justification	B. Dose, route, frequency	Score	Feedback/justification
1. PIPERACILLIN/ TAZOBACTAM	4	This patient has a severe, hospital-acquired pneumonia. He has been an inpatient for more than 5 days (i.e. he is 'late-onset') indicating that he needs piperacillin with tazobactam, a broad spectrum cephalosporin or a quinolone (see BNF section 5.1). The CURB65 score is reserved for community-acquired pneumonia so cannot be directly used; however, the presence of septic shock (systolic BP < 90 mmHg with evidence of infection) alone should make this stand out as severe. Many doctors (incorrectly) prescribe this as 'Tazocin®' but technically the trade name should not be written and the full piperacillin/ tazobactam (or piperacillin with tazobactam) should be written instead.	4.5 G IV 8-HOURLY MUST include an indication (i.e. hospital-acquired pneumonia/ pneumonia) MUST include a review/ stop date (in the majority of cases with IV antibiotics one should review after no more than 3 days as most patients will be able to step down to oral antibiotics)	4	
2. GENTAMICIN	0	While a useful additional treatment for pneumonia due to *Pseudomonas*, the question requests one drug and this would be inappropriate as monotherapy. The absence of a weight makes dosing difficult (and unsafe) so this in not an appropriate answer.	(5 MG/KG IV DAILY)	N/A	Note: in real life one must write the calculated dose not just 5 mg/kg (i.e. in this example we do not know the weight).
3. CIPROFLOXACIN *OR* ANY CEPHALOSPORIN	1	If no other drug options were available, then the risk of causing further diarrhoea might be worth taking given the life-threatening pneumonia; however, this is not the case (piperacillin/tazobactam is suitable) rendering this answer inappropriate.	CORRECT DOSE ACCORDING TO BNF	4	
4. VANCOMYCIN	1	Not indicated as first-line monotherapy when piperacillin/ tazobactam is viable; usually given if there is concern of MRSA (not mentioned here).	500 MG IV 12-HOURLY *OR* 1 G IV DAILY MUST include an indication (hospital-acquired pneumonia/ pneumonia) MUST include a review/ stop date	4	In the elderly, the BNF recommends these doses (while in other adults 1–1.5 g BD IV is recommended).

Question 10.41 Answer *(Cont'd)*

Marking guide for A and B.
4 marks: for an optimal answer that cannot be improved.
3 marks: for an answer that is good but is suboptimal on some grounds (e.g. cost-effectiveness, likely adherence).
2 marks: for an answer that is likely to provide benefit but is clearly suboptimal for more than one reason.
1 mark: for an answer that has some justification and deserves some credit.

C. Timing. Candidates will also be given **1 mark for correctly dating** (and timing) the prescription

D. Signature. Candidates will also be given **1 mark for signing** the prescription

For example, the prescription should appear as:

ANTIBIOTICS

	Date					
	Time					
Drug (Approved name) PIPERACILLIN/TAZOBACTAM	⑥					
	8					
Dose 4.5 G | Frequency 8-HOURLY | Route IV	12					
Prescriber – sign + print *YOUR NAME AND SIGNATURE* | Start date *TODAY'S DATE*	14					
	⑱					
Indication HOSPITAL-ACQUIRED PNEUMONIA | Review/stop date *TODAY'S DATE PLUS 3 DAYS*	㉒					

Question 10.42 Answer

A. Drug choice	Score	Feedback/justification	B. Dose, route, frequency	Score	Feedback/justification
1. SENNA	4	A stimulant laxative is an appropriate choice (i.e. no colitis or cramps which are the main contraindications).	2–4 TABLETS ORAL NIGHTLY (15–30 MG ORAL NIGHTLY)	4	May be prescribed as number of tablets or total dose. NOTE: you must select one dose rather than putting a range.
2. BISACODYL	4	As above	5–10 MG ORAL NIGHTLY	4	NOTE: you must select one dose rather than putting a range.
3. SODIUM PICOSULFATE	0	This stimulant laxative is a slightly extreme option for first-line therapy: it is typically used for bowel evacuation before surgery and endoscopy.	N/A		
4. DANTRON®	0	Dantron®, a stimulant laxative, is potentially carcinogenic so is only prescribed for terminally ill patients.	N/A		
5. ISPHAGULA HUSK *OR* METHYL-CELLULOSE *OR* STERCULIA	0	While bulking agents (such as isphagula) are appropriate in those without symptoms, they can take days to have any effect making it less appropriate for our patient feeling bloated already.	N/A		

Question 10.42 Answer *(Cont'd)*

A. Drug choice	Score	Feedback/justification	B. Dose, route, frequency	Score	Feedback/justification
6. LACTULOSE	0	The main contraindication to osmotic laxatives is bloating which will worsen with this class of drugs. This is thus an inappropriate choice.	N/A		
7. Any stool softener (e.g. docusate)	0	Whilst this might help the patient, you are told her stool is soft so a stimulant laxative is a better option.	N/A		

Marking guide for A and B.

4 marks: for an optimal answer that cannot be improved.

3 marks: for an answer that is good but is suboptimal on some grounds (e.g. cost-effectiveness, likely adherence).

2 marks: for an answer that is likely to provide benefit but is clearly suboptimal for more than one reason.

1 mark: for an answer that has some justification and deserves some credit.

C. Timing. Candidates will also be given **1 mark for correctly dating** (and timing) the prescription

D. Signature. Candidates will also be given **1 mark for signing** the prescription

For example, the prescription should appear as:

REGULAR MEDICATION

Drug (Approved name) SENNA		Date						
		Time						
		6						
		8						
Dose 2 TABLETS	Route ORAL	12						
Prescriber – sign + print *YOUR NAME AND SIGNATURE*	Start date *TODAY'S DATE*	14						
		18						
Notes	Frequency NIGHTLY	(22)						

Question 10.43 Answer

A. Drug choice	Score	Feedback/justification	B. Dose, route, frequency	Score	Feedback/justification
1. CODEINE	4	This is an appropriately weak opioid; the choice between tramadol and codeine usually rests on the likelihood of side effects. Both cause typical opioid side effects (i.e. respiratory depression, reduced consciousness and pinpoint pupils), but tramadol typically causes agitation/hallucinations (particularly in the elderly) while codeine is more constipating.	30 MG 6-HOURLY *OR* 30 MG 4 HOURLY ORAL REGULARLY *OR* 60 MG 6-HOURLY ORAL REGULARLY	4	This should be on the 'regular' chart because the patient is in constant pain; an additional 'as required' drug would be sensible (such as oral morphine sulphate), but the question only asks for one drug. 240 mg is the maximum daily dose (i.e. 60 mg 6-hourly).
2. CO-CODAMOL 8/500 *OR* CO-CODAMOL 30/500 *OR* CO-DYDRAMOL 10/500 *OR* CO-DYDRAMOL 20/500 *OR* CO-DYDRAMOL 30/500	0	While an appropriate choice because it contains a weak opioid, the question asked for one additional drug. The patient is already taking 4 g of paracetamol per day and therefore no further paracetamol-containing drugs should be given.	If the patient was not taking regular paracetamol: 2 TABLETS 6-HOURLY ORAL (OR 1 TABLET 6-HOURLY ORAL) should be 6-hourly to ensure no analgesia-free periods	0	In these drugs the first number refers to the total codeine (in co-codamol) or dihydrocodeine (in co-dydramol) in each tablet, and the second the amount of paracetamol. Thus, 2 tablets (containing 1 g paracetamol regardless of codeine/ dihydrocodeine dose) can be given up to 6-hourly.
3. TRAMADOL	4	See above	50 MG 6-HOURLY *OR* 4-HOURLY ORAL REGULARLY *OR* 100 MG 6-HOURLY ORAL REGULARLY	4	Patients are rarely prescribed more than 400 mg per day (i.e. 100 mg 6-hourly at most).
4. MORPHINE SULPHATE (not 'ORAMORPH®' (brand name))	0	Using a mild opioid before a strong one is more appropriate; as the question asks for one drug the choice is really between codeine and tramadol.	N/A	0	

Marking guide for A and B.
4 marks: for an optimal answer that cannot be improved.
3 marks: for an answer that is good but is suboptimal on some grounds (e.g. cost-effectiveness, likely adherence).
2 marks: for an answer that is likely to provide benefit but is clearly suboptimal for more than one reason.
1 mark: for an answer that has some justification and deserves some credit.

Question 10.43 Answer *(Cont'd)*

C. Timing. Candidates will also be given **1 mark for correctly dating** (and timing) the prescription

D. Signature. Candidates will also be given **1 mark for signing** the prescription

For example, the prescription should appear as:

REGULAR MEDICATION		Date						
		Time						
Drug (Approved name) CODEINE		⑥						
		8						
Dose 30 MG	Route ORAL	⑫						
Prescriber – sign + print *YOUR NAME AND SIGNATURE*	Start date *TODAY'S DATE*	14						
		⑱						
Notes	Frequency 6-HOURLY	㉒						

Question 10.44 Answer

A. Drug choice	Score	Feedback/justification	B. Dose, route, frequency	Score	Feedback/justification
1. CODEINE	4	This is an appropriately weak opioid; the choice between tramadol and codeine usually rests on the likelihood of side effects. Both cause typical opioid side effects (i.e. respiratory depression, reduced consciousness and pinpoint pupils), but tramadol typically causes agitation/ hallucinations (particularly in the elderly) while codeine is more constipating. In this case, the presence of diarrhoea promotes codeine (as does the patient's age).	30 MG 6-HOURLY *OR* 30 MG 4-HOURLY ORAL AS REQUIRED *OR* 60 MG 6-HOURLY ORAL AS REQUIRED	4	This should be on the 'as required' section because the pain is only occasional. 240 mg is the maximum daily dose (i.e. 60 mg 6-hourly).
2. CO-CODAMOL 8/500 *OR* CO-CODAMOL 30/500 *OR* CO-DYDRAMOL 10/500 *OR* CO-DYDRAMOL 20/500 *OR* CO-DYDRAMOL 30/500	0	While an appropriate choice because it contains a weak opioid, the question asked for one additional drug. The patient is already taking 4 g of paracetamol per day and therefore no further paracetamol-containing drugs should be given.	If the patient was not taking regular paracetamol: 2 TABLETS 6-HOURLY ORAL (*OR* 1 TABLET 6-HOURLY ORAL) should be 6-hourly to ensure no analgesia-free periods	4	In these drugs the first number refers to the total codeine (in co-codamol) or dihydrocodeine (in co-dydramol) in each tablet, and the second the amount of paracetamol. Thus, 2 tablets (containing 1 g paracetamol regardless of codeine/ dihydrocodeine dose) can be given up to 6-hourly.

A. Drug choice	Score	Feedback/justification	B. Dose, route, frequency	Score	Feedback/justification
3. TRAMADOL	4	See above	50 MG 6-HOURLY *OR* 4-HOURLY ORAL AS REQUIRED *OR* 100 MG 6-HOURLY ORAL AS REQUIRED	4	This should be on the 'as required' section because the pain is only occasional. Patients are rarely prescribed more than 400 mg per day (i.e. 100 mg 6-hourly at most).
4. MORPHINE SULPHATE (not 'ORAMORPH®' (brand name))	0	Using a mild opioid before a strong one is more appropriate; as the question asks for one drug the choice is really between codeine and tramadol.		0	
5. IBUPROFEN, NAPROXEN, DICLOFENAC, INDOMETACIN, CELECOXIB/ ETORICOXIB	0	This patient has a history of peptic ulcer disease; NSAIDs are therefore contraindicated. Note: the selective COX2-inhibitors (e.g. celecoxib) still increase the risk of serious upper gastrointestinal side effects (albeit to a smaller degree).	N/A	0	

Marking guide for A and B.
4 marks: for an optimal answer that cannot be improved.
3 marks: for an answer that is good but is suboptimal on some grounds (e.g. cost-effectiveness, likely adherence).
2 marks: for an answer that is likely to provide benefit but is clearly suboptimal for more than one reason.
1 mark: for an answer that has some justification and deserves some credit.

C. Timing. Candidates will also be given **1 mark for correctly dating** (and timing) the prescription

D. Signature. Candidates will also be given **1 mark for signing** the prescription

For example, the prescription should appear as:

AS REQUIRED MEDICATION							
Drug (Approved name) TRAMADOL		Date					
		Time					
Dose 50 MG	Route ORAL	Route					
Prescriber – sign + print *YOUR SIGNATURE AND NAME*	Start date *TODAY'S DATE*	Given by					
Indication PAIN	Frequency 4-HOURLY MAX	Sign					

Question 10.45 Answer

Note: aminophylline is theophylline plus ethylenediamine (added to increase theophylline's solubility).

A	At toxic levels, aminophylline (a bronchodilator) causes tachycardia and can go on to cause fatal tachyarrhythmias. Tachycardia indicates toxicity, rather than being a useful measure of effectiveness. In practice, aminophylline would be stopped in this situation.
B	Aminophylline has little direct effect on blood pressure and a measure of blood pressure would not allow assessment of therapeutic effect.
C	**Correct:** if the aminophylline infusion is effective the patient's saturations should improve.
D	The target serum level for aminophylline (measured as 'theophylline') is 10–20 µg/mL. A level should be taken 18 hours after commencing treatment unless there are concerns regarding toxicity, in which case it should be done sooner. However, a serum level within the reference range does not necessarily represent clinical efficacy and is not the most appropriate choice.
E	Not relevant in the context of treatment with aminophylline.

DECISION OPTIONS

A	HEART RATE	☐
B	BLOOD PRESSURE	☐
C	OXYGEN SATURATION	✓
D	SERUM THEOPHYLLINE LEVEL	☐
E	GLASGOW COMA SCALE (GCS)	☐

Question 10.46 Answer

A	Consolidation on a chest X-ray can take up to 6 weeks to clear; therefore, this would be unhelpful in the acute stage.
B	**Correct:** successful treatment of the pneumonia will improve gas exchange, hypoxia and therefore the respiratory rate. If oxygen saturations or ABG were options these would be more accurate and specific, but in their absence a respiratory rate is a good marker of improvement.
C	Hypotension occurs in severe infection (septic shock). Resolution of hypotension would indeed be in keeping with the response to antibiotics and it is a useful marker, but it is less specific than respiratory parameters – improvement may reflect IV fluid administration while deterioration could be due to a nonseptic cause (e.g. cardiogenic, hypovolaemic or anaphylactic shock).
D	Crepitations on auscultation would take several days to resolve.
E	Not specifically relevant to the assessment of infection resolution.

DECISION OPTIONS

A	CHEST X-RAY	☐
B	RESPIRATORY RATE	✓
C	BLOOD PRESSURE	☐
D	RESOLUTION OF CREPITATIONS ON AUSCULTATION	☐
E	FLUID BALANCE	☐

Question 10.47 Answer

A	A tacrolimus level should be a trough (not a peak) level.
B	Not relevant in this scenario.
C	A raised tacrolimus level can manifest as a tremor. However, this is a subjective method of assessing whether a level is therapeutic/toxic and not the most appropriate of the options provided. The presence of a tremor should prompt a tacrolimus level.
D	**Correct:** measuring a trough level before the morning or evening dose is the correct way to check a tacrolimus level. At this stage after transplant we would be aiming for a level of 6–10 ng/mL.
E	Although a side-effect of ciclosporin (another calcineurin inhibitor), it would not give any indication of whether serum concentration was therapeutic or toxic.

DECISION OPTIONS

A	TACROLIMUS LEVEL ('PEAK' LEVEL 1 HOUR AFTER MORNING DOSE)	☐
B	SERUM ALT	☐
C	PRESENCE OF TREMOR	☐
D	TACROLIMUS LEVEL ('TROUGH' LEVEL PRIOR TO MORNING DOSE)	✓
E	PRESENCE OF GUM HYPERPLASIA	☐

Question 10.48 Answer

A	Not relevant.
B	**Correct:** the use of antidepressants is associated with suicidal thoughts and behaviour, particularly at the beginning of treatment and patients should be counselled as such.
C	A full blood count would not routinely be required in the monitoring of treatment with selective serotonin reuptake inhibitors (SSRIs).
D	Treatment should continue for at least 4 weeks before an assessment of efficacy is considered (his appointment is in 2 weeks according to the question).
E	A measure of renal function specifically is not routinely required in the monitoring of treatment of SSRIs, although if it included an electrolyte screen, this might be useful in detecting hyponatraemia.

DECISION OPTIONS

A	BLOOD PRESSURE	☐
B	ASSESSMENT FOR SIGNS OF SUICIDAL IDEATION	✓
C	FULL BLOOD COUNT	☐
D	ASSESS FOR EFFICACY	☐
E	SERUM CREATININE	☐

Question 10.49 Answer

A	This patient has DKA triggered by pneumonia. Serum glucose normalizes rapidly after commencing an insulin sliding scale, but this does not necessarily suggest resolution of DKA (i.e. may still be acidotic and ketotic which (along with serum potassium) are the more important facets to monitor).
B	Blood pressure is not specifically useful in the assessment of response to treatment of DKA.
C	Urinary glucose will improve as the patient's serum glucose is normalized, but is not effective in monitoring resolution of ketoacidosis.
D	**Correct:** normalization of serum ketones suggests cessation of ketogenesis and therefore accurate reflection of response to treatment.
E	Urinary output will reflect adequate response to rehydration only.

DECISION OPTIONS

A	SERUM GLUCOSE	☐
B	BLOOD PRESSURE	☐
C	URINARY GLUCOSE	☐
D	SERUM KETONES	✓
E	URINARY OUTPUT	☐

Question 10.50 Answer

A	Normally increased respiration ('increased respiratory drive') is triggered by hypoxia or hypercapnoea. In patients with chronic type 2 respiratory failure (and therefore chronic hypercapnoea) such as those with COPD, hypercapnoea no longer stimulates increased respiration, so they rely on hypoxia. This is why these patients should have lower target oxygen saturations (88–92%), because correcting their hypoxia (to >95%) can lead to a reduction in respiratory rate, subsequent increased hypercapnoea (because it is not being exhaled) and thus acidosis and carbon dioxide (CO_2) narcosis. The latter in particular will impair consciousness level. Beware of the 'sleepy' patient with COPD! Although GCS is therefore important it is not a pragmatic way to monitor oxygen response.
B	Once oxygenation has improved respiratory rate will also improve. While useful, this is not the most effective way to measure treatment response, particularly as it is so nonspecific: respiratory rate may be increased by multiple other factors such as anxiety.
C	Not useful in assessing response to oxygen therapy.
D	**Correct:** response to oxygen therapy can be monitored noninvasively with pulse oximetry and titrated appropriately. In patients with known COPD oxygen saturations of 88–92% should be targeted.
E	Although suitable for measuring serum acidosis, VBG would not accurately reflect arterial oxygen or carbon dioxide levels. If an arterial blood gas were offered, this would be the best option as it would enable monitoring of oxygenation but also detect acidosis if worsening hypercapnoea occurred with improving PaO_2.

DECISION OPTIONS

A	GLASGOW COMA SCALE (GCS)	☐
B	RESPIRATORY RATE	☐
C	BLOOD PRESSURE	☐
D	PULSE OXIMETRY	✓
E	VENOUS BLOOD GAS (VBG)	☐

Question 10.51 Answer

A	Liver function is not required as a baseline test before initiation of an ACE-inhibitor.
B	**Correct:** the initial dose of ramipril is dependent on renal function. This should be established at baseline.
C	Serum creatinine is a sufficient measure of renal function. Measuring urine output would not be practical in a primary care setting.
D	Serum calcium need not be checked at baseline.
E	Reduced white blood cell count is a rare side effect of ACE-inhibitors and it is not necessary to measure at baseline.

DECISION OPTIONS

A	SERUM ALT	☐
B	SERUM CREATININE	✓
C	URINE OUTPUT	☐
D	SERUM CALCIUM	☐
E	WHITE BLOOD CELL COUNT	☐

Question 10.52 Answer

A	**Correct:** pre-dose 'trough' concentrations of vancomycin should be 10–15 mg/L. The reported level is within this range so it would be appropriate to assume, based on the information you have, that no dose change is required. If in doubt look it up in the BNF!
B	See justification for Option A.
C	See justification for Option A.
D	'Post' dose levels are not routinely required for vancomycin.
E	Clearance of vancomycin is principally renal and regular monitoring of liver function is not required during therapy with vancomycin.

DECISION OPTIONS

A	1 G TWICE DAILY IS A SUITABLE DOSE FOR THIS PATIENT	✓
B	1 G TWICE DAILY IS TOO HIGH A DOSE AND SHOULD BE REDUCED	☐
C	1 G TWICE DAILY IS TOO LOW A DOSE AND SHOULD BE INCREASED	☐
D	A 'POST' DOSE LEVEL IS REQUIRED IN ORDER TO ASCERTAIN THE SUITABILITY OF THIS DOSE FOR THIS PATIENT	☐
E	LIVER FUNCTION OUGHT TO BE CHECKED REGULARLY DURING THERAPY WITH VANCOMYCIN	☐

Question 10.53 Answer

ACE-inhibitors are known to cause renal impairment, which can be tricky to spot clinically, and often presents only as 'malaise' so a measure of serum creatinine (and potassium) is necessary before any dose titration.

DECISION OPTIONS

A	SERUM CREATININE	✓
B	NEUTROPHIL COUNT	☐
C	SERUM SODIUM	☐
D	SERUM ALBUMIN	☐
E	SERUM MAGNESIUM	☐

Question 10.54 Answer

The correct answer is amlodipine.

Calcium-channel blockers are noted to cause facial flushing in a minority of patients starting new prescriptions. For some these symptoms diminish, but others fail to tolerate the side effects.

CURRENT PRESCRIPTIONS

Drug name	Dose	Route	Freq.	
LISINOPRIL	5 MG	ORAL	DAILY	☐
AMLODIPINE	5 MG	ORAL	DAILY	✓
BENDROFLUMETHIAZIDE	2.5 MG	ORAL	DAILY	☐
PARACETAMOL	1 G	ORAL	6-HOURLY	☐
CODEINE	30 MG	ORAL	6-HOURLY	☐

Question 10.55 Answer

The correct answer is diclofenac.

Diclofenac (and the other NSAIDs) can cause acute kidney injury, usually by affecting renal haemodynamics or through a condition known as acute interstitial nephritis. Again, NSAID-induced nephrotoxicity is more likely to occur in patients with pre-existing renal impairment.

Take care when co-prescribing NSAIDs and ACE-inhibitors.

CURRENT PRESCRIPTIONS				
Drug name	**Dose**	**Route**	**Freq.**	
CO-AMOXICLAV	625 MG	IV	8-HOURLY	☐
PARACETAMOL	1 G	ORAL	6-HOURLY	☐
OMEPRAZOLE	20 MG	ORAL	DAILY	☐
VITAMIN B	1 TABLET	ORAL	DAILY	☐
DICLOFENAC	100 MG	PR	DAILY	✓

Question 10.56 Answer

The correct answer is co-dydramol, which contains dihydrocodeine (an opioid).

All opioids (including codeine, morphine and, to a lesser extent, tramadol) slow transit through the bowel; compounding this constipating effect is the increased time for reabsorption of water from the stool rendering the stool dehydrated and thus less mobile through peristalsis. Postoperative inactivity may have initially contributed to constipation too.

CURRENT PRESCRIPTIONS				
Drug name	**Dose**	**Route**	**Freq.**	
CO-DYDRAMOL 10/500	2 TABLETS	ORAL	6-HOURLY	✓
IBUPROFEN	400 MG	ORAL	8-HOURLY	☐
AMLODIPINE	5 MG	ORAL	DAILY	☐
TRIMETHOPRIM	200 MG	ORAL	12-HOURLY	☐
CYCLIZINE	50 MG	ORAL	AS REQUIRED	☐

Question 10.57 Answer

The correct answer is cyclizine.

These are antimuscarinic side effects which can also include urinary retention, constipation, blurred vision, dry mouth and GI disturbances. Note: she should not really be taking cyclizine as she has heart failure and it can worsen fluid retention; metoclopramide would be a more appropriate choice.

CURRENT PRESCRIPTIONS

Drug name	Dose	Route	Freq.	
LISINOPRIL	5 MG	ORAL	DAILY	☐
CYCLIZINE	50 MG	ORAL	8-HOURLY	✓
MORPHINE SULPHATE 10 MG/5 ML	5 MG	ORAL	8-HOURLY AS REQUIRED	☐
ASPIRIN	75 MG	ORAL	DAILY	☐
CARVEDILOL	6.25 MG	ORAL	DAILY	☐

Question 10.58 Answer

Give vitamin K by slow IV injection is the correct answer.
It could be given by mouth if there was no bleeding.

DECISION OPTIONS

A	CONTINUE WARFARIN	☐
B	GIVE VITAMIN K BY MOUTH	☐
C	GIVE VITAMIN K BY SLOW IV INJECTION	✓
D	WITHHOLD 1–2 DOSES OF WARFARIN AND RESTART AT LOWER DOSE	☐
E	GIVE PROTAMINE BY SLOW IV INJECTION	☐

Question 10.59 Answer

Administration of oral chlorphenamine is correct.

Co-amoxiclav contains penicillin; this patient has had an allergic reaction to another penicillin-containing antibiotic rendering this an unsuitable option.

Inducing emesis would not be effective at relieving symptoms particularly as piperacillin/tazobactam can only be given intravenously.

Administering an antihistamine will alleviate the pruritis and acute presentation of the mild allergic reaction.

As there is no evidence of anaphylaxis the adrenaline and IV steroids are not indicated.

DECISION OPTIONS

A	SWITCH TO CO-AMOXICLAV	☐
B	ATTEMPT TO INDUCE EMESIS	☐
C	ADMINISTER ORAL CHLORPHENAMINE	✓
D	ADMINISTER IV HYDROCORTISONE	☐
E	ADMINISTER IM ADRENALINE	☐

Question 10.60 Answer

A conscious patient should be given 10–20 g of glucose by mouth for example using orange juice or biscuits.

Glucose 50% is not recommended due to the high risk of extravasation injury and because administration is difficult due to the high viscosity.

Drug-induced hypoglycaemia should be managed in hospital as the hypoglycaemic effects of these drugs can persist for many hours.

1 mg of IM/IV/SC glucagon is used with unconscious patients, generally when no IV access is available (precluding the use of IV dextrose).

Metformin is less likely to cause hypoglycaemia than the sulphonylureas.

DECISION OPTIONS

A	A CONSCIOUS PATIENT COULD BE GIVEN ORANGE JUICE	✓
B	AN UNCONSCIOUS PATIENT SHOULD BE GIVEN AN IV INFUSION OF 50% GLUCOSE	☐
C	DRUG-INDUCED HYPOGLYCAEMIA CAN BE MANAGED WITHOUT HOSPITAL ADMISSION	☐
D	UNCONSCIOUS PATIENTS SHOULD BE GIVEN 50 MG OF IV GLUCAGON	☐
E	DRUG-INDUCED HYPOGLYCAEMIA IS LESS LIKELY TO OCCUR IN PATIENTS ON SULPHONYLUREAS THAN IN PATIENTS ON METFORMIN	☐

Question 10.61 Prescription review item worth 4 marks

CASE PRESENTATION

A 76-year-old patient presents to his GP complaining of a cough. He is not short of breath and denies chest pain. Examination is unremarkable. The GP sends routine bloods (see below) and a CXR is normal.

PAST MEDICAL HISTORY

Hypertension, hyperlipidaemia and gout. His current regular medicines are listed (see current prescriptions chart).

	Value	Normal range		Value	Normal range
Na	136 mmol/L	(135–145 mmol/L)	Ur	3.8 mmol/L	(3–7 mmol/L)
K	5.6 mmol/L	(3.5–5.0 mmol/L)	Cr	118 µmol/L	(60–125 µmol/L)
CRP	<3 mg/L				

A: Select the *one* drug that is most likely to cause the cough. Mark it with a tick in column A.

B: Select the *one* drug that is most likely to cause the electrolyte disturbance. Mark it with a tick in column B.

CURRENT PRESCRIPTIONS

Drug name	Dose	Route	Freq.	A	B
SIMVASTATIN	10 MG	ORAL	NIGHTLY	☐	☐
BISOPROLOL	10 MG	ORAL	DAILY	☐	☐
ALLOPURINOL	100 MG	ORAL	DAILY	☐	☐
LISINOPRIL	10 MG	ORAL	DAILY	☑	☑
PARACETAMOL	1 G	ORAL	6-HOURLY	☐	☐
BENDROFLUMETHIAZIDE	2.5 MG	ORAL	DAILY	☐	☐

Question 10.62 Prescription review item worth 4 marks

CASE PRESENTATION

A 58-year-old male with a history of osteoarthritis, hypertension and gout presents to A&E complaining of increasing indigestion over 1 month. His regular medications are listed (see current prescriptions). Examination reveals epigastric tenderness. His bloods are as follows:

	Value	Normal range		Value	Normal range
Na	142 mmol/L	(135–145 mmol/L)	Cr	232 µmol/L	(60–125 µmol/L)
K	5.4 mmol/L	(3.5–5.0 mmol/L)	Hb	85 g/L	(135–175 g/L (male))
Ur	14 mmol/L	(3–7 mmol/L)			

A: Select the *two* prescriptions that are most likely to be contributing to the indigestion. Mark with ticks in column A.

B: Select the *two* prescriptions most likely to be responsible for the renal failure. Mark with ticks in column B.

CURRENT PRESCRIPTIONS

Drug name	Dose	Route	Freq.	A	B
PARACETAMOL	1 G	ORAL	6-HOURLY	☐	☐
IBUPROFEN	200 MG	ORAL	8-HOURLY	☑	☑
PREDNISOLONE	30 MG	ORAL	DAILY	☑	☐
RAMIPRIL	2.5 MG	ORAL	DAILY	☐	☑
ALLOPURINOL	100 MG	ORAL	DAILY	☐	☐

Question 10.63 Prescription review item worth 4 marks

CASE PRESENTATION

You are performing medicines reconciliation with a pharmacist for all new inpatients. A 61-year-old woman has been admitted with cholecystitis and is improving with medical management (i.e. antibiotics and IV fluids). She has a background of Parkinson's disease, hypertension and mild heart failure.
Please review her drug chart.

Question: Please identify the *four* drug errors to address in this patient with ticks in column A.

CURRENT PRESCRIPTIONS

Drug name	Dose	Route	Freq.	A
CO-BENELDOPA 12.5/50	2 TABLETS	ORAL	12-HOURLY	☐
BISOPROLOL	10 MG	ORAL	DAILY	☐
BENDROFLUMETHIAZIDE	2.5 MG	ORAL	NIGHTLY	☑
LISINOPRIL	10 MG	ORAL	NIGHTLY	☐
ASPIRIN	75 MG	ORAL	DAILY	☐
PARACETAMOL	1 G	ORAL	AS REQUIRED UP TO 4-HOURLY	☑
DOMPERIDONE	10 MG	ORAL	6-HOURLY	☐
METOCLOPRAMIDE	10 MG	ORAL	8-HOURLY	☑
CYCLIZINE	50 MG	IV	6-HOURLY	☑

Question 10.64 Prescription review item worth 4 marks

CASE PRESENTATION

A 36-year-old is admitted to hospital with a urinary tract infection. She has a history of rheumatoid arthritis and longstanding atrial fibrillation (AF); she is also allergic to penicillin. The admitting doctor has wisely avoided trimethoprim in light of her concurrent use of methotrexate.

Question: Please identify the *four* drug errors in this patient and mark with ticks in the column provided.

CURRENT PRESCRIPTIONS

Drug name	Dose	Route	Freq.	
CO-CODAMOL 8/500	2 TABLETS	ORAL	4-HOURLY	☐
METHOTREXATE	10 MG	ORAL	DAILY _weekly_	☑
ZOPICLONE	7.5 MG	ORAL	NIGHTLY	☐
LANSOPRAZOLE	30 MG	ORAL	DAILY	☐
ASPIRIN	300 MG	ORAL	DAILY	☑
IBUPROFEN	400 MG	ORAL	8-HOURLY	☑
CO-AMOXICLAV	625 MG	ORAL	8-HOURLY	☑

Question 10.65 Prescription review item worth 4 marks

CASE PRESENTATION

A 72-year-old woman is admitted by her GP as she has not opened her bowels for 5 days. She denies any pain and feels well in herself.

PAST MEDICAL HISTORY

Hypertension, osteoarthritis, hypercholesterolaemia. Her medicines are listed (see current prescriptions chart).

	Value	Normal range		Value	Normal range
Na	136 mmol/L	(135–145 mmol/L)	Ur	4.2 mmol/L	(3–7 mmol/L)
K	2.7 mmol/L	(3.5–5.0 mmol/L)	Cr	73 µmol/L	(60–125 µmol/L)

A: Select the *one* prescription that is the most likely cause of the electrolyte disturbance and mark with a tick in column A.

B: Select the *three* prescriptions which should be stopped and mark with ticks in column B.

CURRENT PRESCRIPTIONS

Drug name	Dose	Route	Freq.	A	B
BENDROFLUMETHIAZIDE	2.5 MG	ORAL	DAILY	☑	☑
PARACETAMOL	500 MG	ORAL	6-HOURLY	☐	☑
SIMVASTATIN	20 MG	ORAL	NIGHTLY	☐	☐
AMLODIPINE	5 MG	ORAL	DAILY	☐	☐
CODEINE	30 MG	ORAL	6-HOURLY	☐	☑
LISINOPRIL	10 MG	ORAL	NIGHTLY	☐	☐
CO-CODAMOL 30/500	2 TABLETS	ORAL	AS REQUIRED UP TO 6-HOURLY	☐	☑

Question 10.66 Prescription review item worth 4 marks

CASE PRESENTATION

A 69-year-old woman presents to A&E complaining of a burning upper abdominal pain for 4 weeks.

PAST MEDICAL HISTORY

Chronic headaches (of undiagnosed cause), hypertension and polymyalagia rheumatica. Her current regular medicines are listed (see current prescriptions chart). Examination reveals epigastric tenderness. Her bloods are as follows:

	Value	Normal range		Value	Normal range
Na	139 mmol/L	(135–145 mmol/L)	Cr	301 µmol/L	(60–125 µmol/L)
K	5.6 mmol/L ↑	(3.5–5.0 mmol/L)	Hb	91 g/L	(135–175 g/L (male))
Ur	13 mmol/L	(3–7 mmol/L)			

A: Select the *two* prescriptions that are most likely to be contributing to the indigestion and mark with ticks in column A.

B: Select the *two* prescriptions most likely to be responsible for the deranged blood results and mark with ticks in column B.

CURRENT PRESCRIPTIONS

Drug name	Dose	Route	Freq.	A	B
BUMETANIDE	2 MG	ORAL	DAILY	☐	☐
NAPROXEN	250 MG	ORAL	8-HOURLY	☑	☐
DEXAMETHASONE	0.5 MG	ORAL	DAILY	☑	☐
RAMIPRIL	2.5 MG	ORAL	DAILY	☐	☑
PARACETAMOL	1 G	ORAL	6-HOURLY	☐	☐

Question 10.67 Prescription review item worth 4 marks

CASE PRESENTATION

An 89-year-old male is admitted with breathlessness, pleuritic chest pain and agitation. His PMH includes mild heart failure, arthritis and 'a bad back'. A CXR confirms pneumonia and he is commenced on co-amoxiclav and clonazepam to control his agitation on the ward. He requests diclofenac for his back which is very painful. The next day he is much better, but he subsequently becomes very drowsy and only rouses to pain. You note his respiratory rate is very slow. You perform some blood tests.

	On admission	Now	Normal range			On admission	Now	Normal range
Na	142 mmol/L	146 mmol/L	(135–145 mmol/L)	Cr		91 µmol/L	398 µmol/L↑	(60–125 µmol/L)
K	3.2 mmol/L	5.2 mmol/L↑	(3.5–5.0 mmol/L)	WCC		13.7 × 10⁹/L	13.1 × 10⁹/L	(4–11 × 10⁹/L)
Ur	7.1 mmol/L	14 mmol/L↑	(3–7 mmol/L)					

A: Please identify which *two* drugs may be responsible for the deteriorating biochemistry results. Mark them with ticks in column A.

B: Please identify which *two* drugs may be responsible for the reduced conscious level after treatment. Mark them with ticks in column B.

CURRENT PRESCRIPTIONS

Drug name	Dose	Route	Freq.	A	B
COCODAMOL 8/500	2 TABLETS	ORAL	6-HOURLY	☐	☑
CLONAZEPAM	2 MG	ORAL	DAILY	☐	☑
LISINOPRIL	10 MG	ORAL	NIGHTLY	☑	☐
ASPIRIN	75 MG	ORAL	DAILY	☐	☐
DICLOFENAC	25 MG	ORAL	8-HOURLY	☑	☐
CO-AMOXICLAV	625 MG	ORAL	8-HOURLY	☐	☐

Question 10.68 Prescription review item worth 4 marks

CASE PRESENTATION

A 71-year-old patient is admitted with shortness of breath and chest tightness. His medical history includes depression and asthma. He has been recently diagnosed with mild hypertension but is not sure which two of his drugs were started a month ago to treat it. He is confident that he has been taking aspirin for years. He is allergic to penicillin and does not smoke. His GP gave him antibiotics and analgesia 3 days ago believing his symptoms were due to a chest infection but none of these have helped.

When you see him his respiratory rate is 32/min, SaO$_2$ 91% (on air) and he is afebrile. He has a widespread expiratory wheeze and a new maculopapular rash over his legs. There is no oedema.

His routine bloods and chest X-ray are unremarkable.

A: Select the *three* drugs that should be stopped to improve his breathing. Mark them with ticks in column A.

B: Select the *one* drug which should be continued at a different dose. Mark it with a tick in column B.

CURRENT PRESCRIPTIONS

Drug name	Dose	Route	Freq.	A	B
CITALOPRAM	40 MG	ORAL	DAILY	☑	☐
AMLODIPINE	5 MG	ORAL	DAILY	☐	☐
ASPIRIN	75 MG	ORAL	DAILY	☐	☐
ENALAPRIL	10 MG	ORAL	DAILY	☐	☑
PROPRANOLOL	40 MG	ORAL	8-HOURLY	☑	☐
AMOXICILLIN	500 MG	ORAL	8-HOURLY	☑	☐
IBUPROFEN	200 MG	ORAL	AS REQUIRED UP TO 8-HOURLY	☑	☐

Question 10.69 Data interpretation item worth 2 marks

CASE PRESENTATION

A 73-year-old patient was admitted with pneumonia earlier today and has started antibiotics. The nurses call you because he has become oliguric (10 mL urine output in the last 2 hours). He is not managing oral intake as he feels nauseated. Blood tests from admission are below:

	Value	Normal range		Value	Normal range
Na	140 mmol/L	(135–145 mmol/L)	Ur	9 mmol/L	(3–7 mmol/L)
K	5.1 mmol/L	(3.5–5.0 mmol/L)	Cr	85 µmol/L	(60–125 µmol/L)

HR 92 b.p.m. BP 132/93 mmHg. SaO$_2$ 100% (on 40% oxygen). RR 26/min. Temp. 38.2°C.

Question: Select the *most appropriate* option and mark it with a tick.

DECISION OPTIONS

A	ENCOURAGE ORAL INTAKE	☐
B	1 L GELOFUSINE IV OVER 1 HOUR	☐
C	500 ML GELOFUSINE IV OVER 1 HOUR	☐
D	1 L 5% DEXTROSE WITH 20 mmol KCL IV OVER 2 HOURS	☐
E	1 L 0.9% SALINE OVER 2 HOURS	☐

Question 10.70 Data interpretation item worth 2 marks

CASE PRESENTATION

An 80-year-old is admitted for a hemicolectomy for bowel cancer. You see him the evening before and have been told he is due surgery at 8 a.m. so should be nil by mouth from midnight. His medical history includes type 2 diabetes (diet controlled) and bowel cancer. His routine blood test results from today are below.

	Value	Normal range		Value	Normal range
Na	146 mmol/L	(135–145 mmol/L)	Ur	5 mmol/L	(3–7 mmol/L)
K	4.1 mmol/L	(3.5–5.0 mmol/L)	Cr	76 µmol/L	(60–125 µmol/L)
Blood glucose (random):	7.2 mmol/L				

Question: Select the *most appropriate* option for the first bag of maintenance fluids to be taken from midnight and mark it with a tick.

DECISION OPTIONS

A	1 L 5% DEXTROSE OVER 4 HOURS	☐
B	1 L 10% DEXTROSE OVER 8 HOURS	☐
C	1 L 5% DEXTROSE WITH 20 MMOL KCL OVER 12 HOURS	☐
D	1 L 0.9% SALINE WITH 20 MMOL KCL OVER 8 HOURS	☐
E	1 L GELOFUSINE OVER 12 HOURS	☐

Question 10.71 Data interpretation item worth 2 marks

CASE PRESENTATION

You see a 62-year-old woman who has complained of increasing constipation. She denies fatigue, dyspnoea, dizziness or chest pain. You perform a digital rectal examination and palpate a hard mass in her anal wall. She reports that her stool contains significant amounts of blood. Her blood results are below.

	Value	Normal range		Value	Normal range
WCC	8×10^9/L	$(4–11 \times 10^9$/L)	Ur	6 mmol/L	(3–7 mmol/L)
Neut.	6×10^9/L	$(2–8 \times 10^9$/L)	Cr	112 µmol/L	(60–125 µmol/L)
Lymph.	1.1×10^9/L	$(1–4.8 \times 10^9$/L)	Na	139 mmol/L	(135–145 mmol/L)
Hb	103 g/L ✓	(120–150 g/L (female))	K	4.5 mmol/L	(3.5–5.0 mmol/L)
MCV	71 fL ↓	(76–99 fL)			

non det.

You explain that she requires sigmoidoscopy and that you are concerned about bowel cancer. You also explain that she has anaemia which may be due to her blood loss. You perform haematinics and review her in clinic with the results:

	Value	Normal range
Ferritin	7 ng/mL	(15–200 ng/mL) ↓
Folate	542 ng/mL	(200–600 ng/mL)
Vitamin B$_{12}$	673 ng/mL	(160–950 ng/L) ✓

She has had a chance to research anaemia and requests a blood transfusion.

Question: Select the *most appropriate* option for management of this patient's anaemia and mark it with a tick.

DECISION OPTIONS

A	TRANSFUSE 1 UNIT OF BLOOD	☐
B	START FERROUS SULFATE 200 MG 8-HOURLY ORAL PLUS LOPERAMIDE	☐
C	START FERROUS SULFATE 200 MG 8-HOURLY ORAL UNTIL HB NORMAL	☐
D	START FERROUS SULFATE 200 MG 8-HOURLY ORAL UNTIL HB NORMAL THEN FOR FURTHER 3 MONTHS	☑
E	GIVE IV IRON	☐

Question 10.72 Data interpretation item worth 2 marks

CASE PRESENTATION

A 77-year-old male is admitted with 3 days of breathlessness and a productive cough. He has motor neurone disease and longstanding diabetes. He is allergic to penicillin. His respiratory rate is 24/min, SaO$_2$ 91% (on air) and he has coarse crepitations at his right base. He has an extensive smoking history.

You have requested a temperature. A CXR is shown here.

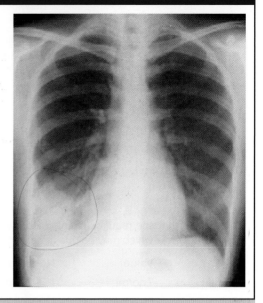

Question: Select the *most appropriate* acute treatment option and mark it with a tick.

DECISION OPTIONS

A	FUROSEMIDE 20 MG ORAL	☐
B	CO-AMOXICLAV 625 MG ORAL	☐
C	BUMETANIDE 1 MG ORAL	☐
D	DOXYCYCLINE 200 MG ORAL	☑
E	PREDNISOLONE 30 MG ORAL	☐

Question 10.73 Data interpretation item worth 2 marks

CASE PRESENTATION

A 73-year-old man is an inpatient following resection of a left temporal glioma. He presented with seizures which transformed to status epilepticus and was loaded with phenytoin preoperatively. He has had no seizures since. He has been on a stable dose (300 mg oral daily) for 3 weeks now. He is also on a reducing course of dexamethasone (currently 4 mg 12-hourly oral). On your ward round today he reports sore gums and his wife thinks his voice has been sounding mildly slurry for the last week. His chest is clear, he has no headache, neck stiffness or dysuria.

You send some routine blood tests:

	Value	Normal range		Value	Normal range
WCC	16×10^9/L	$(4–11 \times 10^9$/L)	Ur	5 mmol/L	(3–7 mmol/L)
Neut.	15×10^9/L	$(2–8 \times 10^9$/L)	Cr	97 µmol/L	(60–125 µmol/L)
Lymph.	1.0×10^9/L	$(1–4.8 \times 10^9$/L)	Na	139 mmol/L	(135–145 mmol/L)
Hb	140 g/L	(135–175 g/L (male))	K	4.1 mmol/L	(3.5–5.0 mmol/L)
MCV	91 fL	(76–99 fL)	CRP	2 mg/L	(<5 mg/L)
Phenytoin	73 µmol/L	(40–80 µmol/L)			

Urinalysis: normal

Question: Select the *most appropriate* treatment option and mark it with a tick.

DECISION OPTIONS

A	CO-AMOXICLAV 625 MG ORAL 8-HOURLY	☐
B	TRIMETHOPRIM 200 MG ORAL 12-HOURLY	☐
C	INCREASE PHENYTOIN TO 350 MG ORAL DAILY	☐
D	DECREASE PHENYTOIN TO 250 MG ORAL DAILY	☒
E	OMIT PHENYTOIN FOR 3 DAYS THEN CONTINUE SAME DOSE	☐

Question 10.74 Data interpretation item worth 2 marks

CASE PRESENTATION

A 73-year-old patient is admitted with diarrhoea and vomiting after a recent course of ciprofloxacin for a urinary tract infection. He is tachycardic (118 b.p.m.), normotensive and has reduced skin turgor.
His blood results are as follows:

	Value	Normal range		Value	Normal range
Na	152 mmol/L	(135–145 mmol/L)	Ur	15 mmol/L	(3–7 mmol/L)
K	3.5 mmol/L	(3.5–5.0 mmol/L)	Cr	119 µmol/L	(60–125 µmol/L)

He has had stool cultures taken. You suspect he has *Clostridium difficile* gastroenteritis following antibiotics, but your registrar advises you to wait for the stool culture results before starting definitive treatment. What treatment would you recommend in the meantime?

DECISION OPTIONS

A	ENCOURAGE ORAL FLUIDS	☐
B	GIVE 1 L 0.9% SALINE WITH 20 MMOL KCL OVER 12 HOURS	☐
C	GIVE 1 L 5% DEXTROSE WITH 20 MMOL KCL OVER 12 HOURS	☐
D	GIVE 1 L 5% DEXTROSE WITH 20 MMOL KCL OVER 4 HOURS	☒
E	GIVE 1 L 5% DEXTROSE WITH 40 MMOL KCL OVER 1 HOUR	☐

CASE PRESENTATION

A 45-year-old obese gentleman attends his GP complaining of feeling tired all the time. His random blood sugar is 11.9 mmol/L. Following this his GP does some blood tests that show the following:

	Value	Normal range		Value	Normal range
Na	135 mmol/L	(135–145 mmol/L)	Cr	85 µmol/L	(60–125 µmol/L)
K	4.5 mmol/L	(3.5–5.0 mmol/L)	Fasting glucose	8 mmol/L	
Ur	6 mmol/L	(3–7 mmol/L)			

Question: Select the *most appropriate* management option at this stage and mark it with a tick.

DECISION OPTIONS

A	GLICLAZIDE 40 MG ORAL ONCE DAILY	☐
B	MIXTARD 30® INSULIN (30% SOLUBLE AND 70% ISOPHANE) S/C TWICE DAILY	☐
C	REVIEW BY DIETICIAN AND WEIGHT LOSS REGIMEN	☑
D	LONG ACTING INSULIN (GLARGINE) S/C ONCE DAILY	☐
E	METFORMIN 500 MG ORAL TWICE DAILY	☐

Question 10.76 Planning management item worth 2 marks

CASE PRESENTATION

A 75-year-old female is admitted under the surgical team with a 12 hour history of rectal bleeding.
On clinical exam her abdomen is soft with very mild left iliac fossa tenderness. There is neither rebound tenderness nor guarding. Bowel sounds were active. Rectal exam reveals fresh blood with no evidence of palpable hemorrhoids. She is pale and clinically dehydrated. Blood pressure is 80/70 mmHg.
Initial blood tests show:

	Value	Normal range		Value	Normal range
Hb	75 g/L	(120–150 g/L (female))	Ur	7 mmol/L	(3–7 mmol/L)
Na	140 mmol/L	(135–145 mmol/L)	Cr	85 µmol/L	(60–125 µmol/L)
K	4.5 mmol/L	(3.5–5.0 mmol/L)	Clotting is normal.		

Blood is being cross-matched and will be ready in 1 hour.

Question: Select the *most appropriate* management option at this stage and mark it with a tick.

DECISION OPTIONS

A	GIVE 2 UNITS OF CROSS-MATCHED PACKED RED CELLS OVER 1 HOUR EACH	☐
B	1 L 5% DEXTROSE IV OVER 4 HOURS	☐
C	1 L 0.9% SALINE IV STAT.	☐
D	4 UNITS OF FRESH FROZEN PLASMA (FFP) IV STAT.	☐
E	1 L 0.9% SALINE IV OVER 12 HOURS	☐

Question 10.77 Planning management item worth 2 marks

CASE PRESENTATION

A 40-year-old female with type 1 diabetes is admitted electively for a vaginal hysterectomy for fibroids. Postoperatively she is commenced back on her standard basal-bolus regimen, but is persistently nauseated and therefore not eating or drinking much. You are asked to see her because the nursing staff notice that she is drowsy.

On clinical exam her GCS is 11/15. The remainder of her clinical examination is unremarkable. Her random blood sugar is 1.5 mmol/L. The nursing staff have inserted a cannula and commenced her on 28% oxygen via a venturi mask and inserted an intravenous cannula.

Question: Select the *most appropriate* management option at this stage and mark it with a tick.

DECISION OPTIONS

A	120 ML LUCOZADE® ORALLY	☐
B	1 MG INTRAMUSCULAR GLUCAGON	☐
C	1 L 5% DEXTROSE IV OVER 8 HOURS	☐
D	40% OXYGEN VIA VENTURI MASK	☐
E	100 ML 20% DEXTROSE INTRAVENOUSLY	☐

Question 10.78 Planning management item worth 2 marks

CASE PRESENTATION

A 25-year-old male is admitted under the gastroenterology team with increasing frequency of stools (more than 6 times per day) with fresh blood mixed within. He has a known history of ulcerative colitis and is usually on mesalazine.

On clinical examination his abdomen is soft and moderately tender in the left iliac fossa. There is no evidence of peritonitis and bowel sounds are scanty but present. He has dry mucous membranes, blood pressure is 100/70 mmHg and heart rate is 105 b.p.m.; he is afebrile. Abdominal X-ray shows a normal bowel gas pattern with no evidence of obstruction or dilatation. Blood tests are unremarkable with normal inflammatory markers.

Question: Select the *most appropriate* management option at this stage and mark it with a tick.

DECISION OPTIONS

A	HYDROCORTISONE 100 MG IV 6-HOURLY	☐
B	ENSURE PATIENT IS DRINKING 4 L/DAY	☐
C	1 L 5% DEXTROSE IV OVER 12 HOURS	☐
D	CEFUROXIME 1.5 G/6-HOURLY AND METRONIDAZOLE 500 MG/8-HOURLY IV	☐
E	PREDNISOLONE 30 MG ONCE DAILY ✓	☐

Question 10.79 Planning management item worth 2 marks

CASE PRESENTATION

A 70-year-old female is admitted to A&E with a 3-day history of diarrhoea and vomiting. Her past medical history includes hypertension for which she takes ramipril 10 mg once daily.

She is clinically dehydrated and the remainder of her clinical examination is unremarkable. An ECG shows tall, tented T-waves. Blood tests show:

	Value	Normal range
Na	140 mmol/L	(135–145 mmol/L)
K	6.5 mmol/L	(3.5–5.0 mmol/L)
Ur	20 mmol/L	(3–7 mmol/L)
Cr	198 µmol/L	(60–125 µmol/L)

She is passing moderate amounts of dark urine.

Question: Select the *most appropriate* management option at this stage and mark it with a tick.

DECISION OPTIONS

A	10 ML OF 10% CALCIUM GLUCONATE IV	☑
B	REDUCE RAMIPRIL TO 5 MG ONCE DAILY	☐
C	CALCIUM RESONIUM 15 MG ORALLY 8-HOURLY	☐
D	10 UNITS ACTRAPID® IN 100 ML OF 20% DEXTROSE	☐
E	1 L 0.9% SALINE IV OVER 6 HOURS	☐

Question 10.80 Planning management item worth 2 marks

CASE PRESENTATION

A 54-year-old female is admitted to A&E with central crushing chest pain with radiation to her left arm and jaw. It started at rest. She smokes 20 cigarettes per day and takes amlodipine 5 mg once daily for hypertension.

Her clinical exam is unremarkable, except for breathlessness at rest. Blood pressure is 170/70 mmHg and heart rate 90 b.p.m.

Chest X-ray is unremarkable with no evidence of pulmonary oedema. ECG reveals ST depression in II, III and a VF with T-wave inversion in V4-V6. A troponin-I is raised at 1.79 ng/mL. Two puffs of GTN are given sublingually and high-flow oxygen administered via facemask. She is now pain free.

Question: Select the *most appropriate* management option at this stage and mark it with a tick.

DECISION OPTIONS

A	ISOSORBIDE MONONITRATE 10 MG TWICE DAILY ORAL	☐
B	ASPIRIN 300 MG AND CLOPIDOGREL 300 MG ONCE ORALLY	☑
C	GTN INFUSION 50 MG: 1–10 ML PER HOUR IV	☐
D	MORPHINE SULPHATE 5 MG IV	☐
E	DISCHARGE HOME	☐

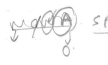

Question 10.81 Planning management item worth 2 marks

CASE PRESENTATION

An 80-year-old female is admitted with acute shortness of breath and palpitations for 3 days. She has no past medical history except hypertension and asthma.

Respiratory examination is unremarkable and no murmurs are heard. Heart rate is approximately 120 b.p.m. Blood pressure is 150/70 mmHg. She is notably breathless at rest. Her ECG is shown.

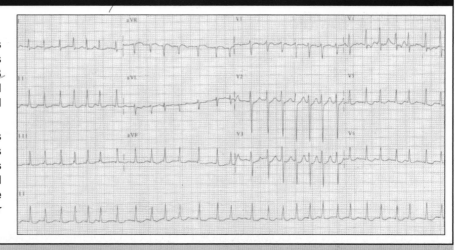

Question: Select the *most appropriate* management option at this stage and mark with a tick.

DECISION OPTIONS

A	FLECAINIDE 50 MG ORALLY	☐
B	DC CARDIOVERSION	☐
C	DIGOXIN 500 MICROGRAMS IV	☐
D	ENOXAPARIN 1.5 MG/KG S/C DAILY	☐
E	BISOPROLOL 5 MG ORALLY	☐

Question 10.82 Planning management item worth 2 marks

CASE PRESENTATION

A 75-year-old female is admitted under the ear, nose and throat team with heavy epistaxis. Her nose is packed. Her past medical history includes atrial fibrillation (AF) for which she takes warfarin.

On clinical examination she looks well, is not breathless and denies fatigue. Blood pressure is 140/70 mmHg and heart rate is 60 b.p.m.

Blood tests reveal:

	Value	Normal range		Value	Normal range
Hb	75 g/L	(135–175 g/L (male))	K	4.5 mmol/L	(3.5–5.0 mmol/L)
Platelets	355 × 10⁹/L	(150–400 × 10⁹/L)	INR	5.3	(2–3)
Cr	85 µmol/L	(60–125 µmol/L)			

Question: Select the *most appropriate* management option at this stage and mark it with a tick.

DECISION OPTIONS

A	VITAMIN K 3 MG IV	☑
B	ONE UNIT PACKED RED CELLS STAT.	☐
C	500 ML COLLOID OVER 30 MINUTES	☐
D	DRIED PROTHROMBIN COMPLEX	☐
E	3 UNITS OF FRESH FROZEN PLASMA (FFP)	☐

Question 10.83 Communicating information item worth 2 marks

CASE PRESENTATION

A 70-year-old lady is seen in A&E for severe lower back pain that has not improved with regular paracetamol. She is commenced on codeine phosphate 30 mg four times daily.

Question: Select the *one* most appropriate piece of information to communicate to the patient and mark it with a tick.

DECISION OPTIONS

A	NO PRECAUTIONS NEED TO BE TAKEN WHILE TAKING CODEINE PHOSPHATE AND DRIVING/OPERATING MACHINERY	☐
B	PRURITIS IS A RARE SIDE EFFECT OF CODEINE PHOSPHATE	☐
C	CONSTIPATION IS A COMMON SIDE EFFECT OF CODEINE AND LAXATIVES SHOULD BE USED IN CONJUNCTION FOR LONG-TERM USAGE	☑
D	CODEINE PHOSPHATE IS A RESPIRATORY STIMULANT AND MAY CAUSE HYPERVENTILATION	☐
E	CODEINE PHOSPHATE CANNOT BE USED IN CONJUNCTION WITH PARACETAMOL	☐

Question 10.84 Communicating information item worth 2 marks

CASE PRESENTATION

A 60-year-old gentleman is admitted under the cardiology team with a non-ST elevation myocardial infarction. Apart from antihypertensives he is also started on simvastatin 40 mg once at night and you are asked to discuss this with him.

Question: Select the *one* most appropriate piece of information to communicate to the patient and mark it with a tick.

DECISION OPTIONS

A	STATINS ARE SAFE TO USE WITH ACTIVE LIVER DISEASE	☐
B	IF MUSCLE CRAMPS DEVELOP THE MEDICATION SHOULD BE STOPPED AND MEDICAL ADVICE SOUGHT	☑
C	STATINS ARE MOST EFFECTIVE WHEN TAKEN IN THE MORNING	☐
D	THERE ARE NO DIETARY RESTRICTIONS WITH STATINS	☐
E	WHEN TAKING CLARITHROMYCIN THE DOSE OF STATINS SHOULD BE DOUBLED	☐

Question 10.85 Communicating information item worth 2 marks

CASE PRESENTATION

An 80-year-old gentleman with known atrial fibrillation and left heart failure is seen in the cardiology clinic for management of his breathlessness. He is commenced on spironolactone 25 mg once daily and you are asked to discuss this medication with him.

Question: Select the *one* most appropriate piece of information to communicate to the patient and mark it with a tick.

DECISION OPTIONS

A	REGULAR BLOOD TESTS ARE REQUIRED WITH SPIRONOLACTONE DUE TO THE RISK OF HYPOKALAEMIA	☐
B	DEHYDRATION IS NOT A SIDE EFFECT OF SPIRONOLACTONE USE	☐
C	A DIET HIGH IN POTASSIUM IS REQUIRED WHEN TAKING SPIRONOLACTONE	☐
D	SPIRONOLACTONE CAN CAUSE EXCESSIVE BREAST TISSUE DEVELOPMENT (GYNAECOMASTIA)	☑
E	SPIRONOLACTONE IS THE FIRST-LINE TREATMENT FOR HEART FAILURE	☐

Question 10.86 Communicating information item worth 2 marks

CASE PRESENTATION

A 50-year-old man is seen by his GP for a 'well-person' check-up and is found to have significantly elevated blood pressure at 190/80 mmHg. He is a smoker with known hypercholesterolaemia. He is commenced on ramipril 2.5 mg once daily and you are asked to discuss this medication with him.

Question: Select the *one* most appropriate piece of information to communicate to the patient and mark it with a tick.

DECISION OPTIONS

A	BLOOD TESTS SHOULD BE PERFORMED REGULARLY DUE TO THE RISK OF HYPOKALAEMIA	☐
B	ACE-INHIBITORS ARE FIRST-LINE THERAPY FOR HYPERTENSION IN PATIENTS WITH AORTIC STENOSIS	☐
C	ANGIO-OEDEMA CAN ONLY BE ATTRIBUTED TO ACE-INHIBITORS IF NEWLY STARTED WITHIN THE LAST 24 HOURS	☐
D	CAUTION SHOULD BE TAKEN WHEN USING ACE-INHIBITORS IN KNOWN CHRONIC KIDNEY DISEASE	☑
E	A DRY COUGH WOULD NOT PRE-EMPT A CHANGE OF MEDICATION	☐

Question 10.87 Communicating information item worth 2 marks

CASE PRESENTATION

A 60-year-old gentleman is admitted under the cardiology team with a non-ST elevation myocardial infarction. Apart from antihypertensives he is also started on simvastatin 40 mg once at night and you are asked to discuss this with him.

Question: Select the *one* most appropriate piece of information to communicate to the patient and mark it with a tick.

DECISION OPTIONS

A	STATINS ARE SAFE TO USE IN ACTIVE LIVER DISEASE	☐
B	IF MUSCLE CRAMPS DEVELOP THE MEDICATION SHOULD BE STOPPED AND MEDICAL ADVICE SOUGHT	☑
C	STATINS ARE MOST EFFECTIVE WHEN TAKEN IN THE MORNING	☐
D	THERE ARE NO DIETARY RESTRICTIONS WITH STATINS	☐
E	WHEN TAKING CLARITHROMYCIN THE DOSE OF STATINS SHOULD BE DOUBLED	☐

Question 10.88 Communicating information item worth 2 marks

CASE PRESENTATION

You are asked to discuss insulin therapy with a patient with a new diagnosis of type 1 diabetes mellitus.

Question: Select the *one* most appropriate piece of information to communicate to the patient and mark it with a tick.

DECISION OPTIONS

A	WHEN UNWELL THE PATIENT'S TOTAL DAILY INSULIN DOSAGE SHOULD BE DECREASED	☐
B	HYPOGLYCAEMIA SHOULD BE TREATED WITH A BOTTLE OF WATER	☐
C	LIPODYSTROPHY IS PREVENTED BY REPEATED USE OF THE SAME INJECTION SITES	☐
D	HBA1C IS A SUITABLE WAY TO MONITOR BLOOD SUGARS FROM DAY TO DAY	☐
E	EXCESSIVE ALCOHOL INTAKE CAN CAUSE HYPOGLYCAEMIA	☑

(handwritten top) 1g u 100 nl
1000 mg u 100 M1

Question 10.89 Calculation skills item worth 2 marks

CASE PRESENTATION

You are asked to give 10 mg chlorphenamine IV to a patient. It is only available as a 1% solution in 1 mL vials.

Calculation: What volume should be administered intravenously? Write your answer in the box.

Answer `1` mL

(handwritten) 1%
1g u 100 mL
1000 g u 100 M1

1 mL

Question 10.90 Calculation skills item worth 2 marks

CASE PRESENTATION

A 78-year-old man was admitted with diverticulitis. On the ward he develops fast atrial fibrillation (AF). You elect to administer a digoxin infusion as a loading dose. It is available as 1 mL vials of 0.025%. You decide to give 500 micrograms as an infusion over 30 minutes.

Calculation: How many vials are in this infusion? Write your answer in the box.

Answer `2 vials / 2mL.`

(handwritten)
1% = 1g
0.025% = 0.025 gms u 100mL

0.025 g = 100 mL
25 mg
25000 mcg = 100 mL
500 mcg = (2 mL)

Question 10.91 Calculation skills item worth 2 marks

CASE PRESENTATION

You use a bleb of lidocaine 2% solution as part of a ring block to anaesthetize a patient's broken finger before attempting a reduction. The nurse records it in the notes and asks you how much lidocaine you have given.

Calculation: How many mg per mL are in a 2% solution of lidocaine?
Write your answer in the box.

Answer `20` mg per mL

(handwritten)
Lido 2%
= 2 g u 100mL
= 2000 mg u 100 mL

20 g 1 mL

You may use a
calculator at any time

Question 10.92 Calculation skills item worth 2 marks

CASE PRESENTATION

A 62-year-old male patient, weighing 75 kg, is given 2 mL of furosemide 50 mg in a 5 mL solution by slow IV injection.

Calculation: What dose (in milligrams) of furosemide was given?

Answer 20 mg

50 mg — 5 mL
? 2 mL

You may use a
calculator at any time

Question 10.93 Calculation skills item worth 2 marks

CASE PRESENTATION

Jean Reed is a 60 kg, 75-year-old patient presenting with symptoms of dysuria and frequency. Her urine dipstick is positive for nitrites, blood and leukocytes. She has a new acute state of confusion and is unable to give a further history, but her daughter thinks she has not passed urine for a few days. Her blood tests indicate normal renal function, a raised white cell count and a CRP of 65. You decide to prescribe one dose of gentamicin before catheterizing her.

Calculation: What dose of gentamicin at 5 mg/kg do you give Jean?

Answer 300 mg

300

You may use a
calculator at any time

Question 10.94 Calculation skills item worth 2 marks

CASE PRESENTATION

You are teaching first year medical students about electrolyte content of intravenous fluids.

Calculation: How many grams of NaCl are in 1000 mL of 0.9% saline?

Answer 9 g/L

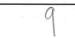

1% = 1 g
0.9 = 0.9 g in 100 mL
9 g 1000 m

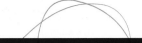

Question 10.95 Calculation skills item worth 2 marks

CASE PRESENTATION

A maxillofacial surgery patient takes 400 mg phenytoin in divided doses daily. After the procedure she is unable to swallow capsules and asks for liquid form. The BNF suggests that 100 mg administered as a capsule is equivalent in therapeutic effect to approximately 92 mg administered as liquid.

Calculation: How many mg of phenytoin liquid do you prescribe?

Answer 435 mg

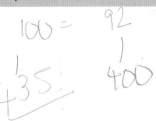

100 = 92

435   400

Question 10.96 Calculation skills item worth 2 marks

CASE PRESENTATION

An 80 kg patient with a diagnosis of Guillain-Barré syndrome is to be commenced on an infusion of intravenous immunoglobulin (IVIg) at 0.4 g/kg/day over 5 days.
The brand the Trust is currently procuring is Flebogamma DIF®; however, it is available in two different concentrations: 5% and 10%.

Calculation: If you were to use the 10% solution, what is the total volume of Flebogamma DIF® that you would need to give to complete this patient's course?

32 g / day for 5 yp ~ 160 g
total.

Answer 1600 mL

10% = 10 g in 100 mL.
160 g ∴ 1600 mL

www.bnf.org

Question 10.97 Prescribing item worth 10 marks

CASE PRESENTATION

You are asked to review a 4-year-old boy who developed otitis media 4 days ago whilst an inpatient awaiting tests for abdominal pain. He is still able to wander around the ward but admits his ear is very sore. He has no allergies. He weighs 20 kg.

Prescribing request: Write a prescription for ONE drug to treat the otitis media. *(Use the hospital antibiotic prescription chart provided.)*

ANTIBIOTICS			Date					
			Time					
Drug (Approved name) AMOXICILLIN			**6**					
			8					
Dose	Frequency	Route PO	**12**					
Prescriber – sign + print		Start date	**14**					
			18					
Indication O.M.		Review/stop date 5 dy	**22**					

You may use the
BNF at any time

BNF

www.bnf.org

Question 10.98 Prescribing item worth 10 marks

CASE PRESENTATION

A 46-year-old patient with myasthenia gravis is diagnosed with moderate severity urge urinary incontinence due to detrusor instability. Pelvic floor exercises have provided partial improvement but she returns to your GP surgery requesting drug therapy.

She has no allergies and is currently taking:

PYRIDOSTIGMINE 30 MG 6-HOURLY ORALLY

PREDNISOLONE 5 MG DAILY ORALLY

Prescribing request: Write a prescription for ONE drug to treat the urge urinary incontinence. *(Use the 'regular drugs' prescription chart.)*

REGULAR MEDICATIONS		Date						
		Time						
Drug (Approved name) *TOLTERODINE*		6						
		8						
Dose *2 mg*	Route *PO*	12						
Prescriber – sign + print	Start date	14						
		18						
Notes	Frequency *bd*	22						

Question 10.99 Prescribing item worth 10 marks

CASE PRESENTATION

An 82-year-old patient complains of constant pain from his arthritic right hip, and has mild diarrhoea after finishing antibiotics for a urinary tract infection. His stool culture is negative and he has no other medical history. His current medication is listed below:

PARACETAMOL 1 G ORAL 6-HOURLY REGULARLY

IBUPROFEN 400 MG ORAL 6-HOURLY REGULARLY

Prescribing request: Write a prescription for ONE additional drug for analgesia. *(Choose between the hospital 'regular medicines' or 'as required' prescription charts provided.)*

REGULAR MEDICATIONS

		Date						
		Time						
Drug (Approved name)		6						
		8						
Dose	Route	12						
Prescriber – sign + print	Start date	14						
		18						
Notes	Frequency	22						

AS REQUIRED

Drug (Approved name)								
		Time						
Dose	Route	Route						
Prescriber – sign + print	Start date	Given by						
Indication	Frequency	Sign						

Question 10.100 Prescribing item worth 10 marks

CASE PRESENTATION

You are the F1 doctor for the ENT surgery. A 3-year-old girl from a traveller family is brought to A&E with stridor, drooling and fever. Your registrar has confirmed the suspicion of epiglottitis and asks you to prescribe appropriate antibiotics. She has no history of any allergies or other medical conditions.

She weighs 20 kg and the A&E doctor has inserted an IV cannula.

Prescribing request: Write a prescription for ONE drug to treat the epiglottitis. *Use the hospital antibiotic prescription chart provided.*

ANTIBIOTICS			Date						
			Time						
Drug (Approved name) *CEFOTAXIME/AMIVIR*			6						
			8						
Dose *1000 mg*	Frequency *8hrly*	Route *IV*	12						
Prescriber – sign + print		Start date	14						
			18						
Indication		Review/stop date	22						

500/kg = 1000

Question 10.101 Prescribing item worth 10 marks

CASE PRESENTATION

A 32-year-old man with no past medical history is seen in A&E following an overdose of paracetamol. The amount was small, he admits it was a 'cry for help' but cannot rule out overdosing again.

He is kept in for a psychiatric review and found to be moderately depressed. He is started on antidepressant therapy while cognitive behavioural therapy is being planned. His partner has agreed to take him home and try to stay with him to ensure he does not self-harm over the next month.

An ECG is normal and his paracetamol level at 5 hours does not require *N*-acetylcysteine treatment.

Prescribing request: Write a prescription for ONE drug to improve his mood. *(Choose between the hospital 'regular medicines' or 'as required' prescription charts provided.)*

REGULAR MEDICATIONS

		Date						
		Time						
Drug (Approved name)		6						
		8						
Dose	Route	12						
Prescriber – sign + print	Start date	14						
		18						
Notes	Frequency	22						

AS REQUIRED MEDICATIONS

		Date						
		Time						
Drug (Approved name)								
		Date						
Dose	Route	Time						
Prescriber – sign + print	Start date	Route						
		Given by						
Indication	Frequency	Sign						

Question 10.102 Prescribing item worth 10 marks

CASE PRESENTATION

A 26-year-old woman has suffered from generalised anxiety disorder (GAD) for 3 years. Education and low-intensity psychological interventions have failed to produce any improvement and she has opted to try drug therapy before trying high intensity psychological intervention.

An ECG is normal.

Prescribing request: Write a prescription for ONE drug for long-term management of anxiety. *(Choose between the hospital 'regular medicines' or 'as required' prescription charts provided.)*

REGULAR MEDICATIONS

		Date						
		Time						
Drug (Approved name) *Sertraline*		**6**						
		8						
Dose *25 mg*	**Route** *PO*	**12**						
Prescriber – sign + print *1 week*	**Start date**	**14**						
		18						
Notes	**Frequency** *OD*	**22**						

AS REQUIRED MEDICATIONS

		Date						
		Time						
Drug (Approved name)								
		Date						
Dose	**Route**	Time						
Prescriber – sign + print	**Start date**	Route						
		Given by						
Indication	**Frequency**	Sign						

You may use the
BNF at any time

BNF

www.bnf.org

TEN

Mock Examinations

Question 10.103 Prescribing item worth 10 marks

CASE PRESENTATION

A 72-year-old woman attends her GP with a painful left calf.

ON EXAMINATION

Her left calf is 4cm larger in circumference than her right calf and has distended superficial veins. The entire left leg is oedematous.

INVESTIGATIONS

Hb and MCV normal. Serum biochemistry normal. A Doppler confirms a left-sided deep vein thrombosis (DVT). She weighs 80kg.

Prescribing request: Write a prescription for ONE drug that will rapidly prevent expansion of the DVT. *(Use the hospital 'once-only medicines' prescription chart provided.)*

ONCE ONLY MEDICINES

Date	Time	Medicine (approved name)	Dose	Route	Prescriber – sign + print	Time given	Given by
		DALTEPARIN		S/C			

Question 10.104 Prescribing item worth 10 marks

CASE PRESENTATION

A 25-year-old man with no medical history is admitted the evening before a colonoscopy. He is extremely anxious about the procedure and is not settling with verbal reassurance. Your consultant asks you to prescribe him an oral anxiolytic for tonight only.

Prescribing request: Write a prescription for ONE drug. *(Choose between the hospital 'regular medicines', 'once-only' and 'as required' prescription charts provided.)*

ONCE ONLY MEDICINES

Date	Time	Medicine (approved name)	Dose	Route	Prescriber – sign + print	Time given	Given by

REGULAR MEDICATIONS

	Date				
	Time				
Drug (Approved name)	**6**				
	8				
Dose / Route	**12**				
Prescriber – sign + print / Start date	**14**				
	18				
Notes / Frequency	**22**				

AS REQUIRED MEDICATIONS

	Date				
	Time				
Drug (Approved name) *M* DIAZEPAM	Date				
Dose 500 mg/kg / Route rectal	Time				
Prescriber – sign + print / Start date	Route				
	Given by				
Indication ACUTE ANX / Frequency 1 hrly	Sign				

Question 10.105 Drug monitoring item worth 2 points

CASE PRESENTATION

An 80-year-old female patient is diagnosed with worsening cardiac failure due to left ventricular systolic dysfunction and is commenced on digoxin 62.5 micrograms daily.

Question: Which *one* of the following parameters would be the most important to monitor during treatment with digoxin? Mark it with a tick in the column provided.

DECISION OPTIONS

A	SERUM CREATININE	☐
B	SERUM ALKALINE PHOSPHATASE	☐
C	CHEST X-RAY	☐
D	SERUM SODIUM	☐
E	BLOOD PRESSURE	☐

Question 10.106 Drug monitoring item worth 2 points

CASE PRESENTATION

A 23-year-old male patient is commenced on sodium valproate for the management of generalized seizures associated with a low-grade glioma.

Question: Before starting treatment, which *one* of the following parameters would be the most important for you to check? Mark it with a tick in the column provided.

DECISION OPTIONS

A	PANCREATIC AMYLASE	☐
B	SERUM VITAMIN D LEVEL	☐
C	SERUM POTASSIUM	☐
D	ALT	☐
E	SERUM CREATININE	☐

Question 10.107 Drug monitoring item worth 2 points

CASE PRESENTATION

A 46-year-old male patient is reviewed by a consultant psychiatrist, who decides that he should be commenced on clozapine for the treatment of his schizophrenia. He has already failed to respond to two other antipsychotic drugs.

The psychiatrist asks you to ensure that the appropriate monitoring is carried out so that therapy can continue.

Question: Regarding the appropriate monitoring of therapy with clozapine, which one of the following statements is correct? Mark it with a tick in the column provided.

DECISION OPTIONS

A	REGISTRATION WITH A CLOZAPINE MONITORING SERVICE IS RESERVED FOR PATIENTS WITH A BASELINE NEUTROPENIA	☐
B	SERUM CREATININE SHOULD BE CHECKED AT REGULAR INTERVALS THROUGHOUT THE DURATION OF THERAPY	☐
C	FULL BLOOD COUNT MUST BE CHECKED WEEKLY FOR THE FIRST 18 WEEKS	☑
D	IF LEUKOCYTE COUNT DROPS TO BELOW 3000/MM^3, THE DOSE SHOULD BE REDUCED	☐
E	IF NEUTROPHIL COUNT DROPS TO BELOW 1500/MM^3, THE DOSE SHOULD BE REDUCED	☐

Question 10.108 Drug monitoring item worth 2 points

CASE PRESENTATION

A 26-year-old male patient needs to be given a 'loading dose' of phenytoin for the treatment of seizures following resection of a high-grade glioma. You prescribe a dose of 1500 mg (20 mg/kg) to be given by IV infusion over 30 minutes.

Question: Which one of the following parameters is the most important to monitor throughout the duration of the infusion? Mark it with a tick in the column provided.

DECISION OPTIONS

A	TEMPERATURE	☐
B	SEIZURE CONTROL	☐
C	ECG	☑
D	PUPIL REACTIVITY	☐
E	PLASMA PHENYTOIN CONCENTRATION	☐

Question 10.109 Drug monitoring item worth 2 points

CASE PRESENTATION

You are asked to review a 45-year-old female on the respiratory ward, admitted with an acute exacerbation of asthma. Despite treatment with nebulized salbutamol and ipratropium she remains symptomatic and is commenced on an aminophylline infusion.

Question: Which *one* option would be most beneficial in checking for signs of aminophylline toxicity? Mark it with a tick in the column provided.

	DECISION OPTIONS	
A	GLASGOW COMA SCORE (GCS)	☐
B	BLOOD PRESSURE	☐
C	OXYGEN SATURATION	☐
D	SERUM THEOPHYLLINE LEVEL	☑
E	RESPIRATORY RATE	☐

Question 10.110 Drug monitoring item worth 2 points

CASE PRESENTATION

A 78-year-old gentleman is commenced on IV Tazocin for severe community-acquired pneumonia.

Question: Which *one* option would most adequately assess response to antibiotics whilst an inpatient? Mark it with a tick in the column provided.

	DECISION OPTIONS	
A	CHEST X-RAY	☐
B	RESPIRATORY RATE	☑
C	BLOOD PRESSURE	☐
D	RESOLUTION OF CREPITATIONS ON AUSCULTATION	☐
E	FLUID BALANCE	☐

Question 10.111 Drug monitoring item worth 2 points

CASE PRESENTATION

A 30-year-old female patient is seen in the transplant clinic 1 month after her renal transplant. Her immunosuppressant regimen, to prevent transplant rejection, is as follows: prednisolone 10 mg daily and tacrolimus (Prograf®) 3 mg twice daily.

Question: Which *one* of the following would best measure/monitor whether her tacrolimus level is within the normal reference range? Mark it with a tick in the column provided.

	DECISION OPTIONS	
A	SERUM CREATININE	☐
B	PRESENCE OF TREMOR	☐
C	TACROLIMUS LEVEL ('TROUGH' LEVEL PRIOR TO MORNING DOSE)	☑
D	PRESENCE OF GUM HYPERPLASIA	☐
E	TACROLIMUS LEVEL ('PEAK' LEVEL 1 HOUR AFTER MORNING DOSE)	☐

Question 10.112 Drug monitoring item worth 2 points

CASE PRESENTATION

A 47-year-old female patient is started on fluoxetine for the treatment of depression after psychosocial and psychological interventions fail to control her symptoms. Her GP asks her to make another appointment in 2 weeks' time to assess how she is getting on with her new prescription.

Question: Which *one* of the following would be the most appropriate for the GP to assess/monitor at her next appointment? Mark it with a tick in the column provided.

	DECISION OPTIONS	
A	MOOD ASSESSMENT	☑
B	PRESENCE OF A RASH	☐
C	FULL BLOOD COUNT	☐
D	ECG	☐
E	SERUM CREATININE	☐

Question 10.113 Adverse drug reactions item worth 2 marks

CASE PRESENTATION

A 28-year-old woman presents to the GP with tachycardia, weight loss and night time waking with 'stress'.

Question: Which *one* medication may be contributing to these symptoms? Mark it with a tick in the column provided.

CURRENT PRESCRIPTIONS

Drug name	Dose	Route	Freq.	
MICROGYNON	1 TABLET	ORAL	DAILY	☐
IBUPROFEN	400 MG	ORAL	8-HOURLY AS REQUIRED	☐
LEVOTHYROXINE	125 MICROGRAMS	ORAL	DAILY	☑
CETIRIZINE HYDROCHLORIDE	10 MG	ORAL	DAILY	☐
PARACETAMOL	1 G	ORAL	AS REQUIRED 6-HOURLY	☐

Question 10.114 Adverse drug reactions item worth 2 marks

CASE PRESENTATION

A 28-year-old woman wants to stop her oral contraceptive and start a family with her long-term partner. You review her recent medications and want to discuss the two most important prescriptions to avoid during pregnancy.

Question: Which *one* medication in addition to her oral contraceptive is most important to counsel her against taking during the first trimester of her pregnancy? Mark it with a tick in the column provided.

CURRENT PRESCRIPTIONS

Drug name	Dose	Route	Freq.	
MICROGYNON	1 TABLET	ORAL	DAILY	☐
IBUPROFEN	400 MG	ORAL	8-HOURLY AS REQUIRED	☑
TRIMETHOPRIM	100 MG	ORAL	AT NIGHT	☑
CETIRIZINE HYDROCHLORIDE	10 MG	ORAL	DAILY	☐
PARACETAMOL	1 G	ORAL	AS REQUIRED 6-HOURLY	☐

Question 10.115 Adverse drug reactions item worth 2 marks

CASE PRESENTATION

A 79-year-old woman presents with a 3-week history of feeling light headed on standing after starting some new medications. Her blood pressure is 105/62 mmHg with a regular pulse of 72 b.p.m. She is otherwise well. You review her recent medications and choose to stop one medication.

Question: Which *one* medication from the list do you stop? Mark it with a tick in the column provided.

RECENT PRESCRIPTIONS

Drug name	Dose	Route	Freq.	
OMEPRAZOLE	20 MG	ORAL	DAILY	☐
LEVOTHYROXINE	125 MICROGRAMS	ORAL	DAILY	☐
SIMVASTATIN	40 MG	ORAL	NIGHTLY	☐
CO-AMILOFRUSE	1 TABLET	ORAL	DAILY	☑
PARACETAMOL	1 G	ORAL	AS REQUIRED 6-HOURLY	☐

Question 10.116 Adverse drug reactions item worth 2 marks

CASE PRESENTATION

A 47-year-old male has not suffered from asthmatic symptoms for 15 years, but feels increasingly short of breath having started a new medication. It has not affected his exercise tolerance, but he presents to the GP worried about this new symptom.

Question: Which *one* prescription from the drug list is the most likely to cause his symptoms? Mark it with a tick in the column provided.

DRUG LIST

Drug name	Dose	Route	Freq.	
OMEPRAZOLE	20 MG	ORAL	DAILY	☐
CARVEDILOL	12.5 MG	ORAL	DAILY	☑
LISINOPRIL	5 MG	ORAL	AT NIGHT	☐
CO-AMILOFRUSE	1 TABLET	ORAL	DAILY	☐
PARACETAMOL	1 G	ORAL	AS REQUIRED 6-HOURLY	☐

Question 10.117 Adverse drug reactions item worth 2 marks

CASE PRESENTATION

An 18-year-old girl has just started university and visits her new GP complaining of weight gain, irritability and new headaches. The GP asks her if she has started any new prescriptions recently.

Question: Which *one* prescription from the drug list is the most likely to cause her symptoms? Mark it with a tick in the column provided.

DRUG LIST

Drug name	Dose	Route	Freq.	
IBUPROFEN	400 MG	ORAL	DAILY AS REQUIRED	☐
DIPROBASE	APPLY	TOP	12-HOURLY	☐
MICROGYNON®	1 TABLET	ORAL	DAILY	☑
SERTRALINE	20 MG	ORAL	DAILY	☐
HYOSCINE BUTYL-BROMIDE	20 MG	ORAL	AS REQUIRED 6-HOURLY	☐

Question 10.118 Adverse drug reactions item worth 2 marks

CASE PRESENTATION

A 52-year-old attends the ward for planned sinus surgery. As advised he did not take his medications today and has new symptoms of tremor, anxiety and insomnia.

Question: Withdrawal of which *one* medication is the most likely cause for his new symptoms? Mark it with a tick in the column provided.

DRUG LIST

Drug name	Dose	Route	Freq.	
IBUPROFEN	400 MG	ORAL	DAILY AS REQUIRED	☐
DIAZEPAM	5 MG	ORAL	12-HOURLY	☐
LABETALOL	200 MG	ORAL	12-HOURLY	☑
SERTRALINE	20 MG	ORAL	DAILY	☐
LORATADINE	10 MG	ORAL	DAILY	☐

Question 10.119 Adverse drug reactions item worth 2 marks

CASE PRESENTATION

A 92-year-old care home resident presents to A&E with a likely case of norovirus. She is tachycardic with a BP of 95/60 mmHg, is oliguric and has vomited 5 times in the waiting room. She has a background of atrial fibrillation (AF), peripheral vascular disease and glaucoma. Her blood results show an isolated hyponatraemia of 125 mmol/L (normal 135–145 mmol/L).

Question: Which *single* prescription would you omit from her drug chart? Mark it with a tick in the column provided.

DRUG LIST

Drug name	Dose	Route	Freq.	
WARFARIN	AS PER INR	ORAL	DAILY	☐
AMLODIPINE	5 MG	ORAL	DAILY	☐
BENDROFLUMETHIAZIDE	2.5 MG	ORAL	DAILY	☑
PARACETAMOL	1 G	ORAL	6-HOURLY	☐
PROPRANOLOL	80 MG	ORAL	12-HOURLY	☐

Question 10.120 Adverse drug reactions item worth 2 marks

CASE PRESENTATION

You review a 67-year-old on the ward round with your registrar 2 days after a cholecystectomy. She is a slight woman of 48 kg and your registrar also asks you to write her eGFR of 45 mL/min in the notes. He asks you to review her drug chart in light of these findings.

Question: Which *one* drug is the most important to amend on this list? Mark it with a tick in the column provided.

CURRENT PRESCRIPTIONS

Drug name	Dose	Route	Freq.	
ENOXAPARIN	40 MG	S/C	DAILY	☑
AMLODIPINE	2.5 MG	ORAL	DAILY	☐
OMEPRAZOLE	20 MG	ORAL	DAILY	☐
PARACETAMOL	500 MG	ORAL	6-HOURLY	☐
PROPRANOLOL	80 MG	ORAL	12-HOURLY	☐

Question 10.61 Answers, see ticks beside current prescriptions chart

A	ACE-inhibitors cause a dry cough through accumulation of bradykinin via reduced degradation by ACE.
B	ACE-inhibitors cause hyperkalaemia through reduced aldosterone production and thus potassium excretion in the kidneys. Remember that loop and thiazide diuretics (including bendroflumethiazide) cause hypokalaemia while aldosterone antagonists and ACE-inhibitors cause hyperkalaemia.

CURRENT PRESCRIPTIONS

Drug name	Dose	Route	Freq.	A	B
SIMVASTATIN	10 MG	ORAL	NIGHTLY	☐	☐
BISOPROLOL	10 MG	ORAL	DAILY	☐	☐
ALLOPURINOL	100 MG	ORAL	DAILY	☐	☐
LISINOPRIL	10 MG	ORAL	DAILY	✓	✓
PARACETAMOL	1 G	ORAL	6-HOURLY	☐	☐
BENDROFLUMETHIAZIDE	2.5 MG	ORAL	DAILY	☐	☐

Question 10.62 Answers, see ticks beside current prescriptions chart

A	Ibuprofen inhibits prostaglandin synthesis needed for gastric mucosal protection from acid: there is therefore a risk of inflammation and ulceration. Oral steroids inhibit gastric epithelial renewal thus predisposing to ulceration.
B	Ibuprofen inhibits prostaglandin synthesis which reduces renal artery diameter (and blood flow) thereby reducing kidney perfusion and function. Ramipril, an ACE-inhibitor, reduces angiotensin-II production necessary for preserving glomerular filtration when the renal blood flow is reduced.

CURRENT PRESCRIPTIONS

Drug name	Dose	Route	Freq.	A	B
PARACETAMOL	1 G	ORAL	6-HOURLY	☐	☐
IBUPROFEN	200 MG	ORAL	8-HOURLY	✓	✓
PREDNISOLONE	30 MG	ORAL	DAILY	✓	☐
RAMIPRIL	2.5 MG	ORAL	DAILY	☐	✓
ALLOPURINOL	100 MG	ORAL	DAILY	☐	☐

Question 10.63 Answer, see ticks beside current prescriptions chart

Bendroflumethiazide (a thiazide diuretic) should not be taken in the evening (such prescribing will make you unpopular with patients who are up all night passing urine!). Lisinopril is appropriately prescribed in the evening (minimizing the daytime effects of postural hypotension).

Paracetamol is prescribed 4 hourly allowing up to 6 g per day (max. 4 g) – whenever you see paracetamol, check the total dose (including the dose in other preparations like co-codamol or co-dydramol).

Metoclopramide should be used with caution in patients with Parkinson's disease (as it is a dopamine antagonist and can worsen parkinsonian features); it should be stopped. Domperidone does not cross the blood brain barrier so is an appropriate choice.

Cyclizine is an effective antiemetic, but is prescribed 6-hourly: the common first-line antiemetics (cyclizine and metoclopramide) are both given up to 8-hourly.

The aspirin has not been stopped as the patient is improving with medical management and is therefore unlikely to require surgery. Most patients with cholecystitis will be managed medically, with an elective cholecystectomy when the acute inflammation has settled.

CURRENT PRESCRIPTIONS

Drug name	Dose	Route	Freq.	A
CO-BENELDOPA 12.5/50	2 TABLETS	ORAL	12-HOURLY	☐
BISOPROLOL	10 MG	ORAL	DAILY	☐
BENDROFLUMETHIAZIDE	2.5 MG	ORAL	NIGHTLY	✓
LISINOPRIL	10 MG	ORAL	NIGHTLY	☐
ASPIRIN	75 MG	ORAL	DAILY	☐
PARACETAMOL	1 G	ORAL	AS REQUIRED UP TO 4-HOURLY	✓
DOMPERIDONE	10 MG	ORAL	6-HOURLY	☐
METOCLOPRAMIDE	10 MG	ORAL	8-HOURLY	✓
CYCLIZINE	50 MG	IV	6-HOURLY	✓

Question 10.64 Answers, see ticks beside current prescription chart

This patient is receiving 6 g of paracetamol per day (1 g 4-hourly, i.e. 6 times per day) and this is more than the maximum normal dose of 4 g per day. Methotrexate should be given weekly not daily. This error can and has led to fatalities.

As her AF is longstanding she should be on a lower dose of aspirin as stroke prophylaxis (75 mg daily); very rarely higher doses may be used but usually warfarin is elected instead.

Co-amoxiclav contains penicillin (co-amoxiclav = clavulanic acid plus amoxicillin), and is therefore contraindicated due to her penicillin allergy.

CURRENT PRESCRIPTIONS

Drug name	Dose	Route	Freq.	
CO-CODAMOL 8/500	2 TABLETS	ORAL	4-HOURLY	✓
METHOTREXATE	10 MG	ORAL	DAILY	✓
ZOPICLONE	7.5 MG	ORAL	NIGHTLY	☐
LANSOPRAZOLE	30 MG	ORAL	DAILY	☐
ASPIRIN	300 MG	ORAL	DAILY	✓
IBUPROFEN	400 MG	ORAL	8-HOURLY	☐
CO-AMOXICLAV	625 MG	ORAL	8-HOURLY	✓

Question 10.65 Answers, see ticks beside current prescriptions chart

A	Bendroflumethiazide, a thiazide diuretic, causes hypokalaemia by increasing potassium excretion in the kidney. Lisinopril (an ACE-inhibitor) causes hyperkalaemia.
B	Bendroflumethiazide should be stopped due to hypokalaemia. As the patient is constipated, all opioid/opioid-containing drugs should be withheld (i.e. codeine and co-codamol). Note that the patient is also taking too much paracetamol (up to 6g per day: 2g regularly and up to 4g as required (within co-codamol), exceeding the daily maximum of 4g). While one could have stopped the regular paracetamol instead of the co-codamol, this would be suboptimal because of the constipation. Furthermore, the patient is pain free so minimal analgesics should be given.

CURRENT PRESCRIPTIONS

Drug name	Dose	Route	Freq.	A	B
BENDROFLUMETHIAZIDE	2.5 MG	ORAL	DAILY	✓	✓
PARACETAMOL	500 MG	ORAL	6-HOURLY	☐	☐
SIMVASTATIN	20 MG	ORAL	NIGHTLY	☐	☐
AMLODIPINE	5 MG	ORAL	DAILY	☐	☐
CODEINE	30 MG	ORAL	6-HOURLY	☐	✓
LISINOPRIL	10 MG	ORAL	NIGHTLY	☐	☐
CO-CODAMOL 30/500	2 TABLETS	ORAL	AS REQUIRED UP TO 6-HOURLY	☐	✓

Question 10.66 Answers, see ticks beside current prescriptions chart

A	Naproxen (an NSAID) inhibits the prostaglandin synthesis needed for gastric mucosal protection from acid. The gastric mucosa is therefore at risk of inflammation and ulceration.
	Oral steroids (including dexamethasone) inhibit gastric epithelial renewal thus predisposing to ulceration. Although prednisolone is typically used for polymyalgia, dexamethasone is also licensed and is included here to reinforce that glucocorticoid side effects can occur with all preparations.
B	Naproxen inhibits prostaglandin synthesis which reduces renal artery diameter (and blood flow) thereby reducing kidney perfusion and function. Ramipril, an ACE-inhibitor, reduces the angiotensin-II production necessary for preserving glomerular filtration when the renal blood flow is reduced.
	Remember bumetanide is a loop diuretic, so whilst it can cause renal failure, it is more likely to cause hypokalaemia (not hyperkalaemia) than the other two options presented will cause hypokalaemia (not hyperkalaemia).

CURRENT PRESCRIPTIONS

Drug name	Dose	Route	Freq.	A	B
BUMETANIDE	2 MG	ORAL	DAILY	☐	☐
NAPROXEN	250 MG	ORAL	8-HOURLY	✓	✓
DEXAMETHASONE	0.5 MG	ORAL	DAILY	✓	☐
RAMIPRIL	2.5 MG	ORAL	DAILY	☐	✓
PARACETAMOL	1 G	ORAL	6-HOURLY	☐	☐

Question 10.67 Answers, see ticks beside current prescriptions chart

This patient has developed acute renal failure; drugs are a common cause. Of the new drugs, diclofenac (an NSAID) is the most likely culprit and should therefore be stopped. While he has acute renal failure (and particularly a raised potassium) the ACE-inhibitor lisinopril (which can cause hyperkalaemia and renal failure anyway) should also be withheld. Remember that while aspirin is an NSAID, it does not cause renal failure and so should be continued.

His drowsiness probably reflects the accumulation of clonazepam (a benzodiazepine) and co-codamol in his blood owing to reduced excretion in the urine due to the new renal failure. While the original dose of clonazepam may have been appropriate, it is now having a significantly excessive effect (i.e. reduced consciousness level and respiratory rate) and should therefore be stopped. Codeine (a weak opioid) should also be stopped as this can cause drowsiness.

CURRENT PRESCRIPTIONS

Drug name	Dose	Route	Freq.	A	B
COCODAMOL 8/500	2 TABLETS	ORAL	6-HOURLY	☐	✓
CLONAZEPAM	2 MG	ORAL	DAILY	☐	✓
LISINOPRIL	10 MG	ORAL	NIGHTLY	✓	☐
ASPIRIN	75 MG	ORAL	DAILY	☐	☐
DICLOFENAC	25 MG	ORAL	8-HOURLY	✓	☐
CO-AMOXICLAV	625 MG	ORAL	8-HOURLY	☐	☐

Question 10.68 Answers, see ticks beside current prescriptions chart

This patient has an exacerbation of asthma triggered by beta-blockers and then worsened by ibuprofen (both of which commonly precipitate bronchospasm; for this reason beta-blockers are contraindicated in asthmatics and NSAIDs should only be used, if strictly necessary and with caution). If an asthmatic patient is already on an NSAID without worsening of asthma then it may be continued.

Despite being an NSAID, aspirin very rarely worsens asthma (less frequently than other NSAIDs), and is thus commonly (though cautiously) used. In this case we are told that he has taken it for years (insinuating without side effects) so it should not be stopped. The patient is allergic to penicillin (including amoxicillin which is probably the cause of the rash and may be worsening the wheeze so should be stopped (it is not indicated anyway: his breathing difficulty is due to the beta-blocker and the clear CXR and normal bloods effectively exclude a chest infection)).

The maximum dose of citalopram for patients over the age of 65 is 20 mg. Higher doses are reserved for younger patients.

CURRENT PRESCRIPTIONS

Drug name	Dose	Route	Freq.	A	B
CITALOPRAM	40 MG	ORAL	DAILY	☐	✓
AMLODIPINE	5 MG	ORAL	DAILY	☐	☐
ASPIRIN	75 MG	ORAL	DAILY	☐	☐
ENALAPRIL	10 MG	ORAL	DAILY	☐	☐
PROPRANOLOL	40 MG	ORAL	8-HOURLY	✓	☐
AMOXICILLIN	500 MG	ORAL	8-HOURLY	✓	☐
IBUPROFEN	200 MG	ORAL	AS REQUIRED UP TO 8-HOURLY	✓	☐

Question 10.69 Answer

This is slightly more tricky because more than one answer is appropriate, but one is more so than the others!

Oliguria is the first sign of a deteriorating patient and usually occurs before the heart rate increases (which in turn usually precedes the onset of hypotension). In this case, hypovolaemia would seem the most likely cause (i.e. reduced oral intake and increased insensible losses through sweating due to fever).

Given that he is not tolerating oral fluid, option A is not appropriate.

As a general rule, colloids (such as gelofusine) are only given to patients who are hypotensive. This is partly because there is a small risk of an anaphylactic reaction, but also because colloids remain in the intravascular space for longer than crystalloids (and as this patient is normotensive a colloid is not indicated).

Either 5% dextrose or normal saline would be appropriate choices here (given that the sodium is mid-range) but the mild hyperkalaemia makes option E a safer one (although one could hypothesize that the reduced intake during the day might need replacing). Always go for the safer option in the PSA and real life.

DECISION OPTIONS

A	ENCOURAGE ORAL INTAKE	☐
B	1 L GELOFUSINE IV OVER 1 HOUR	☐
C	500 ML GELOFUSINE IV OVER 1 HOUR	☐
D	1 L 5% DEXTROSE WITH 20 MMOL KCL IV OVER 2 HOURS	☐
E	1 L 0.9% SALINE OVER 2 HOURS	✓

Question 10.70 Answer

The trick to this question is to remember that maintenance fluids should comprise 3 L (i.e. 8-hourly bags) for most adults, except the elderly or those with low body weight when 2 L per 24 h (i.e. 12-hourly bags) are needed. This limits us to options C and E; gelofusine is never given as maintenance fluids (it is a colloid and therefore given to hypotensive patients).

Option A is too fast – 4-hourly bags would result in 6 L IV fluid (3 times what is required) being given each day with a high risk of fluid overload and subsequent pulmonary oedema.

Option B is inappropriate because 10% dextrose is usually only given to increase blood glucose concentration (i.e. in hypoglycaemia).

Option D is probably the second-best choice but giving saline to a patient with a very mildly increased baseline sodium plus the 8-hourly rate make this less appealing.

Do not be afraid to give 5% dextrose to diabetic patients – by the time the fluid has circulated most of the (tiny!) amount of glucose will have been metabolized so it will have very little affect on the plasma glucose. If a patient is significantly hyperglycaemic then one should opt for 0.9% saline.

DECISION OPTIONS

A	1 L 5% DEXTROSE OVER 4 HOURS	☐
B	1 L 10% DEXTROSE OVER 8 HOURS	☐
C	1 L 5% DEXTROSE WITH 20 MMOL KCL OVER 12 HOURS	✓
D	1 L 0.9% SALINE WITH 20 MMOL KCL OVER 8 HOURS	☐
E	1 L GELOFUSINE OVER 12 HOURS	☐

Question 10.71 Answer

This patient has mild, asymptomatic iron-deficiency anaemia.

Blood transfusion in iron-deficiency anaemia is generally reserved for patients who:

- Are severely symptomatic and cannot tolerate or wait for the effect of iron-replacement (in iron-deficiency anaemia the Hb usually rises by 10 g/L/week on oral iron replacement), *or*
- Have Hb <70 g/L (some recommend using a higher cut-off of 100 g/L in patients with ischaemic heart disease).

Ferrous sulfate/gluconate/fumarate are all used as oral iron supplements. The most common side effect is constipation; by far, the most common reason for treatment failure is poor compliance due to this (plus it also causes black offensive stools). Non-compliance should be considered when the haemoglobin fails to rise on treatment.

Oral iron replacement should be given until the haemoglobin is in the normal range then for a further 3 months to replenish stores.

Loperamide is an antimotility drug used to reduce diarrhoea, and should therefore only be used with non-infective diarrhoea (not constipation). One way to increase compliance with the constipating iron drugs is to provide a laxative.

IV iron is rarely used, and most commonly when the oral route is not possible (or absorption problems necessitate a parenteral route).

DECISION OPTIONS

A	TRANSFUSE 1 UNIT OF BLOOD	☐
B	START FERROUS SULFATE 200 MG 8-HOURLY ORAL PLUS LOPERAMIDE	☐
C	START FERROUS SULFATE 200 MG 8-HOURLY ORAL UNTIL HB NORMAL	☐
D	START FERROUS SULFATE 200 MG 8-HOURLY ORAL UNTIL HB NORMAL THEN FOR FURTHER 3 MONTHS	✓
E	GIVE IV IRON	☐

Question 10.72 Answer

The absence of a temperature means the differential of relatively acute SOB with productive cough should include heart failure and pneumonia. However, the chest X-ray shows right lower-lobe consolidation with no evidence of cardiomegaly, upper-lobe diversion, bat-wing appearance, bilateral pleural effusion or Kerley-B lines to suggest pulmonary oedema. Thus use of furosemide and bumetanide (both diuretics) is not appropriate.

Antibiotics are the definitive treatment for any infection (and certainly the first-line treatment along with supportive measures). Thus doxycycline and co-amoxiclav are the two sensible options. Co-amoxiclav is contraindicated as the patient is allergic to penicillin (and co-amoxiclav contains amoxicillin) making doxycycline the correct choice.

Prednisolone (which may be used for an exacerbation of COPD/asthma) is not indicated (i.e. no wheeze nor history of COPD/asthma).

DECISION OPTIONS

A	FUROSEMIDE 20 MG ORAL	☐
B	CO-AMOXICLAV 625 MG ORAL	☐
C	BUMETANIDE 1 MG ORAL	☐
D	DOXYCYCLINE 200 MG ORAL	✓
E	PREDNISOLONE 30 MG ORAL	☐

Question 10.73 Answer

This patient has leucocytosis because he is on steroids, not because he has an infection (this is most easily determined by the normal CRP).

He has signs of mild phenytoin toxicity despite a normal plasma level. Remember that one should always interpret results in the context of the clinical findings: dysarthria and gum hyperplasia are common side effects of phenytoin, and, in the context of good seizure control, it would be appropriate to reduce the dose (even if it makes the plasma level below the reference range, i.e. the level that reflects the 'normal population'). Option E would only really be appropriate if there was a temporary reason why the level had increased (say addition of a drug that increases phenytoin's level, like chloramphenicol) but this is not the case. Omitting for 3 days might risk seizures too.

DECISION OPTIONS

A	CO-AMOXICLAV 625 MG ORAL 8-HOURLY	☐
B	TRIMETHOPRIM 200 MG ORAL 12-HOURLY	☐
C	INCREASE PHENYTOIN TO 350 MG ORAL DAILY	☐
D	DECREASE PHENYTOIN TO 250 MG ORAL DAILY	✓
E	OMIT PHENYTOIN FOR 3 DAYS THEN CONTINUE SAME DOSE	☐

Question 10.74 Answer

This patient is dry as evidenced clinically (i.e. reduced skin turgor and tachycardia) and biochemically (pre-renal picture of acute kidney injury (raised urea with normal creatinine) and hypernatraemia). Whilst antibiotics will be the definitive treatment in *Clostridium difficile* gastroenteritis, it is usually best to await confirmation from stool cultures to avoid unnecessary further antibiotics.

We are told he is vomiting which precludes reliance on oral intake alone (one should never rely on oral intake for a tachycardic patient as they are too sick!). The U&Es show hypernatraemia and a potassium at the lower end of normal. Given the normal blood pressure (precluding the need for a colloid like gelofusine), one should hunt out an answer using 5% dextrose ideally with some potassium (whilst not hypokalaemic per se, he probably will be after a litre of fluid without any supplementary potassium). This narrows our options to C, D or E. Option C (12-hourly) is a maintenance speed for this age; he requires replacement (i.e. faster fluids). Of the remaining two options, option D is the only appropriate choice because E gives IV potassium at an unsafe speed (i.e. IV potassium should never be given at more than 20 mmol/hour).

DECISION OPTIONS

A	ENCOURAGE ORAL FLUIDS	☐
B	GIVE 1 L 0.9% SALINE WITH 20 MMOL KCL OVER 12 HOURS	☐
C	GIVE 1 L 5% DEXTROSE WITH 20 MMOL KCL OVER 12 HOURS	☐
D	GIVE 1 L 5% DEXTROSE WITH 20 MMOL KCL OVER 4 HOURS	✓
E	GIVE 1 L 5% DEXTROSE WITH 40 MMOL KCL OVER 1 HOUR	☐

Question 10.75 Answer

A	Gliclazide is a sulphonylurea and, although there is no contraindication to using as first line treatment, metformin is a more appropriate first line treatment in the setting of obesity because it is an appetite suppressant and thus assists with weight loss.
B	A standard insulin regimen in type 2 diabetes; however, insulin would not be the first-line management.
C	**Correct:** an essential part of a new diagnosis of diabetes mellitus. Many type 2 diabetics can be managed with diet and weight loss alone.
D	Once-daily regimens can also be used in type 2 diabetes mellitus, but again would not be the first-line treatment.
E	Metformin (a biguanide) is usually the first-line medication in type 2 diabetes mellitus when diet and exercise has proved inadequate, particularly if the patient is overweight as this can facilitate weight loss. However, its use should be limited to when diet and exercise interventions are insufficient.

DECISION OPTIONS

A	GLICLAZIDE 40 MG ORAL ONCE DAILY	☐
B	MIXTARD 30® INSULIN (30% SOLUBLE AND 70% ISOPHANE) S/C TWICE DAILY	☐
C	REVIEW BY DIETICIAN AND WEIGHT LOSS REGIMEN	✓
D	LONG ACTING INSULIN (GLARGINE) S/C ONCE DAILY	☐
E	METFORMIN 500 MG ORAL TWICE DAILY	☐

Question 10.76 Answer

A	This patient is having a significant rectal bleed and is consequently hypotensive. While a blood transfusion is the optimal form of IV replacement it would not be appropriate to wait 1 hour while failing to treat a patient with hypotensive shock. Instead a colloid (such as gelofusine) or 0.9% saline should be administered.
B	Dextrose 5% is not an appropriate fluid for resuscitation particularly when the patient has lost volume. Dextrose 5% is used as a maintenance fluid postsurgery or when not maintaining oral intake. Furthermore, 250 ml per hour is far too slow for hypotensive shock.
C	**Correct:** as explained in option A, in the absence of a colloid, 0.9% saline should be used to resuscitate patients with bleeding. The speed of the infusion is also appropriate.
D	FFP is usually used to correct deranged clotting (where PT/aPTT is >1.5 times the normal limit) and works by replacing clotting factors. With massive transfusions, additional FFP is pre-emptively used due to consumption of coagulation factors. Given that the patient's clotting is normal, FFP would not be an appropriate choice.
E	Although 0.9% saline is an appropriate fluid to use in resuscitation, 1 L over 12 hours is not an appropriate speed when the patient is actively bleeding and hypotensive.

DECISION OPTIONS

A	GIVE 2 UNITS OF CROSS-MATCHED PACKED RED CELLS OVER 1 HOUR EACH	☐
B	1 L 5% DEXTROSE IV OVER 4 HOURS	☐
C	1 L 0.9% SALINE IV STAT.	✓
D	4 UNITS OF FRESH FROZEN PLASMA (FFP) IV STAT.	☐
E	1 L 0.9% SALINE IV OVER 12 HOURS	☐

Question 10.77 Answer

A	Oral carbohydrates are appropriate if the patient is conscious; however, with impaired consciousness the risk of aspiration is too great.
B	As there is intravenous access, IV glucose is preferred over IM glucagon initially.
C	Not only are IV fluids not indicated here, the 5% dextrose will be metabolized within minutes of administration and will have very little (if any) influence on the blood glucose.
D	In the acute setting, unless contraindicated by type 2 respiratory failure, unwell patients should be commenced on high-flow (100% (15 L via non-rebreather mask)) oxygen.
E	**Correct:** in a patient with hypoglycaemia and reduced conscious level, administration of IV glucose is the first choice of treatment. However, if IV access is unavailable or they fail to respond to this then glucagon should be used.

DECISION OPTIONS

A	120 ML LUCOZADE® ORALLY	☐
B	1 MG INTRAMUSCULAR GLUCAGON	☐
C	1 L 5% DEXTROSE IV OVER 8 HOURS	☐
D	40% OXYGEN VIA VENTURI MASK	☐
E	100 ML 20% DEXTROSE INTRAVENOUSLY	✓

Question 10.78 Answer

A	**Correct:** this is a severe flare of ulcerative colitis (>6 bowel motions/day and systemically unwell). Therefore IV steroids (and fast IV fluids) are required.
B	This patient has evidence of a severe flare of his colitis, and should be rehydrated intravenously. In the acute setting 0.9% saline is an appropriate fluid for resuscitation from diarrhoea and in the initial stages over 1–4 hours would be satisfactory. A 500 mL IV fluid challenge would be an alternative given he is tachycardic. Careful attention should be paid to electrolyte replacement.
C	This patient is clearly dehydrated and in need of fluid resuscitation (i.e. dry mucous membranes and tachycardic); 5% dextrose would not be first-line treatment nor would it be appropriate to give 1 L over 12 hours given the frequency of diarrhoea.
D	Antibiotics should only be used if there is evidence of raised inflammatory markers or temperature.
E	In a severe flare of ulcerative colitis IV hydcortisone is the first-line treatment. Oral prednisolone is used in mild flares, i.e. when bowels are opened fewer than 6 times per day without any other symptoms. The dose would be 30 mg per 24 hours.

DECISION OPTIONS

A	HYDROCORTISONE 100 MG IV 6-HOURLY	✓
B	ENSURE PATIENT IS DRINKING 4 L/DAY	☐
C	1 L 5% DEXTROSE IV OVER 12 HOURS	☐
D	CEFUROXIME 1.5 G/6-HOURLY AND METRONIDAZOLE 500 MG/8-HOURLY IV	☐
E	PREDNISOLONE 30 MG ONCE DAILY	☐

Question 10.79 Answer

A	**Correct:** in the event of ECG changes calcium gluconate is important in stabilizing myocardium. This should be repeated every 15 min up to 50 mL until the ECG normalizes. Note it has no effect on potassium levels but prevents (potentially fatal) arrhythmias so must be the first drug treatment with ECG changes (or when ECG not performed).
B	Ramipril (an ACE-inhibitor) worsens acute kidney injury and can even precipitate it in susceptible individuals. It causes hyperkalaemia directly and through reducing renal function. However, it is a useful adjunct in chronic renal failure. Ramipril should be stopped until acute renal dysfunction and hyperkalaemia has normalized. Sick day rules should be explained (i.e. stopping ACE-inhibitors/angiotensin-receptor blockers if diarrhoea or vomiting occurs).
C	Calcium resonium should be used if there is persistent hyperkalaemia despite insulin/dextrose and salbutamol nebulizers. Calcium resonium will take several days to work, and if treatment-resistant hyperkalaemia needs urgent correction then dialysis is the next treatment.
D	Insulin will acutely reduce plasma levels of potassium (as insulin causes uptake of potassium into cells), but only temporarily. Adequate rehydration in addition to hyperkalaemia management will also be required. This patient clearly has ECG changes and stabilization of the myocardium would be your first priority.
E	Adequate rehydration is important to treat dehydration but also to enable urinary excretion of potassium. Given the ECG changes, stabilizing the myocardium and reducing serum potassium acutely are the priority. Furthermore, 6-hourly fluids are far too slow for this very dehydrated patient.

DECISION OPTIONS

A	10 ML OF 10% CALCIUM GLUCONATE IV	✓
B	REDUCE RAMIPRIL TO 5 MG ONCE DAILY	☐
C	CALCIUM RESONIUM 15 MG ORALLY 8-HOURLY	☐
D	10 UNITS ACTRAPID® IN 100 ML OF 20% DEXTROSE	☐
E	1 L 0.9% SALINE IV OVER 6 HOURS	☐

Question 10.80 Answer

A	Oral nitrates are helpful in chronic angina but this patient is pain free so nitrates (which are used for symptomatic relief of ischaemic chest pain) would offer little benefit.
B	**Correct:** this patient has evidence of a non-ST elevation myocardial infarction (NSTEMI), and initial treatment is with aspirin and clopidogrel as antiplatelet agents (plus heparin).
C	GTN infusion is used for ongoing chest pain despite maximal sublingual GTN.
D	This option is used acutely for ischaemic chest pain; however, the patient is pain free so it is not indicated.
E	This patient has had a NSTEMI. She should not be discharged home without treatment.

DECISION OPTIONS

A	ISOSORBIDE MONONITRATE 10 MG TWICE DAILY ORALLY	☐
B	ASPIRIN 300 MG AND CLOPIDOGREL 300 MG ONCE ORALLY	✓
C	GTN INFUSION 50 MG: 1–10 ML PER HOUR IV	☐
D	MORPHINE SULPHATE 5 MG IV	☐
E	DISCHARGE HOME	☐

Question 10.81 Answer

A	The ECG shows fast atrial fibrillation (AF). Given that this patient has had AF for over 48 hours, chemical cardioversion would not be appropriate due to the risk of thromboembolism. Also her age makes rate control a more attractive option, and her history of hypertension (which increases the risk of dilated cardiomyopathy) may preclude use of flecainide (which is contraindicated in structural heart disease).
B	See above: electrical or chemical cardioversion is not indicated due to her age and risk of thromboembolism. If it were pursued she would require full anticoagulation with warfarin and echo (to exclude mural thrombus (which could cause stroke) or structural heart disease (which would make risk of recurrence prohibitively high)).
C	**Correct:** IV or oral digoxin would be an appropriate choice to treat this patient's fast AF in the setting of known asthma. While the maintenance dose is 62.5–125 micrograms daily, a loading dose is required initially in this case.
D	Given that this is an acute event the cardiology team may wish to cardiovert electively after ruling out a mural thrombus or structural heart disease and in this setting anticoagulation should be commenced. However rate control would be the first-line intervention.
E	Beta-blockers are first-line treatment for haemodynamically stable fast AF; however, this is contraindicated in this patient with asthma.

DECISION OPTIONS

A	FLECAINIDE 50 MG ORALLY	☐
B	DC CARDIOVERSION	☐
C	DIGOXIN 500 MICROGRAMS IV	✓
D	ENOXAPARIN 1.5 MG/KG S/C DAILY	☐
E	BISOPROLOL 5 MG ORALLY	☐

Question 10.82 Answer

A	**Correct:** reversal of warfarin will be important in acquiring haemostasis. As this is for AF there are relatively few risks to reversal short term. Any bleeding in the setting of excessive anticoagulation (INR > 5) requires IV (rather than oral) vitamin K.
B	The patient is anaemic presumably from a large epistaxis. However, given that she is asymptomatic from her anaemia and haemodynamically stable, transfusion (particularly at this rate) is inappropriate and certainly not as important as reversing the warfarin (and omitting it for 2 days).
C	The patient is haemodynamically stable and does not require fluid resuscitation. A blood transfusion would be the only choice of IV fluid in this scenario if she was symptomatic.
D	The absence of a major bleed (i.e. one causing hypotension or into a confined space (skull or eye)) precludes use of prothrombin complex.
E	FFP may be used in a major bleed when dried prothrombin complex is unavailable (but it is less effective); as alluded to, this is not the case.

DECISION OPTIONS

A	VITAMIN K 3 MG IV	✓
B	ONE UNIT PACKED RED CELLS STAT.	☐
C	500 ML COLLOID OVER 30 MINUTES	☐
D	DRIED PROTHROMBIN COMPLEX	☐
E	3 UNITS OF FRESH FROZEN PLASMA (FFP)	☐

Question 10.83 Answer

A	Codeine can cause drowsiness, particularly at higher doses, and thus caution should be taken while using machinery or driving.
B	Pruritis is a common side effect associated with codeine and all opioid medications.
C	**Correct:** constipation is a common side effect of any opioid-based medication. Patients should be informed of this risk and advised to take additional laxatives.
D	Opioids are respiratory depressants and can cause hypoventilation, particularly at high doses.
E	Codeine can be used along with paracetamol; however, caution should be taken when using dual preparations.

DECISION OPTIONS

A	NO PRECAUTIONS NEED TO BE TAKEN WHILE TAKING CODEINE PHOSPHATE AND DRIVING/OPERATING MACHINERY	☐
B	PRURITIS IS A RARE SIDE EFFECT OF CODEINE PHOSPHATE	☐
C	CONSTIPATION IS A COMMON SIDE EFFECT OF CODEINE AND LAXATIVES SHOULD BE USED IN CONJUNCTION FOR LONG-TERM USAGE	✓
D	CODEINE PHOSPHATE IS A RESPIRATORY STIMULANT AND MAY CAUSE HYPERVENTILATION	☐
E	CODEINE PHOSPHATE CANNOT BE USED IN CONJUNCTION WITH PARACETAMOL	☐

Question 10.84 Answer

A	Statins should not be used in those with active liver disease as this may affect its metabolism.
B	**Correct**: myositis is a potentially serious complication if left unaddressed; therefore, patients should be warned to seek medical assistance if they develop unusual aches or pains.
C	Most cholesterol metabolism occurs overnight, so conventionally most statins are taken at night.
D	Grapefruit should be avoided in those taking statins as they contain polyphenolic compounds that inhibit CYP3A4 and thus increase statin toxicity.
E	Statins should be stopped while taking clarithromycin (also a CYP3A4 inhibitor) as they increase toxicity and associated side effects.

DECISION OPTIONS

A	STATINS ARE SAFE TO USE WITH ACTIVE LIVER DISEASE	☐
B	IF MUSCLE CRAMPS DEVELOP THE MEDICATION SHOULD BE STOPPED AND MEDICAL ADVICE SOUGHT	✓
C	STATINS ARE MOST EFFECTIVE WHEN TAKEN IN THE MORNING	☐
D	THERE ARE NO DIETARY RESTRICTIONS WITH STATINS	☐
E	WHEN TAKING CLARITHROMYCIN THE DOSE OF STATINS SHOULD BE DOUBLED	☐

Question 10.85 Answer

A	Regular blood tests should be performed while taking spironolactone; however, patients are at risk of hyperkalaemia.
B	Spironolactone functions as a diuretic so dehydration is a possible side effect, particularly when unwell.
C	Spironolactone is an aldosterone antagonist and thus causes potassium retention; therefore, a diet high in potassium should be avoided because of the risk of hyperkalaemia.
D	**Correct**: as well as anti-mineralocorticoid effects spironolactone also has potent anti-androgen effects, resulting in gynaecomastia.
E	ACE-inhibitors and beta-blockers are used first-line in heart failure. Spironolactone, angiotensin receptor blockers, hydralazine and nitrates are used when first-line agents fail (see Chapter 4).

DECISION OPTIONS

A	REGULAR BLOOD TESTS ARE REQUIRED WITH SPIRONOLACTONE DUE TO THE RISK OF HYPOKALAEMIA	☐
B	DEHYDRATION IS NOT A SIDE EFFECT OF SPIRONOLACTONE USE	☐
C	A DIET HIGH IN POTASSIUM IS REQUIRED WHEN TAKING SPIRONOLACTONE	☐
D	SPIRONOLACTONE CAN CAUSE EXCESSIVE BREAST TISSUE DEVELOPMENT (GYNAECOMASTIA)	✓
E	SPIRONOLACTONE IS THE FIRST-LINE TREATMENT FOR HEART FAILURE	☐

Question 10.86 Answer

A	Blood tests should be performed following initiation of therapy, as well as after dose increments due to the risk of hyperkalaemia and renal impairment.
B	ACE-inhibitors should be avoided in aortic stenosis, particularly in severe or symptomatic cases.
C	Angio-oedema-like reactions to ACE-inhibitors can occur many months after initiation of therapy.
D	**Correct**: ACE-inhibitors can be used in CKD, but with caution. Renal function should be checked following any dose increment given the risks of worsening renal function or hyperkalaemia (both of which are more likely in known CKD).
E	Dry cough is a very common side effect of ACE-inhibitors; if intolerable then patients should be converted to an angiotensin II receptor antagonist or other antihypertensive agent.

DECISION OPTIONS

A	BLOOD TESTS SHOULD BE PERFORMED REGULARLY DUE TO THE RISK OF HYPOKALAEMIA	☐
B	ACE-INHIBITORS ARE FIRST-LINE THERAPY FOR HYPERTENSION IN PATIENTS WITH AORTIC STENOSIS	☐
C	ANGIO-OEDEMA CAN ONLY BE ATTRIBUTED TO ACE-INHIBITORS IF NEWLY STARTED WITHIN THE LAST 24 HOURS	☐
D	CAUTION SHOULD BE TAKEN WHEN USING ACE-INHIBITORS IN KNOWN CHRONIC KIDNEY DISEASE	✓
E	A DRY COUGH WOULD NOT PRE-EMPT A CHANGE OF MEDICATION	☐

Question 10.87 Answer

A	Statins should not be used in those with active liver disease as this may potentially affect its metabolism.
B	**Correct:** myositis is a potentially serious complication if left unaddressed; therefore, patients should be warned to seek medical assistance if they develop unusual aches or pains.
C	Most cholesterol metabolism occurs overnight, so conventionally statins are taken at night.
D	Grapefruit should be avoided in those taking statins as it contains polyphenolic compounds that inhibit CYP3A4 and thus increase statin toxicity.
E	Statins should be stopped while taking clarithromycin (a CYP3A4 inhibitor) as they increase toxicity and associated side effects.

DECISION OPTIONS

A	STATINS ARE SAFE TO USE IN ACTIVE LIVER DISEASE	☐
B	IF MUSCLE CRAMPS DEVELOP THE MEDICATION SHOULD BE STOPPED AND MEDICAL ADVICE SOUGHT	✓
C	STATINS ARE MOST EFFECTIVE WHEN TAKEN IN THE MORNING	☐
D	THERE ARE NO DIETARY RESTRICTIONS WITH STATINS	☐
E	WHEN TAKING CLARITHROMYCIN THE DOSE OF STATINS SHOULD BE DOUBLED	☐

Question 10.88 Answer

A	When unwell basal blood glucose increases necessitating higher insulin doses. Failing to do so will increase the risk of diabetic ketoacidosis.
B	In the conscious patient, hypoglycaemia should be treated with glucose tablets, a sugary snack or glucose gel.
C	Failing to rotate injection sites will result in lipodystrophy which can be uncomfortable and vary the quantity of insulin absorbed.
D	HbA1c gives average glucose control over a 3 month period. In diabetic patients an HbA1c of less than 48 mmol/mol is targeted.
E	**Correct:** excessive alcohol intake can result in life-threatening hypoglycaemia, and is a common cause of hypoglycaemia in young adults.

DECISION OPTIONS

A	WHEN UNWELL THE PATIENT'S TOTAL DAILY INSULIN DOSAGE SHOULD BE DECREASED	☐
B	HYPOGLYCAEMIA SHOULD BE TREATED WITH A BOTTLE OF WATER	☐
C	LIPODYSTROPHY IS PREVENTED BY REPEATED USE OF THE SAME INJECTION SITES	☐
D	HBA1C IS A SUITABLE WAY TO MONITOR BLOOD SUGARS FROM DAY TO DAY	☐
E	EXCESSIVE ALCOHOL INTAKE CAN CAUSE HYPOGLYCAEMIA	✓

Question 10.89 Answer

Correct answer and working

A 1% solution contains 1 g in 100 mL. There is 10 mg in 1 mL.

Answer | 1 mL

Question 10.90 answer

Correct answer and working

In patients with AF, it might be necessary to administer the cardiac glycoside, digoxin, by the IV route. The IV preparation contains 250 micrograms/mL. Express this as a percentage.

250 micrograms/mL is equivalent to 0.025%. Therefore 250 mg × 2 mL = 500 micrograms.

Answer | 2 vials

Question 10.91 Answer

Correct answer and working

By convention 1 mL is equivalent to 1 g, and so 1% lidocaine means 1 g in 100 mL
This means 1000 mg = 100 mL
1 mL of 1% lidocaine contains 1000/100 mg of lidocaine
2% lidocaine is equivalent to 20 mg/mL

Learning point

A 1% solution is equivalent to 1 g in 100 mL. You can always use this to estimate your answers elsewhere.

Answer | 20 mg per mL

Question 10.92 Answer

Correct answer and working

50 mg/5 mL = 10 mg/1 mL – this is the dose in 1 mL
2(mL) × 10(mg) = 20 mg

Answer | 20 mg

Question 10.93 Answer

Correct answer and working

She has normal renal function and a likely (severe) UTI for which gentamicin is an appropriate antibiotic. One-off doses of gentamicin can be used with good effect alongside catheterization to prevent further spread of infection, i.e. to either blood or further along the urinary tract.

$5\,mg/kg \times 60\,kg = 300\,mg$

Answer | 300 mg

Question 10.94 Answer

Correct answer and working

By convention 1 mL is equivalent to 1 g, and so 1% means 1 g in 100 mL.

It means 10 g in 1000 mL.

0.9% = 0.9 g in 100 mL or 9 g in 1000 mL

The solution is 9 g of salt dissolved in water up to a volume of 1000 mL.

For interest:

5 g of salt = one level teaspoon

Answer | 9 g/L

Question 10.95 Answer

Correct answer and working

$400\,mg \times 0.92 = 368\,mg$

Learning point

As above. Note that the answer is in mg not mL.

Answer | 368 mg

Question 10.96 Answer

Correct answer and working

First, calculate the dose (in g) required for the course:

$(80\,kg \times 0.4\,g) \times 5\,days = 160\,g$

We know that 10% = 10 g in 100 mL, so now we can use our equation, ensuring χ is the numerator:

$$\frac{100\,mL}{10\,g} = \frac{\chi\,mL}{160\,g}$$

Answer | 1600 mL (or 1.6 L)

Question 10.97 Answer

A. Drug choice	Score	Feedback/ justification	B. Dose, route, frequency	Score	Feedback/justification
1. AMOXICILLIN	4	This is the first-line antibiotic for otitis media (see BNF section 12.1.2). NOTE: if you do not know which antibiotic to prescribe look up the condition in the BNF index and it will give you advice on the antibiotic choice for each condition.	125 MG 8-HOURLY ORAL FOR 5 DAYS MUST have an indication (otitis media) MUST have an end/ review date (5 days from now)	4	5 DAYS in this age range (1–5 years) NOTE: the BNF gives you all the information needed here.
2. CO-AMOXICLAV 125/31	2	This tends to be reserved for unresponsive or severe infection. As the patient is mobilizing around the ward the latter is not the case. Note: the 125/31 means 125 mg amoxicillin and 31 mg clavulanic acid.	5 ML 8-HOURLY ORAL FOR 5 DAYS MUST have an indication (i.e. otitis media) MUST have an end/ review date (5 days from now)	4	NOTE: whether you calculated the dose by weight (0.25 mL/kg, i.e. 0.25 mL × 20 kg = 5 mL) or by the age estimate in the BNF (age 1–6 years = 5 mL 8-hourly) the answer is the same.
3. CLARITHROMYCIN	2	Clarithromycin is typically reserved for patients with penicillin allergy.	187.5 MG 12-HOURLY ORAL FOR 5 DAYS MUST have an indication (i.e. otitis media) MUST have an end/ review date (5 days from now)	4	

Marking Guide
4 marks: for an optimal answer that cannot be improved.
3 marks: for an answer that is good but is suboptimal on some grounds (e.g. cost-effectiveness, likely adherence).
2 marks: for an answer that is likely to provide benefit but is clearly suboptimal for more than one reason.
1 mark: for an answer that has some justification and deserves some credit.

C. Timing. 1 mark for correctly dating (and timing) the prescription.

D. Signature. 1 mark for signing the prescription.

For example, the prescription should appear as:

ANTIBIOTICS			Date					
			Time					
Drug (Approved name) AMOXICILLIN			⑥					
			8					
Dose 125 MG	Frequency 8-HOURLY	Route ORAL	12					
Prescriber – sign + print YOUR NAME AND SIGNATURE		Start date TODAY'S DATE	⑭					
			18					
Indication OTITIS MEDIA		Review/stop date TODAY'S DATE PLUS 5 DAYS	㉒					

Question 10.98 Answer

A. Drug choice	Score	Feedback/ justification	B. Dose, route, frequency	Score	Feedback/justification
1. OXYBUTYNIN	0	Oxybutynin (an antimuscarinic, i.e. anti-cholinergic) should be avoided in myasthenia gravis (where antibodies already block the acetylcholine receptor and thus neuromuscular transmission) as it will worsen the myasthenia.	N/A		
2. TOLTERODINE	0	See above	N/A		
3. SOLIFENACIN	0	See above	N/A		
4. TROSPIUM	0	See above	N/A		
5. ANY OTHER MUSCARINIC ANTAGONIST	0	See above	N/A		
6. DULOXETINE	4	Duloxetine is an inhibitor of serotonin and noradrenaline re-uptake; as it has no anticholinergic effect it may be used in myasthenia gravis. Remember, if you do not know how to treat a condition then look it up in the BNF!	40 MG 12-HOURLY ORAL	4	This is the correct starting dose; 20 mg 12-hourly may be used if worried about side effects, but none are likely here.

Marking guide for A and B.
4 marks: for an optimal answer that cannot be improved.
3 marks: for an answer that is good but is suboptimal on some grounds (e.g. cost-effectiveness, likely adherence).
2 marks: for an answer that is likely to provide benefit but is clearly suboptimal for more than one reason.
1 mark: for an answer that has some justification and deserves some credit.

C. Timing. 1 mark for correctly dating (and timing) the prescription.

D. Signature. 1 mark for signing the prescription.

For example, the prescription should appear as:

REGULAR MEDICATIONS		Date						
		Time						
Drug (Approved name) DULOXETINE		⑥						
		8						
Dose 40 MG	Route ORAL	12						
Prescriber – sign + print *YOUR NAME AND SIGNATURE*	Start date *TODAY'S DATE*	14						
		⑱						
Notes	Frequency 12-HOURLY	22						

A. Drug choice	Score	Feedback/justification	B. Dose, route, frequency	Score	Feedback/justification
1. CODEINE	4	This is an appropriately weak opioid; the choice between tramadol and codeine usually rests on the likelihood of side effects. Both cause typical opioid side effects (i.e. respiratory depression, reduced consciousness and pinpoint pupils), but tramadol typically causes agitation/hallucinations (particularly in the elderly) while codeine is more constipating. In this case, the presence of diarrhoea promotes codeine (as does his age).	30 MG 6-HOURLY *OR* 30 MG 4 HOURLY ORAL REGULARLY *OR* 60 MG 6-HOURLY ORAL REGULARLY	4	This should be on the 'regular' chart because the patient is in constant pain; an additional 'as required' drug would be sensible (such as oral morphine sulphate) but the question only asks for one drug. 240 mg is the maximum daily dose (e.g. 60 mg 6-hourly).
2. CO-CODAMOL 8/500 *OR* CO-CODAMOL 30/500 *OR* CO-DYDRAMOL 10/500 *OR* CO-DYDRAMOL 20/500 *OR* CO-DYDRAMOL 30/500	0	While an appropriate choice because it contains a weak opioid, the question asked for one additional drug. The patient is already taking 4 g paracetamol per day and therefore no further paracetamol-containing drugs should be given.	N/A	0	In these drugs the first number refers to the total codeine (in co-codamol) or dihydrocodeine (in co-dydramol) in each tablet, and the second the amount of paracetamol. Thus, 2 tablets (containing 1 g paracetamol regardless of codeine/dihydrocodeine dose) can be given up to 6-hourly.
3. TRAMADOL	3	See above	50 MG 6-HOURLY ORAL REGULARLY *OR* 50 MG 4-HOURLY ORAL REGULARLY *OR* 100 MG 6-HOURLY ORAL REGULARLY	4	This should be on the 'regular' chart because the patient is in constant pain; an additional 'as required' drug would be sensible (such as oral morphine sulphate) but the question only asks for one drug. Patients are rarely prescribed more than 400 mg per day (i.e. 100 mg 6-hourly at most).
4. MORPHINE SULPHATE (not Oramorph® which is a (trade name))	1	Using a mild opioid before a strong one is more appropriate. As the question asks for one drug the choice is really between codeine and tramadol.	2.5 MG UP TO 1-HOURLY ORAL AS REQUIRED *OR* 5 MG UP TO 1-HOURLY ORAL AS REQUIRED MUST include a maximum frequency (as above) MUST include an indication (i.e. pain) MUST NOT include a dose range, e.g. 5–10 mg	4	Morphine sulphate is usually given as-required until one can see how much a patient requires in one day; when it may be converted to a regular long-acting preparation which are taken 12-hourly.

Question 10.99 Answer *(Cont'd)*

Marking Guide for A and B.
4 marks: for an optimal answer that cannot be improved.
3 marks: for an answer that is good but is suboptimal on some grounds (e.g. cost-effectiveness, likely adherence).
2 marks: for an answer that is likely to provide benefit but is clearly suboptimal for more than one reason.
1 mark: for an answer that has some justification and deserves some credit.

C. Timing. 1 mark for correctly dating (and timing) the prescription.

D. Signature. 1 mark for signing the prescription.

For example, the prescription should appear as:

REGULAR MEDICATIONS		Date						
		Time						
Drug (Approved name) CODEINE		⑥						
		8						
Dose 30 MG	Route ORAL	⑫						
Prescriber – sign + print *YOUR NAME AND SIGNATURE*	Start date *TODAY'S DATE*	14						
		⑱						
Notes	Frequency 6-HOURLY	㉒						

Question 10.100 Answer

A. Drug choice	Score	Feedback/justification	B. Dose, route, frequency	Score	Feedback/justification
1. CEFOTAXIME	4	This is the first-line antibiotic for epiglottitis. Again, if you did not know this, look up epiglottitis in the BNF which will be available to you during the exam.	1 G 6-HOURLY IV *OR* 1 G 6-HOURLY IV INFUSION *OR* 2 G 12-HOURLY IV *OR* 2 G 12-HOURLY IV INFUSION MUST have an indication (i.e. epiglottitis) MUST have an end/review date (at most 3 days from now)	4	As epiglottitis is a life-threatening infection, the severe infection dose is selected (i.e. for a child 200 mg/kg daily in 2–4 divided doses). It may be given IM, by IV injection or IV infusion; the presence of a cannula should steer you away from the IM route (unnecessary pain for the child). Remember, if unsure about stop/review date select 5 days for oral antibiotics or 3 for IV (as the latter should be stepped down to oral as soon as possible).
2. CHLORAMPHENICOL	3	This tends to be reserved for patients with immediate hypersensitivity reaction to penicillin or cephalosporins.	250 MG 6-HOURLY IV *OR* 500 MG 6-HOURLY IV MUST have an indication (i.e. epiglottitis) MUST have an end/review date (at most 3 days from now)	4	

Marking Guide for A and B.
4 marks: for an optimal answer that cannot be improved.
3 marks: for an answer that is good but is suboptimal on some grounds (e.g. cost-effectiveness, likely adherence).
2 marks: for an answer that is likely to provide benefit but is clearly suboptimal for more than one reason.
1 mark: for an answer that has some justification and deserves some credit.

C. Timing. 1 mark for correctly dating (and timing) the prescription.

D. Signature. 1 mark for signing the prescription.

For example, the prescription should appear as:

ANTIBIOTICS			Date						
			Time						
Drug (Approved name) CEFOTAXIME			⑥						
			8						
Dose 1 G	Frequency 6-HOURLY	Route IV	⑫						
Prescriber – sign + print *YOUR NAME AND SIGNATURE*		Start date *TODAY'S DATE*	14						
			⑱						
Indication EPIGLOTTITIS		Review/stop date *TODAY'S DATE PLUS 3 DAYS*	㉒						

Question 10.101 Answer

A. Drug choice	Score	Feedback/justification	B. Dose, route, frequency	Score	Feedback/justification
1. CITALOPRAM	4	This is a selective serotonin reuptake inhibitor (SSRI) which is the first choice of antidepressant and has a lower toxicity in overdose than tricyclics or venlafaxine.	20 MG ORAL DAILY	4	Remember, even if you do not know how to treat depression, the BNF (which will be with you in the exam) will tell you – if in doubt, look it up! Antidepressants should be given regularly and not as-required.
2. ESCITALOPRAM	4	See above	10 MG ORAL DAILY	4	See above
3. FLUOXETINE	4	See above	20 MG ORAL DAILY	4	See above
4. FLUVOXAMINE MALEATE	4	See above	50 MG ORAL DAILY *OR* 100 MG ORAL DAILY	4	See above
5. PAROXETINE	4	See above	20 MG ORAL (IN THE MORNING)	4	Should be taken in the morning.
6. SERTRALINE	4	See above	50 MG ORAL DAILY	4	
7. VENLAFAXINE	0	While an effective antidepressant, venlafaxine is highly toxic in overdose which this patient is at risk of (i.e. previous deliberate self-harm and reports continued risk).	N/A		
8. ANY TRICYCLIC ANTIDEPRESSANT	1	While effective, tricyclic antidepressants are more toxic in overdose than SSRIs.	CORRECT DOSE ACCORDING TO BNF	4	
9. ANY MONOAMINE OXIDASE INHIBITORS	1	These are reserved for prescription by specialists only.	CORRECT DOSE ACCORDING TO BNF	4	
10. ST JOHN'S WORT	0	Doctors should never prescribe or recommend St John's Wort because it interacts with a large number of prescribed medications through enzyme induction, and the amount of active ingredient in different preparations varies significantly.	N/A		

Marking Guide for A and B.
4 marks: for an optimal answer that cannot be improved.
3 marks: for an answer that is good but is suboptimal on some grounds (e.g. cost-effectiveness, likely adherence).
2 marks: for an answer that is likely to provide benefit but is clearly suboptimal for more than one reason.
1 mark: for an answer that has some justification and deserves some credit.

C. Timing. 1 mark for correctly dating (and timing) the prescription.

D. Signature. 1 mark for signing the prescription.

Question 10.101 Answer *(Cont'd)*

For example, the prescription should appear as:

REGULAR MEDICATIONS		Date						
		Time						
Drug (Approved name) CITALOPRAM		**6**						
		⑧						
Dose 20 MG	Route ORAL	**12**						
Prescriber – sign + print *YOUR NAME AND SIGNATURE*	Start date *TODAY'S DATE*	**14**						
		18						
Notes	Frequency DAILY	**22**						

Question 10.102 Answer

A. Drug choice	Score	Feedback/justification	B. Dose, route, frequency	Score	Feedback/justification
1. CITALOPRAM	2	This is a selective serotonin reuptake inhibitor (SSRI) which is the first-choice group of drugs for managing GAD in this situation (see NICE clinical guideline 113, (2011)). The only licensed SSRIs for GAD are escitalopram and paroxetine, although NICE advocates first-line use of the (more cost-effective) sertraline.	20 MG ORAL DAILY	4	Remember, even if you do not know how to treat GAD, the BNF (which will be with you in the exam) will tell you. If in doubt, look it up.
2. ESCITALOPRAM	3	See above.	10 MG ORAL DAILY	4	
3. FLUOXETINE	2	See above.	20 MG ORAL DAILY	4	This is the dose for the only other anxiety-related disorder (OCD) for which fluoxetine is licensed.
4. FLUVOXAMINE MALEATE	2	See above.	50 MG ORAL DAILY	4	
5. PAROXETINE	3	See above.	20 MG ORAL IN THE MORNING	4	Should be taken in the morning.
6. SERTRALINE	4	This is the most cost-effective SSRI (but is no more effective than the others) and hence should be selected first despite not being licensed for GAD (this is because NICE recommended it.)	25 MG ORAL DAILY	4	This is the dose for non-OCD anxiety disorders and thus should be followed.
7. VENLAFAXINE M/R	2	This is second-line treatment for GAD.	75 MG ORAL DAILY	4	This is the correct dose for GAD.
8. ANY BENZODIAZEPINE	0	This is reserved for acute treatment of anxiety, not long-term use.	N/A		

Question 10.102 Answer *(Cont'd)*

Marking Guide for A and B.
4 marks: for an optimal answer that cannot be improved.
3 marks: for an answer that is good but is suboptimal on some grounds (e.g. cost-effectiveness, likely adherence).
2 marks: for an answer that is likely to provide benefit but is clearly suboptimal for more than one reason.
1 mark: for an answer that has some justification and deserves some credit.

C. Timing. 1 mark for correctly dating (and timing) the prescription.

D. Signature. 1 mark for signing the prescription.

For example, the prescription should appear as:

REGULAR MEDICATIONS

		Date					
		Time					
Drug (Approved name) SERTRALINE		**6**					
		⑧					
Dose 25 MG	Route ORAL	**12**					
Prescriber – sign + print *YOUR NAME AND SIGNATURE*	Start date *TODAY'S DATE*	**14**					
		18					
Notes	Frequency DAILY	**22**					

Question 10.103 Answer

A. Drug choice	Score	Feedback/justification	B. Dose, route, frequency	Score	Feedback/justification
1. DALTEPARIN	4	LMW heparin is needed to prevent the clot enlarging while the body breaks it down; it does not thrombolyse the clot itself. Factor V Leiden is the most commonly inherited thrombophilia (i.e. increased likelihood of thromboembolism).	15 000 UNITS S/C ONCE DAILY	4	This is the treatment dose (i.e. LMW heparin may be used for treatment or prophylaxis). It should be continued until warfarin has achieved a therapeutic INR (i.e. >2). Use the BNF to calculate dose according to weight.
2. ENOXAPARIN	4	See above.	120 MG *OR* 12 000 UNITS S/C ONCE DAILY (CAN BE PRESCRIBED EITHER WAY)	4	As above. (It does not matter which of the three LMW heparins you selected; in real life it reflects hospital policy and dalteparin is cheapest at present.)
3. TINZAPARIN	4	See above.	14 000 UNITS S/C ONCE DAILY	4	As above.
4. ALTEPLASE	1	Thrombolytics activate plasminogen to form plasmin, which degrades fibrin and so breaks up thrombi. Thrombolysis is never indicated in DVT.	10 MG IV OVER 1–2 MIN	4	Correct dose for initial therapy; then requires infusion.

Question 10.103 Answer *(Cont'd)*

A. Drug choice	Score	Feedback/justification	B. Dose, route, frequency	Score	Feedback/justification
5. ASPIRIN	0	Aspirin is an antiplatelet and has no role in the treatment of PE or DVT.	N/A	0	300 mg is the treatment dose for acute coronary syndrome or stroke; 75 mg is the prophylactic dose for IHD, stroke, peripheral vascular disease and thromboembolism from AF.
6. WARFARIN	1	Warfarin is the oral anticoagulant of choice. It antagonizes the effect of vitamin K, preventing formation of the vitamin K-dependent clotting factors (II, VII, IX and X), and hence prolonging the PT/INR. Its anticoagulant effects occur after 48–72 h , so concomitant heparin must be given. This question specifically asked for a drug that will rapidly prevent expansion of the DVT (and hence also reduce the risk of pulmonary embolus), i.e. LMW heparin, although warfarin will probably be started concomitantly.	10 MG ORAL	4	Follow local policy, but most hospitals give patients 10 mg on the first day and then check the INR to direct following days. (Most patients will require 2–3 days of 10 mg daily before the INR increases from 1).

Marking Guide for A and B.
4 marks: for an optimal answer that cannot be improved.
3 marks: for an answer that is good but is suboptimal on some grounds (e.g. cost-effectiveness, likely adherence).
2 marks: for an answer that is likely to provide benefit but is clearly suboptimal for more than one reason.
1 mark: for an answer that has some justification and deserves some credit.

C. Timing. 1 mark for correctly dating (and timing) the prescription.

D. Signature. 1 mark for signing the prescription.

For example, the prescription should appear as:

ONCE ONLY MEDICINES

Date	Time	Medicine (approved name)	Dose	Route	Prescriber – sign + print	Time given	Given by
01/02/13	13 00	DALTEPARIN	15 000 UNITS	S/C	*YOUR NAME AND SIGNATURE*		

Question 10.104 Answer

A. Drug choice	Score	Feedback/justification	B. Dose, route, frequency	Score	Feedback/justification
1. DIAZEPAM	4	Benzodiazepines are the mainstay of short-term management of severe anxiety.	2 MG ORAL on the once-only chart at a stated time before midnight	4	Your consultant has asked for one dose and this should therefore go on the once-only chart. The oral route is indicated because again this is what your boss requested.
2. ALPRAZOLAM	4	See above.	250 MICROGRAMS ORAL *OR* 500 MICROGRAMS ORAL on the once-only chart at a stated time before midnight	4	If in doubt look it up in the BNF.
3. CHLORDIAZEPOXIDE	4	See above.	10 MG ORAL on the once-only chart at a stated time before midnight	4	Although usually used to treat and prevent alcohol withdrawal it is licensed for short-term management of anxiety.
4. LORAZEPAM	4	See above.	1 MG ORAL *OR* 2 MG ORAL *OR* 3 MG ORAL *OR* 4 MG ORAL on the once-only chart at a stated time before midnight	4	
5. OXAZEPAM	4	See above.	15 MG ORAL *OR* 30 MG ORAL on the once-only chart at a stated time before midnight	4	
6. ANY BETA-BLOCKER	0	Beta-blockers reduce the autonomic symptoms of anxiety but have no effect on psychological symptoms.	N/A		

Question 10.104 Answer *(Cont'd)*

A. Drug choice	Score	Feedback/justification	B. Dose, route, frequency	Score	Feedback/justification
7. HALOPERIDOL	0	Haloperidol is licensed as a short-term adjunct for severe anxiety (although it is more typically used in the elderly). It should be actively avoided in young patients (particularly females) due to the risk of dystonic reactions. As a general rule, if you have no choice but to give drugs for managing agitation use benzodiazepines in the young and haloperidol in the elderly. Either way give small doses orally (if possible) and give each one at least 30 minutes (but ideally longer) to take effect before considering a further dose.	N/A		

Marking Guide for A and B.
4 marks: for an optimal answer that cannot be improved.
3 marks: for an answer that is good but is suboptimal on some grounds (e.g. cost-effectiveness, likely adherence).
2 marks: for an answer that is likely to provide benefit but is clearly suboptimal for more than one reason.
1 mark: for an answer that has some justification and deserves some credit.

C. Timing. 1 mark for correctly dating (and timing) the prescription.

D. Signature. 1 mark for signing the prescription.

For example, the prescription should appear as:

ONCE ONLY MEDICINES							
Date	Time	Medicine (approved name)	Dose	Route	Prescriber – sign + print	Time given	Given by
01/02/13	13 00	DIAZEPAM	2 MG	ORAL	*YOUR NAME AND SIGNATURE*		

Question 10.105 Answer

A	**Correct**: digoxin is predominantly renally excreted and patients with renal dysfunction are at increased risk of toxicity.
B	Not required at baseline.
C	Not specifically required for patients on digoxin.
D	Not specifically required for patients on digoxin. A measure of serum potassium is much more relevant owing to the fact that hypokalaemia increases the risk of digoxin toxicity.
E	Not specifically required for patients on digoxin.

DECISION OPTIONS

A	SERUM CREATININE	✓
B	SERUM ALKALINE PHOSPHATASE	☐
C	CHEST X-RAY	☐
D	SERUM SODIUM	☐
E	BLOOD PRESSURE	☐

Question 10.106 Answer

A	Pancreatitis is a known side effect of sodium valproate, but a measurement of pancreatic amylase would only be required if a patient were to report symptoms of pancreatitis while on therapy.
B	Vitamin D supplementation should be considered for patients on sodium valproate and at risk of osteoporosis; however, a vitamin D level would not be routinely checked at baseline.
C	Not required.
D	**Correct**: sodium valproate therapy is associated with hepatotoxicity and liver function should be measured at baseline as well as at regular intervals throughout the duration of therapy.
E	A measure of renal function is not routinely required prior to commencing treatment with sodium valproate. It is neither significantly cleared renally nor nephrotoxic. In patients with severe renal impairment, it might be necessary to adjust the dose based on careful monitoring, but we are not given any indication that this gentleman has severe renal impairment.

DECISION OPTIONS

A	PANCREATIC AMYLASE	☐
B	SERUM VITAMIN D LEVEL	☐
C	SERUM POTASSIUM	☐
D	ALT	✓
E	SERUM CREATININE	☐

Question 10.107 Answer

A	Registration with a clozapine monitoring service is required for all patients.
B	Not routinely required in patients on clozapine.
C	**Correct**: owing to the risk of neutropenia and potentially fatal agranulocytosis, routine monitoring of full blood count is required at regular intervals and throughout the duration of treatment as dictated by the product license.
D	No! Clozapine must be immediately stopped under these circumstances.
E	No! Clozapine must be immediately stopped under these circumstances.

DECISION OPTIONS

A	REGISTRATION WITH A CLOZAPINE MONITORING SERVICE IS RESERVED FOR PATIENTS WITH A BASELINE NEUTROPENIA	☐
B	SERUM CREATININE SHOULD BE CHECKED AT REGULAR INTERVALS THROUGHOUT THE DURATION OF THERAPY	☐
C	FULL BLOOD COUNT MUST BE CHECKED WEEKLY FOR THE FIRST 18 WEEKS	✓
D	IF LEUKOCYTE COUNT DROPS TO BELOW 3000/MM^3, THE DOSE SHOULD BE REDUCED	☐
E	IF NEUTROPHIL COUNT DROPS TO BELOW 1500/MM^3, THE DOSE SHOULD BE REDUCED	☐

Question 10.108 Answer

A	Not relevant in this scenario.
B	Although important, this is not specifically related to the phenytoin infusion.
C	**Correct**: IV administration is associated with cardiac arrhythmias.
D	Not specifically relevant to monitoring of IV phenytoin infusion.
E	It would be appropriate to check a plasma phenytoin concentration 2–4 hours after the end of the infusion.

DECISION OPTIONS

A	TEMPERATURE	☐
B	SEIZURE CONTROL	☐
C	ECG	✓
D	PUPIL REACTIVITY	☐
E	PLASMA PHENYTOIN CONCENTRATION	☐

Question 10.109 Answer

A	Glasgow coma score is not directly affected in the setting of aminophylline toxicity.
B	Aminophylline has little direct effect on blood pressure and therefore is not the correct answer.
C	If the aminophylline infusion is working the patient's oxygen saturation should improve; however, this would have no reflection on whether the level was too high (suggesting toxicity).
D	**Correct**: the ideal level for theophylline is 10–20 mg/L. A level should be taken 18 hours after commencing treatment unless there are concerns regarding toxicity, in which case it should be done sooner. It is worth noting that it is not an 'aminophylline' level that is checked, but a 'theophylline' level. Aminophylline is a simply a stable mixture of combined theophylline and ethylenediamine.
E	Similar to the situation with oxygen saturation, as the aminophylline takes effect, the patient's respiratory rate will improve, but this provides no information on potential toxicity.

DECISION OPTIONS

A	GLASGOW COMA SCORE (GCS)	☐
B	BLOOD PRESSURE	☐
C	OXYGEN SATURATION	☐
D	SERUM THEOPHYLLINE LEVEL	✓
E	RESPIRATORY RATE	☐

Question 10.110 Answer

A	Consolidation on a chest X-ray can take up to 6 weeks to clear, therefore would be unhelpful for an inpatient (as the question asks).
B	**Correct**: successful treatment of the pneumonia will improve gas exchange, hypoxia and therefore the respiratory rate. If oxygen saturations or ABG were options these would be more accurate and specific, but in their absence a respiratory rate is a good marker of improvement.
C	Hypotension occurs in severe infection (septic shock). Resolution of hypotension would indeed be in-keeping with response to antibiotics and it is a useful marker, but it is less specific than temperature. Improvement may reflect IV fluid administration while deterioration could be due to nonseptic causes (e.g. cardiogenic, hypovolaemic or anaphylactic shock).
D	Resolution of crepitations on auscultation will take several days to occur.
E	Not specifically relevant to the assessment of infection resolution.

DECISION OPTIONS

A	CHEST X-RAY	☐
B	RESPIRATORY RATE	✓
C	BLOOD PRESSURE	☐
D	RESOLUTION OF CREPITATIONS ON AUSCULTATION	☐
E	FLUID BALANCE	☐

Question 10.111 Answer

A	Creatinine is an objective way of measuring whether a current tacrolimus level is therapeutic as a raised creatinine can indicate rejection, and thus an insufficient tacrolimus level. (Note that rejection can also occur at a therapeutic level). It is not, however, the most appropriate parameter to monitor.
B	A raised tacrolimus level can manifest as a tremor. However, this is a subjective method of assessing whether a level is therapeutic/toxic and not the most appropriate answer from the options provided. The presence of a tremor should prompt a tacrolimus level check.
C	**Correct**: measuring a trough level before the morning or evening dose is the correct way to check a tacrolimus level. At this stage after transplant we would be aiming at a level of 6–10 ng/mL.
D	Although a side-effect of ciclosporin (another calcineurin inhibitor), it would not give any indication of whether serum concentration was therapeutic or toxic.
E	Timing of the level should be as stated in Option C.

	DECISION OPTIONS	
A	SERUM CREATININE	☐
B	PRESENCE OF TREMOR	☐
C	TACROLIMUS LEVEL ('TROUGH' LEVEL PRIOR TO MORNING DOSE)	✓
D	PRESENCE OF GUM HYPERPLASIA	☐
E	TACROLIMUS LEVEL ('PEAK' LEVEL 1 HOUR AFTER MORNING DOSE)	☐

Question 10.112 Answer

A	Treatment should continue for at least 4 weeks before an assessment of efficacy is considered (her appointment is in 2 weeks according to the question).
B	**Correct**: any rash should prompt consideration of discontinuing fluoxetine as it may be a sign of an impending serious systemic reaction.
C	A full blood count would not routinely be required in the monitoring of treatment with SSRIs.
D	Not relevant in the monitoring of SSRIs.
E	A measure of renal function specifically is not routinely required in the monitoring of treatment of SSRIs, although if it included an electrolyte screen, this might be useful in detecting hyponatraemia.

	DECISION OPTIONS	
A	MOOD ASSESSMENT	☐
B	PRESENCE OF A RASH	✓
C	FULL BLOOD COUNT	☐
D	ECG	☐
E	SERUM CREATININE	☐

Question 10.113 Answer

The correct answer is levothyroxine.

Levothyroxine replaces the endogenous hormone thyroxine, and has a narrow therapeutic margin. Small dosing errors can induce hyperthyroid side effects like tremor, tachycardia, weight loss, insomnia and anxiety.

CURRENT PRESCRIPTIONS

Drug name	Dose	Route	Freq.	
MICROGYNON	1 TABLET	ORAL	DAILY	☐
IBUPROFEN	400 MG	ORAL	8-HOURLY AS REQUIRED	☐
LEVOTHYROXINE	125 MICROGRAMS	ORAL	DAILY	✓
CETIRIZINE HYDROCHLORIDE	10 MG	ORAL	DAILY	☐
PARACETAMOL	1 G	ORAL	AS REQUIRED 6-HOURLY	☐

Question 10.114 Answer

The correct answer is trimethoprim.

Trimethoprim is a folate antagonist. Folate is essential for cellular synthesis and base pair generation. Limiting this activity diminishes resources available for the developing foetus, and theoretically can lead to birth defects. It is therefore strictly contraindicated in the first trimester of pregnancy and ideally avoided throughout. The prescribed dose is a prophylactic dose (to prevent urinary tract infections).

Ibuprofen is an NSAID and inhibits prostaglandin synthesis. In general, NSAIDs should be avoided in pregnancy unless the benefits outweigh the potential harms: the greatest risk of harm is in the third trimester when prostaglandin activity maintains a patent ductus arteriosus (enabling blood from the right ventricle to bypass the fluid-filled lungs and join the 'left-sided' circulation). If pregnant women take NSAIDs they risk narrowing or early closure of the ductus arteriosus.

The question specifically asks for the one medication that is most important to counsel against taking during the first trimester and, from the above, the answer is thus trimethoprim.

CURRENT PRESCRIPTIONS

Drug name	Dose	Route	Freq.	
MICROGYNON	1 TABLET	ORAL	DAILY	☐
IBUPROFEN	400 MG	ORAL	8-HOURLY AS REQUIRED	☐
TRIMETHOPRIM	100 MG	ORAL	AT NIGHT	✓
CETIRIZINE HYDROCHLORIDE	10 MG	ORAL	DAILY	☐
PARACETAMOL	1 G	ORAL	AS REQUIRED 6-HOURLY	☐

Question 10.115 Answer

The correct answer is co-amilofruse.

The only hypotensive agent here is the antihypertensive co-amilofruse. It is an older agent combining amiloride and furosemide. This woman's presentation and history are consistent with postural hypotension. Witholding the agent and retesting her blood pressure in 7 days is a suitable first step. You might also recheck her electrolytes as both amiloride and furosemide act on the renal parenchyma and salt exchange to control fluid balance.

RECENT PRESCRIPTIONS

Drug name	Dose	Route	Freq.	
OMEPRAZOLE	20 MG	ORAL	DAILY	☐
LEVOTHYROXINE	125 MICROGRAMS	ORAL	DAILY	☐
SIMVASTATIN	40 MG	ORAL	NIGHTLY	☐
CO-AMILOFRUSE	1 TABLET	ORAL	DAILY	✓
PARACETAMOL	1 G	ORAL	AS REQUIRED 6-HOURLY	☐

Question 10.116 Answer

The correct answer is carvedilol.

The adverse effects associated with beta adrenergic receptor agonists include bronchospasm. The cardio-selective (B1 agonists) are theoretically less likely to cause respiratory side effects, although in high doses their selectivity diminishes. ACE-inhibitors may cause a dry cough, but the question specifically states he is short of breath, which ACE-inhibitors should not cause.

DRUG LIST

Drug name	Dose	Route	Freq.	
OMEPRAZOLE	20 MG	ORAL	DAILY	☐
CARVEDILOL	12.5 MG	ORAL	DAILY	✓
LISINOPRIL	5 MG	ORAL	AT NIGHT	☐
CO-AMILOFRUSE	1 TABLET	ORAL	DAILY	☐
PARACETAMOL	1 G	ORAL	AS REQUIRED 6-HOURLY	☐

Question 10.117 Answer

The correct answer is Microgynon®.

The adverse effects associated with oestrogen-containing oral contraceptives include weight gain, irritability and new headaches. For some women hypertension is a feature and regular pill checks should be part of GP monitoring programmes, because it changes their cardiovascular risk profile.

DRUG LIST

Drug name	Dose	Route	Freq.	
IBUPROFEN	400 MG	ORAL	DAILY AS REQUIRED	☐
DIPROBASE	APPLY	TOP	12-HOURLY	☐
MICROGYNON®	1 TABLET	ORAL	DAILY	✓
SERTRALINE	20 MG	ORAL	DAILY	☐
HYOSCINE BUTYL-BROMIDE	20 MG	ORAL	AS REQUIRED 6-HOURLY	☐

Question 10.118 Answer

The correct answer is diazepam.

These are withdrawal symptoms of benzodiazapines. They might also be confused with the side effects of labetalol, but the question states that normal drugs were not given. This means these are symptoms in the absence of a drug, consistent with withdrawal, not dose-related side effects. Further, beta-blockers would not be withdrawn preoperatively (see Chapter 2).

DRUG LIST

Drug name	Dose	Route	Freq.	
IBUPROFEN	400 MG	ORAL	DAILY AS REQUIRED	☐
DIAZEPAM	5 MG	ORAL	12-HOURLY	✓
LABETALOL	200 MG	ORAL	12-HOURLY	☐
SERTRALINE	20 MG	ORAL	DAILY	☐
LORATADINE	10 MG	ORAL	DAILY	☐

Question 10.119 Answer

The correct answer is bendroflumethiazide.

Thiazides are a class of diuretics that prevent sodium absorption early in the renal pathway (at the beginning of the distal convoluted tubule). Water is lost because more sodium reaches the collecting ducts. Side effects include postural hypotension/hyponatraemia/hypokalaemia/hypercalcaemia.

Withholding this prescription during a period of dehydration (vomiting/diarrhoea) protects the patient from acute kidney injury, worsening hyponatraemia and dehydration.

While her low BP would probably also mean her calcium and beta-blockers should be withheld, you are asked for the single prescription and withholding the diuretic is more important.

DRUG LIST

Drug name	Dose	Route	Freq.	
WARFARIN	AS PER INR	ORAL	DAILY	☐
AMLODIPINE	5 MG	ORAL	DAILY	☐
BENDROFLUMETHIAZIDE	2.5 MG	ORAL	DAILY	✓
PARACETAMOL	1 G	ORAL	6-HOURLY	☐
PROPRANOLOL	80 MG	ORAL	12-HOURLY	☐

Question 10.120 Answer

The correct answer is enoxaparin.

Enoxaparin is dose-adjusted in low eGFRs (<30 mL/min) but also in adults under 50 kg to prevent excessive anticoagulation. This woman is 48 kg and qualifies for dose adjustment on this basis (and not on her eGFR). Note that patients under 50 kg should also have lower dose paracetamol (as prescribed here) to prevent hepatotoxicity.

CURRENT PRESCRIPTIONS

Drug name	Dose	Route	Freq.	
ENOXAPARIN	40 MG	S/C	DAILY	✓
AMLODIPINE	2.5 MG	ORAL	DAILY	☐
OMEPRAZOLE	20 MG	ORAL	DAILY	☐
PARACETAMOL	500 MG	ORAL	6-HOURLY	☐
PROPRANOLOL	80 MG	ORAL	12-HOURLY	☐

Index